The Biological Foundations of Clinical Psychiatry

KH Blacker MD
February 1988

The Biological Foundations of Clinical Psychiatry

Edited by

A. James Giannini, M.D.

Professor and Vice-Chairman, Department of Psychiatry, Northeastern Ohio Universities College of Medicine, Rootstown; *Associate Clinical Professor,* Department of Psychiatry, Ohio State University, Columbus; *Director of Psychiatry and Toxicology Services,* Youngstown Hospital Association, Youngstown, Ohio

MEDICAL EXAMINATION PUBLISHING CO.

Main entry under title:

The Biological foundations of clinical psychiatry.

　　Includes bibliographies and index.
　　1.　Biological psychiatry.　I.　Giannini, A. James,
1947-　　　.　[DNLM: 1.　Biological Psychiatry.
WM 100　B6144]
RC343.B47　　1985　　　　616.89　　　　　　85-10541
ISBN　0-87488-449-7

To my other and most favored projects,

Jocelyn Danielle Giannini
and
Juliette Nicole Giannini

Contents

Contributors

HENRY R. BLACK, M.D.
Associate Professor of Internal Medicine
Yale University
New Haven, Connecticut

SAM CASTELLANI, M.D.
Associate Professor of Psychiatry
University of Kansas
Kansas City

CHARLES A. DACKIS, M.D.
Staff Psychiatrist
Fair Oaks Hospital
Summit, New Jersey

ANA E. DVOREDSKY, M.D.
Associate Professor of Psychiatry and Medicine
Chicago Medical School
Illinois

IRL L. EXTEIN, M.D.
Medical Director
Falkirk Hospital
Central Valley, New York

A. JAMES GIANNINI, M.D.
Professor of Psychiatry
Northeastern Ohio College of Medicine
Rootstown
Associate Clinical Professor of Psychiatry
Ohio State University
Columbus

ROBERT L. GILLILAND, M.D.
Associate Professor of Neurology
Northeastern Ohio College of Medicine
Rootstown

MARK S. GOLD, M.D.
Director of Research
Psychodiagnostic Laboratories of America
Fair Oaks Hospital
Summit, New Jersey

RICHARD J. GOLDBERG, M.D.
Associate Professor of Psychiatry
Brown University
Providence, Rhode Island

CARY L. HAMLIN, M.D.
Staff Psychiatrist
Fair Oaks Hospital
Summit, New Jersey

RICHARD L. HAUGER, M.D.
Research Psychiatrist
National Institute of Mental Health
Rockville, Maryland

JONATHAN HIMMELHOCH, M.D.
Professor of Psychiatry
University of Pittsburgh
Pennsylvania

DANIEL W. HOMMER, M.D.
Research Psychiatrist
National Institute of Mental Health
Rockville, Maryland

STEVEN M. KALAVSKY, M.D.
Associate Professor of Neurology and Pediatrics
Northeastern Ohio College of Medicine
Rootstown

RONALD J. LEINEN, Ph.D.
Associate Professor of Psychiatry
Northeastern Ohio College of Medicine
Rootstown

JULIAN LIEB, M. D.
Associate Professor of Psychiatry
Yale University
New Haven, Connecticut

JAMES R. MERIKANGAS, M. D.
Assistant Professor of Psychiatry
Yale University
New Haven, Connecticut

KATHLEEN R. MERIKANGAS, Ph. D.
Assistant Professor of Psychiatry
Yale University
New Haven, Connecticut

STEVEN PAUL, M. D.
Director
Clinical Neuroscience Branch
National Institute of Mental Health
Rockville, Maryland

A. L. CARTER POTTASH, M. D.
Medical Director
The Regent Hospital
New York, New York

WILLIAM PRICE, M. D.
Clinical Fellow in Psychiatry
University of Pittsburgh
Pennsylvania

ANDREW E. SLABY, M. D., Ph. D., M. P. H.
Professor of Psychiatry and Medicine
Brown University
Providence, Rhode Island

DUANE G. SPIKER, M. D.
Associate Professor of Psychiatry
University of Pittsburgh
Pennsylvania

DAVID E. STERNBERG, M. D.
Associate Professor of Psychiatry
Yale University
New Haven, Connecticut

CONRAD SWARTZ, M.D., Ph.D.
Associate Professor of Psychiatry
Chicago Medical School
Illinois

KARL VEREBEY, M.D.
Director
New York State Substance Abuse Laboratory
Associate Professor of Psychiatry
Downstate Medical School
Brooklyn, New York

Acknowledgments

In editing this book, I wish to acknowledge my debt to my contributing authors who endured my letters, telephone calls, threats, and cajolery in completing this book. I wish to also thank Dr. Robert L. Miller of the University of Pittsburgh for his assistance in bringing cohesion to this broad topic. I want to also thank my colleagues at Northeastern Ohio Medical College for their support: Drs. Robert H. Loiselle, James Hodge, and Matthew Giannini.

Many institutions also gave support to the contributing authors and their assistance merits noting. These include Truckee Meadows Hospital of Reno, Nevada; Fair Oaks Hospital in Summit, New Jersey; Regent Hospital in New York City; and Falkirk Hospital of Central Valley, New York.

Resource assistance was given by Professor Judith Giannini of Youngstown State University, my office manager, Amy Takach, and my secretary, Marian Flaviani. Finally, a large debt is hereby acknowledged to my tireless and uncomplaining typist, Jeanne DiThomas.

Introduction

Much as the antibiotic age changed the character and focus of internal medicine, forcing it into the scientific mold, the biochemical age is revolutionizing the practice of psychiatry. The empirical and often random pattern of drug therapy has been overtaken by the discovery of specific neurotransmitters and receptors. While techniques and theories of psychotherapy retain an important niche in medical school and residency curricula, a distinct shift toward psychobiology is evident. This has led to a more complete understanding of the effects and side effects produced by psychotropic medication as well as guidelines for more judicious prescribing. Development of biochemical models for many psychiatric disorders is leading to a more complete understanding of the actual pathology being treated as well as generating diagnostic tests. This development has also allowed for specific antidotal, rather than palliative, treatment for the detoxification of drug overdoses and addictions.

This revolution with a rarified terminology and exotic modeling to express psychobiological processes has separated many practicing psychiatrists from advances in this specialty. It is for this reason that my colleagues and I have put together this compendium of biological psychiatry. The focus is upon conditions actually seen in the hospital or office setting. The neuronal biology discussed in the first section has been limited to those concepts whose mastery is essential for understanding the conditions discussed later in the book. These latter topics include disease processes most seen, diagnostic tests, and commonly used and abused psychoactive drugs. All are discussed from a biochemical perspective. The focus is upon clinical mastery of underlying principles. It is hoped that not only will this book assist residents and attending psychiatrists in understanding and applying biological techniques to their practice but that it will serve as a guide to future developments in this field.

AJG

notice _____

Part I

PSYCHOPHYSIOLOGY

Chapter 1

THE NEURONAL MEMBRANE

A. James Giannini, M.D.

The outer membrane of a neuron is a three-layered structure approximately 5 nm thick. A protein layer, the intrinsic pro-tein, is sandwiched between two layers of lipid. The inner and outer lipid layers resemble each other and do not vary in com-position from neuron to neuron. Each lipid layer is composed of a single large lipid molecule whose hydrophobic end points inward toward the intrinsic protein and whose hydrophilic end points away from the intrinsic protein. If the lipid molecule is in the top or outer layer of the "sandwich," its hydrophobic end points toward and comes in contact with the external milieu while the hydrophilic end of the bottom or inner layer of the sandwich points toward and limits the cytoplasm.

Embedded in the outer lipid layer are clumps of proteins, the peripheral membrane proteins. These do not form a dis-tinct layer and are considered a part of the lipid layer rather than the intrinsic protein. The intrinsic and peripheral pro-teins vary from neuron type to neuron type and define both the structure and function of each neuron. They act as the key "machinery" of the membrane and perform its actual work. In performing their work they routinely alter the confirmation and in so doing either expend or store energy.

The usual sources for protein energy are the cyclic nucle-otides such as cyclic adenosine monophosphate (cAMP) and cy-clic guanosine monophosphate (cGMP). Many drugs function by enhancing or diminishing the activity of these cyclic nucleo-tides. Caffeine increases cAMP activity while lithium carbon-ate has the opposite effect. Most of the general anticonvulsants such as phenobarbital and carbamezine decrease cGMP activ-ity.

3

The membrane proteins which are of major interest to psychiatrists belong to the intrinsic layer. This layer can be divided into six groups depending upon function. These briefly include:

Channel proteins: These provide a "hole" in the membrane through which ions can selectively diffuse.

Enzyme proteins: This type of protein catalyzes membrane chemical reactions.

Pump proteins: The action of this group serves to maintain necessary ion concentrations by using chemical energy to pump ions against a gradient.

Recognition proteins: Proteins in this group form metastable complexes with carbohydrate molecules. These are of prime importance during early development and growth during which time they direct proper synaptic connections.

Receptor proteins: These proteins recognize and react to neurotransmitters from other cells.

Structural proteins: This last group maintains the structural integrity of the individual cells and serves to connect other similar neurons to form tissues and organs.

Channel proteins regulate the internal ionic milieu of the neuron. They regulate opening and closing of actual pores in the membrane. These pores usually have a radius of less than 0. 5 nm and are filled with an aqueous solution in which ions flow in and out of cytoplasm. Dealing with these ultramicroscopic dimensions, the stacking of individual water molecules becomes important in the regulation of ion flow. In addition to this stacking and regulation of pore radius, direct interactions with the pore and the channel and changes in the shape of the channel protein maintain the rate and specificity of ion flow through each channel.

The actual opening or closing of the channel gate is an event that can be regulated by either receptor proteins or changes in voltage differentials. No channel has yet been discovered which responds in a significant degree to both voltage-gating and chemical- (i. e. , receptor) gating. This specificity of gating mechanism extends to the geographic distribution on the neuronal membrane. Voltage gates are highly concentrated on axons but only sparsely distributed in the dendritic membranes. Chemical gates are found almost exclusively on dendrites. As a generalization, voltage-gated channels may be considered the media of the intraneuronal transmission of "messages" while chemically gated channels receive interneuronal messages and transmit them through their own neurons.

Voltage-gated channels can be categorized according to the type of ion that is most easily shunted through it (e. g. , a sodium channel). As an impulse is activated in the dendrite or soma of a cell, the area of the axon most nearly adjacent to the soma has its voltage-gated channels opened. This opening causes a drop in the maintained gradient in the immediate area of the inner face of the membrane. As the gradient drops, so does the voltage potential. This spread of voltage drop is called the propagation of the neuronal impulse. Each voltage drop in a discrete area opens voltage-gated channels in the next distally adjacent area. In this way, these types of channels are affected by the neuronal impulse and help to propagate it along the axon.

In contrast, chemically gated channels can initiate an impulse but are only minimally affected by such an impulse. Each channel of this type can be considered to be a door composed of channel protein and water. A receptor protein is the lock that holds it shut, while a neurotransmitter protein or peptide functions as the key. Since each of these channels can be opened by only one type of key per lock (i. e. , receptor), they are named after the neurotransmitter key (e. g. , noradrenergic channels). This specificity, which is referred to as the "Dale hypothesis," is nearly absolute in vivo.

Enzyme proteins serve many purposes but the most important from a psychiatric perspective is the activation of cyclic ribonucleotides. The best understood of the enzyme proteins is adenylate cyclase. This protein is made up of two functional subunits. The catalytic subunit has one function only, the ongoing production of cAMP. The regulatory subunit binds to a specific neurotransmitter to regulate the production of cAMP by the catalytic unit. Each type of adenylate cyclase is named after the neurotransmitter to which the regulatory subunit binds.

Pump proteins are exchange mechanisms by which ions in the cytoplasm are exchanged by fixed ratio for ions in the external milieu. As in the case of channel proteins, this is done against a gradient. Pumps are named after the ions exchanged (e. g. , sodium-potassium pump, sodium-bicarbonate pump, etc.). Energy for this exchange is obtained during the breaking of the phosphate bonds of cyclic nucleotide molecules associated with the pump. The rate of pumping is variable. There appears to be a cybernetic mechanism which adjusts to neuronal ionic concentration levels.

Though there are many pumps, the most important is the sodium-potassium pump. It exchanges three cytoplasmic sodium ions for two potassium ions in the external milieu. In this way the neuron can maintain a potassium ion concentration of 10:1 compared to the external milieu. The exact reverse concentration is maintained with sodium. This causes the cytoplasm to have a -70 mV potential when compared to the surface of the membrane. It is this potential difference that is altered during the propagation of a neuronal impulse.

Recognition proteins are most important during the growth phase of a neuron. During embryonic development most neurons originate near the ventricular lining of the neural tube and then migrate after mitosis. Specific types of cells migrate to specific regions in the developing brain. It is at this point that the recognition proteins are most necessary. They appear to be able to "recognize" the recognition proteins of other similar neurons and cause these to stick together. This stickiness is specific and exists only between similar cells. As these neurons come together, the recognition proteins cause them to align in certain directions.

Receptor proteins will be discussed in Chapter 3. Receptors tend to be specific, at least in vivo, for a single neurotransmitter. Each neuron, furthermore, appears to have only one type of receptor, which is named after the neurotransmitter which reversibly binds to it (e. g. , noradrenergic receptors, dopaminergic receptors, etc.). Also, there are different subtypes of each receptor which appear to mediate different actions of a single type of neurotransmitter (e. g. , alpha-1 and alpha-2 noradrenergic receptors and dopaminergic (DA)-1 and DA-2 dopaminergic receptors). In addition, at least one type of receptor, the gamma-aminobutyric acid (GABA)-receptor, has been found to be associated with coreceptors which enhance its actions.

The action of a receptor depends on location. Presynaptic receptors or autoreceptors are found on the axon and act as a part of the negative, feedback loop which regulates neurotransmitter release. Postsynaptic receptors are found on the dendrite and serve to continue the impulse generated in a previous neuron and transformed into a chemical message by the neurotransmitter. To continue this impulse the neurotransmitter-receptor complex releases the energy of a cyclic nucleotide, either cAMP or cGMP. This is done through the action of an effector, an enzyme that breaks apart the nucleotide ring. This energy, in turn, activates kinases. These kinases are protein enzymes that act to increase membrane permeability to ions and thus to regenerate the impulse.

BIBLIOGRAPHY

Almers, W. , and Stirling, C.: Distribution of transport proteins over animal cell membranes. J Membr Biol 77(3):169-186, 1984.

Bastiani, M. J. , and Goodman, C. S.: Neuronal growth cones: specific interactions mediated by filopidial insertion and induction of coated vesicles. Proc Natl Acad Sci 81(6): 1849-1853, 1984.

Carley, L. R. , and Raymond, S. A.: Threshold measurement: applications to excitable membranes of nerve and muscle. J Neurosci Methods 9(4):309-333, 1983.

Fossier, P. , Tauc, L. , and Baux, G.: Side effects of phosphorylated acetylcholinesterase reactivators on neuronal membrane and synaptic transmission. Pfluegers Arch 396(1): 8-14, 1983.

Game, C. J.: BVP models of nerve membrane. Nature 23: 299(5881):375, 1983.

Gonatas, N. K.: Presidential address. The role of neuronal Golgi apparatus in a centripetal membrane vesicular traffic. J Neuropathol Exp Neurol 41(1):6-17, 1982.

Goto, K.: Transmembrane macromolecule rotation model—molecular hypothesis of membrane excitation. Tohoku J Exp Med 139(2):159-164, 1983.

Holden, A. V. , Haydon, P. G. , and Winlow, W.: Multiple equilibria and exotic behavior in excitable membranes. Biol Cybern 46(3):167-172, 1983.

Kostyuk, P. G.: Basic principles of the organization of ion channels determining the electric stimulation of the neuronal membrane. Zh Evol Biokhim Fiziol 19(4):333-340, 1983.

Kostyuk, P. G.: Intracellular perfusion of nerve cells and its effects on membrane currents. Physiol Rev 64(2):435-454, 1984.

Kostyuk, P. G.: The main principles of the organization of ionic channels which determine the excitability of the neuronal membrane. Acta Morphol Hung 31(1-3):63-72, 1983.

Levitt, P.: A monoclonal antibody to limbic system neurons. Science 223(4633):299-301, 1984.

Marsocci, V. A.: Electrical network modeling of active membranes of nerves. Crit Rev Biomed Eng 8(2):135-194, 1982.

Marx, J. L.: Organizing the cytoplasm. Science 222:1109-1112, 1983.

Mathers, D. A., and Barker, J. L.: Chemically-induced ion channels in nerve cell membranes. Int Rev Neurobiol 23:1-34, 1982.

Petito, C. K., and Pulsinelli, W. A.: Sequential development of reversible and irreversible neuronal damage following cerebral ischemia. J Neuropathol Exp Neurol 43(2):141-153, 1984.

Yawo, H., and Kuno, M.: How a nerve fiber repairs its cut end. Science 222:1351, 1983.

Chapter 2

NEUROTRANSMITTERS AND MENTAL DISORDERS

Mark S. Gold, M.D. and Cary L. Hamlin, M.D.

Neurotransmitters are chemicals that are stored in the boutons of nerves and that are released, by depolarization of the
bouton, to stimulate other neurons. Recent models of mental
illness assert that many mental disorders result from problems in the regulation of specific neurotransmitter systems
(i. e. , all the neurons that use a given transmitter). There is,
e. g. , a developing body of data that associates catecholamine
neuron dysfunction with several major neuropsychiatric syndromes including Parkinson's disease, depression, panic disorders, and schizophrenia. Drugs that ameliorate clinical
symptoms in these syndromes normalize catecholamine activity. The assumption made by extrapolation from these examples is that if one knew which neurotransmitter dysfunctions
were associated with a particular mental disorder, then one
could find a pharmacologic approach to control the dysfunction
and thus the disorder. Thus, the road to a rational psychopharmacology is paved with neurotransmitter systems.
    "The gain in brain lies mainly in the stain" (Floyd Bloom)
(see Cooper and associates work in the Bibliography at the end
of this chapter). The information currently available cannot
suffice to create a rational psychopharmacology. Psychiatrists
are only beginning to systematically apply the knowledge that
is arising in the field of molecular neurology to the study and
treatment of mental disorders, and knowledge of the molecular physiology of the nervous system is still small compared
to its potential extent. However, quite a lot of knowledge about
neurotransmitter dynamics in the brain has been developed in
the last decade. This information can be clinically useful, and
it may be necessary to the modern practice of psychiatry.
There is a time in the history of all sciences when technology
becomes equal to the complexities under study. Myth and

magic yield to truth: alchemy became chemistry, vitalism became biology, witch doctoring became medicine. Recent developments in neuroscience, particularly histochemistry, immunohistochemistry, and radioligand binding have opened new areas to exploration, and promise to bring an increasingly scientific approach to psychiatry. It is the purpose of this chapter to introduce the reader to these new frontiers. Information about what is currently clinically useful will be discussed in subsequent chapters on dexamethasone suppression testing (Chapter 1), thyrotropin-releasing hormone (TRH) (Chapter 19) stimulation testing, and specific psychotropics (Chapters 21-34).

There are approximately 20 billion neurons in the human nervous system, and there are as many as 500 thousand synapses per neuron. Each synapse stores at least one chemical neurotransmitter which upon release diffuses to several types of local receptors and modifies the activity of next neurons. Even if the identity of all the neurotransmitters in the million billion of synapses were known, and it is not, then the tasks of understanding how their activities are coordinated with each other to produce thought, emotions, and adaptive behavior is awesomely complex. So far the highly useful molecular biological techniques have been restricted to animal behavior studies by ethical constraints. Exceptions to this are studies of cerebrospinal fluid (CSF), blood, and urine neurotransmitter metabolites which give a gross idea of the activities of a few neurotransmitter systems in healthy and diseased individuals. Other exceptions are studies of the responses of these systems to stress, selective drugs, and clinical improvement. The techniques of positron emission tomography and nuclear magnetic resonance tomography hold great promise to bring the dynamics of synaptic activity as a function of specific brain nuclei, stressors, and drugs to light in Homo sapiens.

A large number of neurochemicals have been proposed to be neurotransmitters. Putative neurotransmitters must go through a series of demonstrations to prove that they are neurotransmitters. These property demonstrations are called Bloom's criteria and are named after the great Salk Institute scientist Floyd Bloom who proposed them. These properties that reflect neurotransmitter function include the following items: the neurochemical is present in some brain nuclei and absent in others, the neurochemical is located within synaptosomes, it is released by plasma membrane depolarization, it has a synthetic mechanism capable of replenishing synaptosomal stores and has a catabolic mechanism available in the nuclei where it is found, and it exerts physiologic effects at physiologic concentrations. If a neurochemical passes all of

Bloom's criteria, then it is very likely to be a neurotransmitter.

The number of neurochemicals that have satisfied all or most of Bloom's criteria is becoming large. Some of these have become generally familiar to physicians; acetylcholine; nicotinic or muscarinic receptors; adrenaline or noradrenaline; alpha-1 or alpha-2 or beta-1 or beta-2 receptors; dopamine and dopamine-1-, -2-, and -3-receptors; serotonin; 5-hydroxy-tryptamine (5-HTP)-1-, -2-, or -3-receptors; histamine and histamine-1- or -2- receptors; gamma-aminobutyrate (GABA) and GABA-receptors; glutamate and glutamate-receptors; aspartate and its receptors; and glycine and glycine-receptors. Other of these are less generally known: the peptides, beta-endorphin, enkephalin, adrenocorticotropic hormones (ACTH), antidiuretic hormone (ADH), oxytocin, substance P, corticotropin-releasing factor (CRF), somatostatin, insulin, lutinizing hormone-releasing hormone (LHRH), vasoactive intestinal peptide (VIP), calcitonin, angiotensin II, neurotensin, melanocyte inhibitory factor (MIF), and neuropeptide Y, the purine adenosine, and beta-carboline. Although this list is long it is probably not exhaustive. The student's necessary task of learning how these 30 neurotransmitters or probable neurotransmitters are distributed among the nuclei in the brain's million billion or so synapses, and what their anabolic and catabolic mechanisms are, is in itself formidable. Given that almost none of this information identifying neurotransmitter systems in the nervous system was available 20 years ago, knowledge about them is a growth industry. Since knowledge about the dynamic relationships among those neurotransmitter systems and their activity states in response to changing environments and adaptational demands in health and disease is meager, there is plenty of work available for aspiring investigators to do for the forseeable future.

A complete discussion of these topics for the 30 neurotransmitter systems listed is beyond the scope of this chapter. The goal of this chapter is to identify some of the neurotransmitter systems in the reticular formation and limbic system areas, and to report the results of certain animal studies that define some of their interrelationships and effects upon behavior. It is assumed, that since these brain areas are little different in mice or men, that similar neurons, interrelationships, and effects upon behavior occur in men also.

IDENTIFICATION OF NEUROTRANSMITTER SYSTEMS

As the identification of the catecholamine neurotransmitter
systems using adrenaline, noradrenaline, and dopamine is
dealt with in Chapter 4, their anatomic relations are
presented there. This section will concern itself with defining
the anatomy of systems using beta-endorphin, enkephalin,
acetylcholine, serotonin, GABA, TRH, histamine, substance
P, and neurotensin that are within the reticular formation and
limbic system.

BETA-ENDORPHIN

The 20-μm neurons that stain with antibody to beta-endorphin,
and by other studies probably use it as a neurotransmitter
agent, are located as a band in the dorsal arcuate nucleus of
the hypothalamus and adjacent lateral hypothalamus. These
are distinctly separate from adjacent cell bodies that stain
with LHRH antibodies. However, they are precisely the same
cells that stain with anticorticotropin antibodies. The biosynthesis of beta-endorphin from proopiocorticotropin in their
neurons is likely to be the same as that occurring in the pituitary cells: the proopiocorticotropin molecule contains
ACTH's 39 amino acids as one sequence and beta-endorphin's
31 as another, and peptidases leave the precursor molecule to
produce the two hormones. It is possible that ACTH is also a
neurotransmitter in those beta-endorphinergic neurons that
project from the lower-middle hypothalamus.
    The synaptic terminal areas of beta-endorphin that re-
ceive the 5-μm-diameter boutons includes a variety of hypothalamic, thalamic, basal forebrain amygdala, and reticular
formation sites. Hypothalamic projection sites include the
median eminence, supraoptic nucleus, periventricular nucleus, paraventricular nucleus, and lateral anterior nucleus. The
thalamic projection field is the dorsomedial nucleus which is
directly interconnected to prefrontal cortex. Basal forebrain
sites include the lateral septal nucleus, nucleus accumbens,
and the red nucleus of the striae terminalis. The amygdala's
projection field is restricted to the corticomedial group. The
reticular nuclei projected to are the locus coeruleus and the
raphe. Endorphinergic and probably also corticotropinergic
neurons are strategically located within the limbic system to
exert a profound effect upon emotional life. Direct connections
between beta-endorphin and enkephalinergic, serotonergic,
adrenergic, and dopaminergic neurons are conceivable based
upon known anatomic relationships among them.

ENKEPHALINS

Enkephalinergic systems are more extensive than endorphinergic. Immunohistochemistry reveals cell bodies located in the widespread areas of the central nervous system. The areas that receive primary nociceptive and visceroceptive afferents—the substantia gelatinosa of the spinal cord, spinal trigeminal nucleus, and the nucleus solitarius—contain enkephalin cell bodies. Visual centers, part of the lateral geniculate and superior colliculus, contain them. Dopaminergic midbrain nuclei, the nigra and ventral tegmental area, contain them. They are found at widespread locations in the limbic system; the posterior and dorsal nuclei of the thalamus, the habenula in the epithalamus, the red nucleus of the striae terminalis, the septum, and the central nucleus of the amygdala. The neostriatium has the largest number of enkephalin cell bodies of any other nucleus in the brain. Finally, a gustatory to hypothalamic relay nucleus, the parabrachialis, contains enkephalin-staining cells.

Projection sites of enkephalin neurons include all of the nuclei that contain cell bodies and several other sites. The neocortex receives a few. The globus pallidus receives many. There are projections to the dorsomedial, ventromedial, periventricular, and preoptic hypothalamus nuclei. Particularly noteworthy are enkephalin terminals, derived from the cells in the parabrachialis, which terminate in the ventral median and adjacent lateral hypothalamus in close proximity to the endorphin-corticotropin cell bodies. This pathway supports intracranial self-stimulation. There are projections to the nucleus ambiguus and near the adrenergic neurons by the lateral reticular nucleus.

There is some basis for speculation that delta-receptor subtypes are the enkephalinergic receptors, whereas mu-receptor subtypes are the endorphinergic receptors. This is based upon the preferential affinity of enkephalins for delta-receptors and of endorphins for mu-receptors, and it is based upon the distribution of delta-receptors and mu-receptors to exclusively enkephalin or endorphin bouton areas. However, other receptors, sigma and kappa, have been described as well. How many different receptors of opiates there are and whether some may have agonist preference or antagonist preference allosteric forms, is currently the object of scrutiny in the literature.

ACETYLCHOLINE

The greatest density of neurons that stain with antibodies to acetylcholinesterase and choline-acetyltransferase is found in the interneurons of the neostriatum and accumbens. These are the very same neurons that receive the A_9- and $A_{8,10}$-dopaminergic projections, respectively. There is also a dense staining of medial septal nucleus and these cells project acetylcholine synapses to the hippocampus and dentate gyrus. Stained cells in the anterior ventral and anterior dorsal nuclei of the thalamus project to the habenula and to the anterior and posterior cingulate gyrus, respectively, and these same locations also receive an $A_{8,10}$-dopaminergic projection. Stained cells in the lateral preoptic hypothalamus nucleus project to the nucleus accumbens, to the septal nuclei, and to the magnocellular division of the dorsomedial thalamic nucleus. Stained cells in the medial septal nucleus project to the intralaminar thalamic nuclei and the habenula. Stained cells in the midbrain reticular formation in the nucleus cuniformis project to the intralaminar thalamus, raphe, and interpeduncular and caudal brain stem reticular formation. Stained cells in ventral tegmental area project to the premammillary, supraoptic, paraventricular, lateral hypothalamus, and globus pallidus areas, and to the basal nucleus of the amygdala. Stained cells in the globus pallidus project to the neostriatum, and diffusely to the neocortex.

SEROTONIN

Fluorescence histochemistry shows serotonin cell bodies in the caudal brain stem reticular formation (i. e. , B_1-B_6 Dahlstrom and Fuxe) which project to the intermediolateral columns and ventral horns of the spinal cord and to the brain stem's preganglionic autonomic centers. Fluorescent cells in the dorsal raphe nucleus (B_7) project to the suprachiasmatic mammillary, dorsomedial, arcuate, periventricular, and anterior hypothalamic nuclei. Fluorescent cells in the medial raphe nucleus project to the perifornical nucleus, lateral preoptic area, accumbens, and lateral septal nucleus, corticomedial amygdaloid group, and neostriatum. There are also heavy projections to the thalamic nuclei and to cingulate gyrus.

GAMMA-AMINOBUTYRATE

Hokfelt's group has shown retrograde labeling of the magnocellular medial mammillary hypothalamic cell bodies from all over the neocortex neostriatum and amygdala. This is the first demonstration of a projection of the medial mammillary hypothalamus to neocortex and each neuron projects to widely different neocortical areas (diffuse projection). All of the magnocellular neurons are strongly stained by antibody to glutamate decarboxylase (GAD) which is the synthetic enzyme for gamma-aminobutyrate (GABA). The magnocellular medial mammillary hypothalamic neurons that project to the neostriatum, amygdala, and neocortex are GABA-ergic.

The concentration of GAD has a good correlation with the number of GABA synapses in a brain area. There are high concentrations of GAD within the preoptic, anterior, and dorsomedial hypothalamic nuclei. Medium concentrations are found within the paraventricular nucleus and the ventromedial nucleus. Most of the cells responsible for these GABA terminals are within the hypothalamus.

There are GABA cells in the neostriatum and accumbens that terminate in the substantia nigra and ventral tegmental area, respectively. These two projections synapse upon the dopaminergic cell bodies or dendrites in A9 (striatonigral pathway). The technique of amino acid autoradiography reveals projections to the preoptic, anterior, paraventricular, and dorsomedial hypothalamic nuclei as well as to the ventral tegmental area. The likelihood is that some of the GABA synapses in these hypothalamic nuclei originate from nucleus accumbens. The GABA cells in the neostriatum provide terminals to the globus pallidus as they pass through enroute to the substantia nigra.

THYROTROPIN-RELEASING HORMONE

Since we know no role for TRH except that it is released in the median eminence of the hypothalamus to stimulate TSH secretion from the anterior pituitary, it would come as some surprise to know that about 67% of all whole-brain TRH content lies outside the hypothalamus. Although the hypothalamus at 0.25 ng TRH/mg tissue has the highest density of TRH in the forebrain, only about 30% of that total is located within the median eminence. The arcuate nucleus, ventromedial nucleus, periventricular nucleus, and medial preoptic area contain the majority of the rest. Studies suggest that the cells that supply TRH to the median eminence are located in the ventromedial area, preoptic area, periventricular nucleus in the anterior, parvocellular portion of the paraventricular nuclei, and in the arcuate. There is probably a TRH pathway from the corticomedial amygdala to the ventromedial hypothalamus. The lateral septal nucleus has a density to TRH enervation comparable to the ventromedial hypothalamus.

The majority of the rest of the TRH portion of the brain is found within the thalamus where it is about 20% as dense as in the hypothalamus. However, given the relative sizes of the two nuclear masses involved, there is about as much thalamic TRH as hypothalamic. Whether thalamic TRH is found in one particular nucleus or scattered throughout is presently not known.

Thyrotropin-releasing hormone is released from brain synaptosome preparations by depolarizing stimuli. In concentrations of about 10^{-8} M, TRH produced inhibition of about 33% of cells in the preoptic hypothalamic nuclei, but it produced no inhibition of cortical neurons. Luteinizing hormone-releasing hormone also inhibited about 33% of preoptic cells, but they belonged to a different group from those inhibited by TRH. Oxytocin in doses of 10^{-3} M did not effect any preoptic hypothalamic neurons. Whereas efforts to define the mechanism of synthesis of TRH have thus far not succeeded because of methodologic problems, TRH appears to function as a limbic system neurotransmitter.

HISTAMINE

Histamine is present in brain and together with its synthetic enzyme, 1-histidine decarboxylase, is found localized within synaptic boutons. The number of such boutons is only about one-tenth that of noradrenaline. Histamine is most densely concentrated in the hypothalamus, although significant amounts are found in the midbrain and nonhypothalamic forebrain, particularly in the paraventricular nuclear areas and in the hippocampus. Within the hypothalamus, the densest histamine projections are present in the median eminence, however, significant amounts are found in the arcuate nucleus, premammillary nucleus, suprachiasmatic nucleus, dorsomedial nucleus, paraventricular nucleus, and supraoptic nucleus. The precise localization of cell bodies and projection by immunohistochemistry has not been accomplished, however, lesion studies suggest the posterior hypothalamus, perhaps the premammillary nuclei, as the cell body site. Ligand binding studies for histamine-1- and -2-receptors give roughly the same distribution as that for histamine or histidine decarboxylase.

SUBSTANCE P

In the caudal brain stem reticular formation the majority of the B_1-B_6 serotonin-containing cells also stain with antibody to substance P. Substance P in the ventral horns of the spinal cord declines with declines in serotonin subsequent to 5, 7-dihydroxytryptamine-induced lesions of these neurons. Substance P levels in the dorsal horn substantia gelatinosa decline after dorsal root section, suggesting a role for substance P as a neurotransmitter in primary nociceptive afferents. Significant amounts of substance P are found in the substantia nigra and ventral midbrain, scattered throughout the hypothalamus and thalamus, and in the central amygdaloid nucleus. That substance P exists in neurons besides those of the raphe is suggested by the observation of a 70% decline in substantia nigra substance P after globus pallidus lesion.

NEUROTENSIN

Cell bodies staining with antibody to neurotensin are found in the periventricular nucleus, medial preoptic area, the paracellular part of the paraventricular nucleus, the arcuate nucleus, and the perifornical area in the hypothalamus. The parvocellular paraventricular nucleus is distinguished from the magnocellular part which contains ADH and oxytocin cells, and receives input of angiotensin II and cholecystokinin synapses. The parvocellular neurotensin neurons project to the posterior pituitary as do the magnocellular neurons. Neurotensin cells in the arcuate nucleus project to the median eminence.

Neurotensin cells in the central nucleus of the amygdala project to the red nucleus of the striae terminalis.

The substance gelatinosa receives boutons containing neurotensin as does the spinal nucleus of the trigeminal. The locus coeruleus receives neurotensin boutons, and iontophoretic application there results in inhibition of noradrenergic neuron firing.

The periaqueductal gray area of the midbrain has moderate densities of neurotensin terminals, cell bodies, and receptors. The dorsal raphe contains neurotensin cells, terminals, and receptors. The medial raphe contains moderate densities of terminals and receptors but no cells. The ventral tegmental area contains high densities of cells, terminals, and receptors. Neurotensin fibers and receptors are found within the substantia nigra. Lesions within 6-OH-dopamine show a loss of neurotensin receptors which presumably means they are located upon dopaminergic neurons.

NEUROTRANSMITTER INTERRELATIONSHIPS
AND EFFECTS ON BEHAVIOR

There has been considerable study by physiologic psychologists of the relationships of hypothalamic neurotransmitters to feeding and drinking behavior in animals, and these studies have shed important light upon relationships of hypothalamic neurotransmitters to one another. Endocrinologists studying the control of the pituitary gland by the hypothalamus have also discovered interesting relationships among hypothalamic neurotransmitters. Neuropharmacologists have also contributed to this knowledge.

The adrenergic synaptic fields in the hypothalamus include the periventricular, paraventricular (PVN), supraoptic, dorsomedial, perifornical, and median eminence nuclear areas. Mapping studies by Sarah Liebowitz reveal that local injection of about 2 ng norepinephrine or epinephrine into the paraventricular field produces feeding in a satiated rat within 1 min after injection and potentiates feeding in a hungry rat. These animals eat larger meals at greater rates than normal animals. Meteraminol or clonidine injection into the paraventricular nucleus can produce feeding, however, this effect is attenuated in animals with lesions of the adrenergic inputs to this nucleus. Hypoglycemia is associated with increased paraventricular adrenergic turnover and feeding. Systemic or local PVN injection of alpha- but not beta-adrenergic antagonists is associated with blockade of this alpha-agonist-induced feeding response. The alpha-adrenergic feeding response requires cortisol.

In contrast to alpha-adrenergic-induced feeding, injection of epinephrine or isoproterenol into the perifornical area suppresses eating in a hungry rat. This anorexic effect of epinephrine is potentiated by amphetamine or desipramine if the adrenergic enervation of the perifornical region is intact. The effect can be blocked by beta-adrenergic blockade, but alpha-adrenergic antagonists, serotonin antagonists, and muscarinic antagonists are without effect. Beta-adrenergic stimulation decreases frequency of meals.

Noradrenaline, adrenaline, or alpha-adrenergic agonists that are injected into the paraventricular hypothalamus suppress drinking in a thirsty rat or one given hypertonic saline, and this drinking suppression is blocked by alpha-adrenergic antagonists. The drinking response to hypertonic saline is blocked by periventricular hypothalamic lesion. The alpha-adrenergic enervation of the periventricular nucleus inhibits the cells there.

The alpha-adrenergic paraventricular injection released feeding is associated with enhanced insulin release and peripheral parasympathetic drive. Locus coeruleus lesions cause hyperdypsia and decreased periventricular noradrenaline.

Lateral ventricle injections of adrenergic agonists cause an increased release of ADH from cells in the paraventricular hypothalamus. This ADH release is blocked by alpha-adrenergic antagonists, and also the ADH release evoked by electrical pulse stimulation of the supraoptic or paraventricular hypothalamus is similarly blocked. Antagonists to serotonin, or muscarinic receptors do not effect this ADH release.

Injection of serotonin into the paraventricular hypothalamic nucleus results in suppression of feeding in a hungry rat, and it blocks the alpha-adrenergic feeding response from there. Systemic (5-HTP) or 1-tryptophan similarly causes suppression of feeding by decreasing meal size and rate of eating without affecting meal frequency. 5-Hydroxytryptophan-induced suppression of alpha-adrenergic feeding is blocked by methlysergide. Methylsergide itself produces increased appetite and weight gain. These data suggest that serotonin is excitatory and noradrenaline inhibitory in the paraventricular hypothalamus.

There is evidence for two catecholamines being involved in perifornical feeding suppression. Amphetamine stimulation of the perifornical hypothalamus can be blocked by neuroleptics or by beta-adrenergic blockers. Perifornical injection or dopamine (30 ng) or apomorphine suppresses feeding, and this effect is blocked by neuroleptics. Selective midbrain lesion of the A_8-dopaminergic cells partially blocks amphetamine-induced feeding suppression but increases dopamine agonist-induced suppression. These data have been used to argue for the existence of two separate catecholaminergic suppressions of feeding in the perifornical hypothalamus: one beta-adrenergic and the other dopaminergic.

Acetylcholine agonists (2 ng) produce drinking when injected into the anterior medial hypothalamus. This response can be blocked by antimuscarinics or by lesion of the periventricular nucleus. This phenomenon seems motivationally like thirst because animals will perform operant tasks to obtain water. These injections increase release of ADH, and cause antidiuresis and naturesis. Hypertonic saline causes similar effects, and antimuscarinics block the drinking and the increased ADH release caused by this hyperosmolar load.

Histamine injection into the rostral hypothalamus, particularly the paraventricular nucleus, produces drinking, and this response can be blocked by a combination of histamine-1- and

-2-receptor antagonists. This phenomenon apparently depends upon stimulation of that nucleus because microiontophoretic application produced excitation postsynaptic potentials. The histamine injections also cause antidiuresis. Alpha-adrenergic antagonists block the ADH release but not the drinking. On the other hand, neuroleptics, beta-adrenergic blockers, serotonin blockers, and antimuscarinics did not block histamine-induced antidiuresis. It has been proposed that histamine antidiuresis requires alpha-adrenergic stimulation of the paraventricular hypothalamus.

Gamma-aminobutyrate agonists injected into the medial rostral hypothalamus produce feeding, and again the most sensitive site is the paraventricular hypothalamic nucleus. This feeding can be blocked by bicuculline, an GABA antagonist. Alpha-adrenergic antagonists fail to block this feeding response. On the other hand, GABA agonists suppress feeding if they are injected into the perifornical area. Catecholaminergic feeding suppression can be blocked by GABA antagonists in this area.

Intraventricular injection of angiotensin II and substance P produce drinking and antidiuresis. Similarly ADH and neurotensin injections fail to produce drinking. Substance P stimulates adrenergic activity.

Beta-endorphin injection into the ventromedial hypothalamic nucleus produces a dose-dependent feeding response.

Roles for serotonin, acetylcholine, nicotinic, and alpha-adrenergic receptors in the control of CRF secretron have been reported. Specifically, serotonin excites acetylcholine release which acts on nicotinic receptors to stimulate CRF release, and alpha-adrenergic stimulation inhibits CRF release. Central administration of CRF causes low motor hyperactivity and sympathetic nervous system arousal.

The tridecapeptide neurotensin produces effects upon nociception avoidance behavior and thermoregulation when it is applied intracerebrally. Specifically, when injected into the caudal pontine reticular formation, central amygdaloid nucleus, midbrain periaqueductal gray area, medial preoptic hypothalamus, or midline thalamus, there is a decreased response to painful stimuli. This is similar to the responses observed for intracerebral injections of endorphin and enkephalin, however, unlike them the effects are not blocked by naloxone. Conversely, intracerebral application of antibodies to neurotensin caused increased responses to painful stimuli. The decreased pain sensitivity was blocked by intracerebral TRH administration. Neurotensin injections into fourth ventricle, medial preoptic, or anterior hypothalamus, and ventral tegmental area produced a decreased core body temperature. Ventral tegmental area injections, consistent with evidence discussed for the presence of neurotensin receptors on A_{10}-dopamine neurons, resulted in increased dopamine turnover in the nucleus accumbens. Lateral ventricle injections of neurotensin in nanogram amounts produced deficits in active and passive avoidance behavior and decreased muscle tone. Thyrotropin-releasing hormone antagonizes the relaxing effects of neurotensin.

Enkephalin neurons have known functional relationships with several other neurotransmitter systems. Specifically functional interrelations among them and acetylcholine neurons, dopamine neurons, GABA-neurons, and adrenaline neurons have been demonstrated.

Analagous interrelationships among the enkephalinergic, dopaminergic, cholinergic, and GABAergic systems have been found in two sets of brain nuclei: the substantia nigra and neostriatum, and the ventral tegmental area and accumbens. In both these sets, dopaminergic neurons synapse upon the dendrites of cholinergic interneurons and produce inhibitory postsynaptic potentials in them. Also in both sets, GABAergic neurons synapse upon the dendrites of dopaminergic neurons and produce inhibitory postsynaptic potentials in them. Enkephalinergic (delta-) transmission produces inhibitory postsynaptic potentials in the cholinergic neurons. Cholinergic transmission (muscarinic) produces inhibitory postsynaptic potentials in GABAergic neurons. The increase in dopamine turnover that is produced by neuroleptic can be blocked by potentiating GABA neurotransmission, presumably by blocking a decrease in it. Neuroleptic potentiates cholinergic neurotransmission. Antimuscarinics block the increase in dopamine turnover which is induced by neuroleptics, presumably by blocking neuroleptic-induced increases in cholinergic neurotransmission and thus by preventing neuroleptic-induced decreases in GABA neurotransmission. Thus, in series, dopaminergic neurotransmission inhibits cholinergic, cholinergic inhibits GABAergic, and GABAergic inhibits dopaminergic neurotransmission. Arvid Carlsson hypothesized this neuronal negative feedback loop in 1963 to account for his observation of neuroleptic-induced increased in striatial dopamine turnover. Enkephalinergic potentiation in striatum and accumbens also increased dopaminergic turnover, however, unlike neuroleptic it decreased cholinergic turnover. Presumably this happens because enkephalin inhibits GABAergic neurotransmission. Neuroleptics increase enkephalin turnover, presumably by dopamine inhibiting enkephalin directly.

NEUROTRANSMITTER IMBALANCE
AND PSYCHOPATHOLOGY

The role of noncatecholamine neurotransmitter systems in human mental disorders has not been thoroughly studied. However, a few provocative observations portend the future development of such knowledge. Studies of subgroups of major depressed patients suggest the presence of corticotropin release factor excess, TRH excess, endorphin excess, and acetylcholine excess in some of them. Studies of patients with chronic pain suggest that serotonin and endorphin deficiency states are associated with symptoms of anxiety and guilt. The premorbid personalities of opiate-dependent persons are characterized by frequent states of rage, guilt, shame, and anxiety which perhaps leave them predisposed to excessively value the antiaggressive, antidepressant, and antianxiety properties of opiates. Improvement in anxiety associated with obsessive-compulsive disorders is correlated with increases in central serotonin turnover. Finally, panic-disordered patients have increased sensitivity to pain, and they have evidence of increased hypothalamic TRH activity. Future research will refine and extend these observations to better clarify the role of neurotransmitter imbalances in the mental disorders.

BIBLIOGRAPHY

Cooper, J. , Bloom, F. , and Roth, R. : The Biochemical Basis of Neuropharmacology, 3d ed. Oxford University Press, Toronto, 1978.

Fuxe, K. , Hokfelt, T. , and Luft, R. : Central Regulation of the Endocrine System. Plenum Press, New York, 1979.

Harris, I. , and Usden, E. : Animal Models in Psychiatry and Neurology. Pergamon Press, Oxford, Toronto, 1977

Morgane, P. , and Panksepp, J. : Handbook of Hypothalamus, Vol. 3. Marcel Dekker, New York, 1980.

Nemeroff, C. , and Prange, A. : Neurotensin, a brain and gastrointestinal peptide, Ann NY Acad Sci 400:1982.

Serotonin. Year Book Medical Publishers, Chicago, 1968.

Verebey, K.: Opioids in mental illness. Ann NY Acad Sci 398; 217-219, 1982.

Chapter 3

NEURORECEPTORS

Sam Castellani, M.D.

INTRODUCTION

A "receptor" is conceptualized as a molecular entity which upon stimulation by a hormone, neurotransmitter, or drug initiates a sequence of cellular processes leading to a biological response. Considerable progress, especially spurned by radiolabeled ligand binding techniques in the last two decades, has been made in identifying and characterizing receptors since the concept was first used by Langley in 1905. Neuroreceptors are of paramount importance in biological psychiatry since an understanding of their functioning is central to an understanding of central nervous system (CNS) mechanisms underlying psychotropic drug action and psychopathology. Indeed, biological psychiatry appears to be entering a phase in which the study of neuroreceptor dynamics is challenging if not superseding classical studies of neurotransmitter synthesis, turnover, and metabolism. In this review the basic concepts of neuroreceptor functioning will be presented along with practical and heuristic applications relevant to psychiatric illness.

RECEPTOR CRITERIA

The following interrelated properties are considered essential to validly define a receptor:

1. High-affinity binding. Receptors should bind with high affinities to their respective ligands.
2. Reversibility of binding. It is assumed, since hormones, neurotransmitters, and drugs usually show reversible biological actions, that binding of a receptor to its ligand should be reversible.

3. Saturability of binding. Biologically relevant or "specific" (see below) ligand binding occurs at sites that have a finite number per cell and are thus saturable.
4. Specificity. This most important criterion consists of three types: (1) molecular specificity – a receptor should have high affinity for a specific molecule or chemical class of molecules, including specific isomers (stereospecificity); (2) pharmacospecificity – potency of agonist and antagonist binding should correlate with potency in relevant physiologic or behavioral response systems; (3) tissue specificity – anatomic localization of ligand binding should exist in CNS areas rich in specific neurotransmitter levels and nerve terminals.

The majority of these criteria have been satisfied for the following CNS neurotransmitters: acetylcholine, dopamine, norepinephrine, serotonin, opiates (enkephalins, endorphins), and gamma-aminobutyric acid (GABA).

MODEL AND MECHANISMS

The basic model for receptor functioning which fits a large body of data accumulated during the last decade consists of a "recognition" component which involves specific ligand binding, and a "translation" component which modulates the initial receptor-ligand interaction to produce a biological response. A summary of this model with its functional aspects for neuroreceptors is illustrated schematically in Figure 3-1.

RECOGNITION

It is generally accepted that neurotransmitter receptors consist of macromolecules located on the outside of a plasma membrane and due to conformational properties selectively binding to their specific endogenous neurotransmitter and structurally similar agonists and antagonists (drugs). Although no neuroreceptor molecule has been fully purified and characterized, there is substantial evidence that they consist of protein molecules with or without carbohydrate and/or lipid constituents. The recognition or binding process is established using the receptor criteria mentioned above.

TRANSLATION

Binding of neurotransmitter to receptor is generally followed

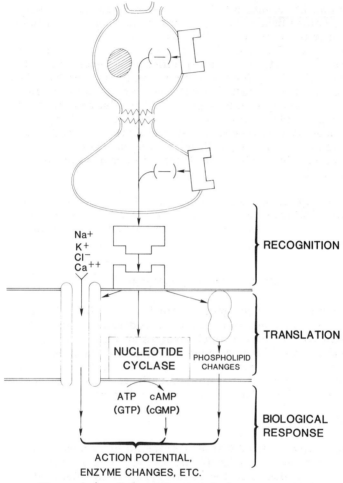

Figure 3-1   Schematic model of a neuroreceptor.

by functional changes within the plasma membrane in ion channels and/or membrane-bound enzymes. Ion channel alterations consist of opening or closing of channels to influence the passage of ions (sodium, potassium, chloride, calcium) along electrochemical gradients. The classical example of this mechanism is the nicotinic acetylcholine receptor, which activates the opening of sodium and potassium channels. Ionic channel regulation has been implicated in other neurotransmitter receptor actions: GABA and benzodiazepines-CNS chloride; serotonin-molluscan neurons, sodium, potassium, chloride; enkephalins-CNS potassium. Enzymes most commonly linked to receptor action are the cyclases, which catalyze formation of the cyclic nucleotides, cyclic adenosine monophosphate (cAMP), and guanosine monophosphate (cGMP). The cyclic nucleotides in turn regulate intracellular processes, such as activation of cellular enzymes (protein kinases, which catalyze phosphorylate proteins) and are thus termed "second messengers." Substantial evidence indicates that neurotransmitter receptors functionally linked to the activation of cyclases are: beta-norephinephrine (increases cAMP), dopamine (increases cAMP), acetylcholine (muscarinic, increases cGMP), serotonin (increases cAMP), GABA (increases cGMP), and opiates (decrease cAMP).

Two other plasma membrane mechanisms thought to be important in receptor translation are phospholipid methylation (beta-adrenergic) and calcium-mediated stimulation of phospholipids (alpha-norepinephrine, muscarinic cholinergic). Phospholipid methylation has been postulated to change membrane fluidity and affect coupling of the receptor to adenylate cyclase.

MULTIPLE RECEPTORS

Mathematical models have been developed using mass action equations to derive equilibrium or affinity constants for receptor-ligand interactions. However, binding studies have revealed that many ligand-receptor reactions do not follow simple mass action concepts. Moreover, binding studies using displacement of radiolabeled ligand from brain membranes reveal that some pharmacologic agonists differ from antagonists in pharmacospecificity, regional localization, and/or affinity for respective agonist or antagonist site. These data call into question early notions of a simple one-to-one relationship between ligand-receptor occupation and biological response ("occupation theory"), and have led to the following concepts of multiple receptor classes for a single neurotransmitter.

1. Two-state model. This hypothesis states that receptors exist in two conformational states that are in dynamic equilibrium: an "activated" or agonist state and a "nonactivated" or antagonist state, each of which responds selectively to its respective ligand. This model tends to fit the data for dopamine, acetylcholine, and opiate receptors but remains speculative.

2. Multiple postsynaptic receptors. Numerous studies have
demonstrated evidence for the existence of multiple functionally and anatomically distinct receptors for individual
neurotransmitters. Table 3-1 illustrates examples of these
with distinguishing characteristics.

PRESYNAPTIC RECEPTORS (AUTORECEPTORS)

Extensive data also exist demonstrating the presence of receptors on neuronal cell bodies and nerve terminals that decrease release of neurotransmitters and thereby modulate
neuronal functioning by negative feedback regulation (hence the
term "autoreceptors") (Fig. 3-1). Presynaptic CNS receptors
have been found for the following neurotransmitters: acetylcholine, norepinephrine, dopamine, serotonin, and GABA.

RECEPTOR SENSITIVITY CHANGES THROUGH TIME

Neurotransmitter receptors are in a dynamic state such that
they are constantly being degraded and synthesized. Decrease
in receptor stimulation due to a variety of means – chemical
or mechanical interruption of presynaptic input, depletion of
presynaptic neurotransmitter, or blockade of receptor stimulation – leads to enhanced receptor responsiveness or "supersensitivity." This may reflect increased receptor sites and/or
affinity and has been shown by biochemical (increased adenylate cyclase activity), electrophysiologic (increased response
to microiontophoretic application of neurotransmitter), and
behavioral (enhanced apomorphine- and amphetamine-induced
stereotypy in animals) response systems. Conversely, receptor activation leads to decreased sensitivity or "subsensitivity." These phenomena may be important underlying mechanisms for production of drug effects and various pathologic
states (see below).

RELEVANCE OF RECEPTORS TO PSYCHOPHARMACOLOGY
AND PSYCHIATRIC ILLNESS

Data from biochemical, electrophysiological, and behavioral
studies provide substantial evidence that many psychotropic
drugs exert their actions by interacting with crucial CNS neurotransmitter receptor sites. If the milligram potency of a
drug for producing pharmacologic effects is positively

Table 3-1 Multiple Postsynaptic Receptors[a]

Neurotransmitter	Localization	Agonist(s)	Antagonist(s)	Other
Norepinephrine				
Alpha-1	Heart, vas deferens Brain, widespread	Epinephrine, norepinephrine	Prazocin, WB-4101	Not affected by guanine nucleotides Not affected by sodium ion
Alpha-2	Rabbit duodenum Brain, less wide-spread	Clonidine, imidazolines	Piperoxan, yohimbine	Agonist binding decreased by guanosine triphosphate Agonist binding decreased by sodium ion Mainly associated with presynaptic receptors
Beta-1	Brain, variable distribution	Epinephrine equal to norepinephrine	Practalol	Supersensitivity (increased receptors) with presynaptic lesions
Beta-2	Brain, even distribution	Epinephrine more than norepinephrine	—	No supersensitivity with presynaptic lesions

Table 3-1 (Continued)

Neurotransmitter	Localization	Agonist(s)	Antagonist(s)	Other
Dopamine D1	Striatum, intrinsic	Dopamine, apomorphine	Ergots	Associated with adenylate cyclase Agonist binding decreased by guanine nucleotides
D2	Striatum, from cortex Pituitary	Dopamine, ergots	Butryroph-enones	Not associated with adenyl-ate cyclase, Not affected by guanine nucleotides Mediates antischizo-phrenic and extrapyra-midal effects of neuro-leptics(?)
Serotonin 5HT1	Brain, wide-spread	Serotonin, lysergic acid diethylamide	Metergoline	Associated with adenylate cyclase Agonist binding decreased by guanine nucleotides

5HT$_2$	Frontal cortex, caudate	Serotonin	Lysergic acid diethylamide, neuroleptics	Labeled selectively by 3H spiroperidol Not affected by guanine nucleotides Not associated with adenylate cyclase
Opiates Mu	Brain, guinea pig ileum(?)	Morphine	Naloxone	Agonist binding decreased by sodium ion and guanine nucleotides Probably most associated with CNS analgesia-producing areas
Kappa	Brain(?)	Ethylketazocine	Naloxane (less than m)	General Note: mu, kappa, and sigma show different response patterns in many physiologic effects in the chronic spinal dog, and discriminative stimulus test in the rat.
Delta	Brain: striatum, limbic nuclei, frontal cortex; mouse vas deferens	Enkephalins	Naloxone (less than m)	

Table 3-1 (Continued)

Neurotransmitter	Localization	Agonist(s)	Antagonist(s)	Other
Sigma	Brain (?)	SKF, 10, 047	Naloxone (less than mu)	

[a] Major differences between receptor types are presented.

Source note: Adapted from Snyder and Goodman (1980) and Adler (1981).

Table 3-2 Receptor Measures as Indices of Psychotropic Drug Effects

Drug Class	Drug Action		Receptor Measure[a]
	Therapeutic Effect	Side Effects	
Neuroleptics	Antipsychotic		Inhibition of ^{3}H haloperidol binding in striatum Blockade of amphetamine-induced depression ventral tegmental dopamine neuronal firing Inhibition of apomorphine and amphetamine stereotypy in rat
		Extrapyramidal Parkinson-like	Inhibition of muscarinic cholinergic ([^{3}H] quinuclidinyl benzilate) binding in striatum. Increased firing of substantia nigra dopamine neurons and blockade of amphetamine-induced depression of same
		Tardive dyskinesia	Increased [^{3}H] haloperidol striatal binding following chronic treatment Increased apomorphine stereotypy following chronic treatment

Table 3-2   (Continued)

Drug Class	Drug Action Therapeutic Effect	Drug Action Side Effects	Receptor Measure[a]
		Sedation and hypotension	Increased ratio of inhibition of alpha-adrenergic ([3H] WB-4101) to [3H] haloperidol binding in rat brain
Tricyclic antidepressant[a]	Antidepressant		With chronic treatment: decreased beta-adrenergic binding in rat brain. Decreased norepinephrine-stimulated cAMP accumulation in rat brain slices. Decreased $5HT_2$ binding in rat cerebral cortex
			Single-cell neuronal firing: decreased (beta responses) and increased (alpha response) to norepinephrine, increased to serotonin
			Increased norepinephrine – (locomotor activity, aggression) and serotonin – (body shakes, sleep) mediated behaviors
		Sedation and hypotension	Inhibition of alpha-adrenergic binding to rat brain
			Inhibition of histamine (H_1) in vitro binding

Benzodiazepines	Muscle relaxant	Anticholinergic	Inhibition of muscarinic binding in rat brain	Displacement of $[^3H]$ diazepam brain binding

[a] All measures are positively correlated with drug actions except inhibition of muscarinic cholinergic binding and Parkinsonian effects, which are negatively correlated.

Abbreviations: $5HT_2$, 5-hydroxytryptamine-2.

correlated with its potency in a CNS receptor assay system, then support is given that the drug acts by means of the particular CNS receptor in question. Table 3-2 illustrates psychotropic drug classes for which receptor assay systems strongly support action at CNS receptor sites. The value of obtaining a "receptor profile" for psychotropic drugs is three-fold. First, it provides a tool for studying the mechanisms involved in the therapeutic and side effects of a drug and for screening the pharmacologic activities of novel agents. Second, it provides a method for measuring clinical levels of drugs in biological fluids. Third, it points to hypotheses of underlying pathogenetic mechanisms in psychiatric illnesses.

The case is most clear regarding the therapeutic effects of neuroleptic drugs, where strongly positive correlations are found between milligram potencies for antipsychotic efficacy and blockade of amphetamine-induced depression of ventral tegmental dopamine neuronal firing, inhibition of $[^3H]$ haloperidol binding, and blockade of apomorphine/amphetamine stereotypy in animals (a dopamine-mediated behavior). These measures are currently considered valid tests for antipsychotic action. Furthermore, they are regarded as powerful supportive evidence for the dopamine hypothesis of schizophrenia (see Chapter 15). While the correlations are not as robust for receptor measures and tricyclic antidepressants, they provide interesting stimuli for hypotheses of depressive illness, e. g. , that depression may be due to supersensitivity of CNS beta-adrenergic receptors, and its treatment involves production of subsensitivity or "down-regulation" of CNS beta-adrenergic receptors (see Chapter 22).

The value of receptor measures for predicting side effects is a promising area, especially for the following: extrapyramidal effects of neuroleptics (antimuscarinic, Parkinson-like symptoms; increased dopamine functioning, tardive dyskinesia); and both sedative/hypotensive and anticholinergic side effects of the neuroleptics and tricyclics (Table 3-2). Tardive dyskinesia, which is produced by long-term neuroleptic usage, is thought to be due to dopamine receptor supersensitivity. The potential of a drug for producing tardive dyskinesia may be assessed using dopamine binding and behavioral measures of receptor supersensitivity (Table 3-2).

An interesting new possibility is the discovery by many investigators of high-affinity, saturable $[^3H]$ diazepam binding to brain membranes. The notable positive correlation between binding to diazepam receptors and muscle relaxant effects of benzodiazepines suggest that specific receptors exist which mediate anxiety. A close functional relationship has been found between benzodiazepine and GABA receptors (see Chapter 25). Furthermore, research has been generated to discover whether an endogenous ligand exists for the benzodiazepine receptor, in effect an "anxiety" or "antianxiety" neurotransmitter.

The presynaptic action of drugs is a potentially valuable area for understanding drug mechanism and possibly developing new agents. Presynaptic mechanisms have been implicated in mechanisms of tricyclic antidepressants (decreased presynaptic adrenergic sensitivity with chronic administration – see Chapter 22), antimanic effects of clonidine (see Chapter 29), and antischizophrenic effects of apomorphine.

A fertile area for speculation and further research illuminated by an understanding of receptor functioning is the development of receptor sensitivity changes through time as underlying mechanisms in the development of psychopathology. Repeated usage of amphetamines and cocaine in man lead to a schizophreniform paranoid psychosis, and animal models using chronic administration of these psychostimulants produce enhanced stereotyped behaviors and depletion of CNS catecholamines, both of which are consistent with development of postsynaptic CNS dopamine supersensitivity. Similarly, a supersensitivity mechanism for CNS catecholamines has been postulated for the switch into mania in bipolar illness.

Finally, a provocative recent finding is the discovery of high-affinity, saturable, reversible phencyclidine binding in rat brain membranes. The correlation of binding affinity of phencyclidine and its structural analogs with effects in behavioral tests suggests the interesting hypothesis that this binding represents a specific CNS receptor that mediates the psychopharmacologic actions of phencyclidine (see Chapter 17).

BIBLIOGRAPHY

Adler, M. W. (1981): The in vivo differentiation of opiate receptors: introduction. Life Sci 28:1543-1545.

Aghajanian, G. K.: Tricyclic antidepressants and single-cell responses to serotonin and norepinephrine: a review of chronic studies. In: Neuroreceptors – Basic and Clinical Aspects (Edited by E. Usdin, W. E. Bunny, and J. M. Davis). John Wiley & Sons, New York, 1981, pp. 27-35.

Ariens, E. J., and Rodrigues De Miranda, J. F.: The receptor concept: recent experimental and theoretical developments. In: Recent Advances in Receptor Chemistry (Edited by F. Gualtieri, M. Giannella, and C. Melchiorre). Elsevier/North-Holland Biomedical Press, Amsterdam, 1979, pp. 1-36.

Arienti, G., and Porcellati, G. (1980): Relationship between phospholipids and receptors. In: Receptors for Neurotransmitters and Peptide Hormones (Edited by G. Pepeu, M. J. Kuhar, and S. J. Enna). Raven Press, New York, 1980, pp. 43-49.

Birdsall, N. J. M., Hulme, E. C., Hammer, R. and Stockton, J. S.: Subclasses of muscarinic receptors. In: Psychopharmacology and Biochemistry of Neurotransmitter Receptors (Edited by Yamamura, H.I., Olsen, M.L., and Usdin, E.). Elsevier/North-Holland Biomedical Press, Amsterdam, 1980, pp. 97-100.

Bunney, B. S.: Central dopaminergic systems: two in vivo electrophysiological models for predicting therapeutic efficacy and neurological side effects of putative antipsychotic drugs. In: Animal Models in Psychiatry and Neurology (Edited by I. Hamin and E. Usdin). Pergamon Press, New York, 1977, pp. 91-105.

Bunney, W. E., Post, R. M., Andersen, A. E., and Kopanda, R. T.: A neuronal receptor sensitivity mechanism in affective illness. Commun Psychopharmacol 1:393-405, 1977.

Castellani, S., Ellinwood, E. H., and Kilbey, M. M.: Behavioral analysis of chronic cocaine intoxication in the cat. Biol Psychiat 13:203-215, 1978.

Charney, D. S., Menkes, D. B., and Heninger, G. R.: Receptor sensitivity and the mechanism of action of antidepressant treatment. Arch Gen Psychiat 38:1160-1180, 1980.

Costa, T., Rodbard, D., and Pert, C.: Is the benzodiazepine receptor coupled to a chloride anion channel? Nature 277:315-317, 1979.

Creese, I.: Receptor binding as a primary drug screening device. In: Neurotransmitter Receptor Binding (Edited by H. I. Yamamura, et al.). Raven Press, New York, 1978, pp. 141-190.

Creese, I., Sibley, D., Leff, S., and Hamblin, M.: Dopamine receptors: subtypes, localization and regulation. Fed Proc 40:147-152, 1981.

Dreyer, F.: Acetylcholine receptor. Br J Anaesthesiol 54: 115-130, 1982.

Gerschenfeld, H. M., Paupardin-Tritsch, D., and Deterre, P.: Neuronal responses to serotonin: a second view. In: Serotonin Neurotransmission and Behavior (Edited by B. C. Jacobs and A. Gelperin). MIT Press, Cambridge, MA, 1981, pp. 105-130.

Hirata, F., Tallman, J. F., Henneberry, R. C., Mallorga, P., Strittmatter, W. J., and Axelrod, J.: Regulation of β adrenergic receptors by phospholipid methylation. In: Receptors for Neurotransmitters and Peptide Hormones (Edited by G. Pepeu, M. J. Kuhar, and S. J. Enna). Raven Press, New York, 1980, pp. 91-97.

Kahy, R. C.: Membrane receptors for hormones and neurotransmitters. J Cell Biol 70:261-286, 1976.

Langer, S. Z., Briley, M. S., and Raisman, R.: Regulation of neurotransmission through presynaptic receptors and other mechanisms: possible clinical relevance and therapeutic potential. In: Receptors for Neurotransmitters and Peptide Hormones (Edited by G. Pepeu, M. J. Kuhar, and S. J. Enna). Raven Press, New York, 1980, pp. 203-212.

McGrath, J. C.: Evidence for more than one type of postjunctional α-adrenoceptor. Biochem Pharmacol 31:467-484, 1982.

Miller, R. J., and Dawson, G.: Neuroreceptors: an overview. In: Receptors for Neurotransmitters and Peptide Hormones (Edited by G. Pepeu, M. J. Kuhar, and S. J. Enna). Raven Press, New York, 1980, pp. 11-20.

Molinoff, P. B., Wolfe, B. B., and Weiland, G. A.: Quantitative analysis of drug-receptor interactions: II. Determination of the properties of receptor subtypes. Life Sci 29:427-443, 1981.

Norman, J.: Drug-receptor reactions. Br J Anaesthesiol 51: 595-601, 1979.

Obestreicher, A. B. , Zwiers, H. , and Grispen, W. H. : Synaptic membrane phosphorylation: target for neurotransmitters and peptides. In: Chemical Transmission in the Brain (Edited by R. M. Buijs, P. Pevet, and D. F. Swaab). Elsevier/North/ Holland Biomedical Press, Amsterdam,1982, pp. 349-367.

Overstreet, D. H. , and Yamamura, H. I. : Receptor alterations and drug tolerance. Life Sci 25:1865-1878, 1979.

Palacios, J. M. , and Wamsley, J. K. : Receptors for amines, amino acids and peptides: biochemical characterization and microscopic localization. In: Chemical Transmission in the Brain (Edited by R. M. Buijs, P. Pevet, and D. F. Swaab). Elsevier/North/Holland Biomedical Press, Amsterdam, 1982.

Paul, S. M. , Marangos, P. , and Skolnick, P. : CNS benzodiazepine receptors: is there an endogenous ligand? In: Psychopharmacology and Biochemistry of Neurotransmitter Receptors (Edited by Yamamura, Olsen, and Usdin). Elsevier/ North Holland Biochemical Press, Amsterdam, 1980, pp. 661-676.

Peck, E. J. , and Clark, J. H. : Brain receptors for neurotransmitters. In: Receptors and Hormone Action (Edited by B. W. O'Malley and L. Birnbaumer). Academic Press, New York, 1978, pp. 515-534.

Peroutka, S. J. , and Snyder, S. H. : Recognition of multiple serotonin receptor binding sites. In: Serotonin in Biological Psychiatry (Edited by B. T. Ho, et al.). Raven Press, New York, 1982, pp. 155-172.

Rang, H. P. (1981): Drugs and ionic channels: mechanisms and implications. Postgrad Med J 57:89-97, 1981.

Richelson, E. : Tricyclic antidepressants and neurotransmitter receptors. Psychiatr Ann 9:16-32, 1979.

Richelson, E. : Neuroleptics and neurotransmitter receptors. Psychiatr Ann 10:21-37, 1980.

Richelson, E. , and El-Fakahany, E. : Changes in the sensitivity of receptors for neurotransmitters and the actions of some psychotherapeutic drugs. Mayo Clin Proc 57:576-582, 1982.

Schwartz, J. , Costentin, J. , Martres, M. P. , Protais, P. , and Baudry, M. : Modulation of receptor mechanisms in the CNS: hyper- and hyposensitivity to catecholamines. Neuropharmacology 17:665-685, 1978.

Snyder, S. H. , and Bennett, J. P. : Neurotransmitter receptors in the brain: biochemical identification. Annu Rev Physiol 38:153-175, 1976.

Snyder, S. H. , and Goodman, R. R. (1980): Multiple neurotransmitter receptors. J Neurochem 35:5-15, 1980.

Snyder, S. H. , U'Prichard, D. C. , and Greenberg, D. A. : Neurotransmitter receptor binding in the brain. In: Psychopharmacology: A Generation of Progress (Edited by M. A. Lipton, A. DiMascio, and K. F. Killam). Raven Press, New York, 1978, pp. 361-369.

Tallman, J. F. , Mallorga, P. , Thomas, J. W. , and Gallagher, D. W. : Characterization of benzodiazepine binding sites. In: Psychopharmacology and Biochemistry of Neurotransmitter Receptors (Edited by Yamamura, Olsen, and Usdin). Elsevier/North Holland Biochemical Press, 1980, pp. 619-630.

U'Prichard, D. C. , and Snyder, S. H. : Therapeutic and side effects of psychotropic drugs: the relevance of receptor binding methodology. In: Animal Models in Psychiatry and Neurology (Edited by I. Hamin and E. Usdin). Pergamon Press, New York, 1977, pp. 477-495.

Vetulani, J. , Stawarz, R. J. , Dingell, J. V. , and Sulser, F. : A possible common mechanism of action of antidepressant treatments. Arch Pharmacol 293:109-114, 1976.

Williams, J. T. , Terrance, M. E. , and North, R. A. : Enkephalin opens potassium channels on mammalion central neurons. Nature 299:74-77, 1982.

Zukin, S. R. , and Zukin, R. S. : PCP (Phencyclidine): Historical and Current Perspectives (Edited by E. F. Domino). NPP Books, Ann Arbor, MI, 1981, pp. 105-130.

Chapter 4

CATECHOLAMINES

Mark S. Gold, M.D. and Cary L. Hamlin, M.D.

CATECHOLAMINES AND MENTAL DISORDERS:
AN OVERVIEW

Catecholamines in the general sense of the term refer to the mehtyl-substituted amines of dihydroxy (para, meta) toluene. Important physiologic roles as neurotransmitter substances have only been demonstrated for three catecholamines, dopamine, norepinephrine, and epinephrine. The neurons which utilize these catecholamines as neurotransmitters will be called collectively catecholaminergic. Some neurons are dopaminergic, others are norepinephrinergic, ane still others are epinephrinergic. The locations of the cell bodies and boutons of catecholaminergic neurons predict their physiological role in the regulation of the homeostasis of the internal mileu of the body and in coordinating homeostatic demands with external behaviors. The cell bodies and dendrites of catecholaminergic neurons are located in the brain stem reticular formation; they receive inputs from viceroceptive afferents, pain via the lateral spinothalamic tract downstream from the substantia gelatinosa and vagal and glossopharyngeal inputs via the nucleus solitarius. There are 13 pairs of catecholamine ganglia, called by Dahlstrom and Fuxe A_1 through A_{13}. A_1 through A_7 are norepinephrinergic or epinephrinergic, and A_8 through A_{13} are dopaminergic. Most studies have not clearly differentiated norepinephrinergic from epinephrinergic neuronal pathways, thus the European term adrenergic will be used here to refer collectively to epinephrinergic and norepinephrinergic neurons. Dopaminergic and adrenergic neurons are small and unmyelinated and a single catecholaminergic neuron projects about 500,000 boutons to its projection fields. Ungerstedt has noted that single adrenergic neurons in the locus coeruleua (LC) project boutons to cerebral cortex, thalamus, cerebellar cortex, and brain stem. Thus, catecholamine neurons influence and integrate a wide scope of brain functions. A_6, the LC, projects to the brain stem, thalamus, cerebellum, and cerebral cortex. The other adrenergic reticular nuclei project to the spinal cord diffusely, to the hypothalamus, basal forebrain, and amygdala via the medial forebrain bundle. A_9, the zona compacta of the substantia nigra, projects to the neostriatum and the amygdala. Nigrostriatal dopamine neurons supply boutons within the striatum to diffusely located interneurons, and about 10% of the total boutons in the striatum are dopaminergic. A_{10}, the ventral tegmental area of the midbrain, supplies boutons to basal forebrain nuclei (accumbens, septum), to limbic cortex (cingulate gyrus), and to prefrontal cortex. A_{11} through A_{13} are intrahypothalamic dopaminergic systems. The catecholaminergic neuron's central position in the reticular formation and limbic system suggests a central role in influencing one's emotional life.

The evidence that associates catecholamine neurotransmitter function with emotional state and certain mental disorders comes from studies of animals and humans.

Ungerstedt, having first defined the locations of the catecholamine fiber pathways in the rat and discovered a specific chemical lesioning technique — 6-hydroxydopamine stereotaxic injection — showed that selective bilateral A_9-A_{10} dopaminergic lesions (90% of those neurons) produced animals that fail to respond to hypoglycemia by eating and dehydration by drinking as normal animals do. Marshall subjected these animals to a series of neurobiological tests and concluded that sensory inattention contralateral to the lesions was present and extends across all modalities of stimuli. Such animals are unmotivated to groom themselves, have sex, eat, or drink even though they can move well enough to accomplish these activities. If not force fed, the animals die.

These experiments by Ungerstedt and Marshall were the first to demonstrate a disorder of "reward" mechanisms in dopamine-deficient animals. In contrast, workers (e.g., Antelman, Fibiger, Atrens, and Hoebel) investigating the phenomena of brain self-stimulation noted that the loci that support it include the dopaminergic fiber tracts and synaptic terminal areas. Square-wave pulse stimulation of nucleus accumbens, for example, produces stimulus-bound eating in a satiated rat and produces self-stimulation by biting and licking a lever at fantastic rates. Similar electrical stimulation of the system produces stimulus-bound copulation and also fantastic rates of self-stimulation which often result in ejaculation in males.

Intracerebral self-stimulation at these sites is potentiated by administration of systemic amphetamines or cocaine (Antelman). Finally, intracerebral self-injection of cocaine has been observed (Hernandez and Hoebel) at these sites.

Thus it can be concluded that dopaminergic neurotransmission is somehow related to motivation and attention. As brute fact it is related to interest and orientation. Perhaps it is primarily related to joy. Or perhaps it is related to the inhibition of fear. Or perhaps it is related to anger or at least disgust.

The answers to these speculations can be found in human psychophysiology experiments, and the study of certain human mental disorders and their responses to various specific dopaminergic drugs has to figure prominently in finding the answers to these questions. Such drugs exist and have been used extensively in various mental disorders by psychiatrists.

The neuroleptics block dopamine postsynaptic receptors, and they disinhibit acetylcholinergic interneurons in the neostriatum and accumbens and probably others. Carlsson showed that the dopamine neurons themselves are disinhibited and the turnover of dopamine is increased.

One of the major observations used to support the hypothesis that dopaminergic hyperactivity is associated with schizophrenia is that there is a strong correlation between a drug's potency to reduce symptoms and its affinity for the dopamine receptor. If therefore neuroleptics act by blocking dopamine receptors, then perhaps dopaminergic activity is too high in schizophrenia.

There are a number of potential problems with the second hypothesis, although the first conclusion appears inducible from the observations. The first is the assumption that all specific dopamine binding inhibits dopaminergic activity. Greengard has demonstrated dopamine autoreceptors that when blocked accelerated dopamine turnover. If the increase in CSF dopamine concentration secondary to autoreceptor blockade exceeds the decrease in average postsynaptic receptor availability induced by the other block, then neuroleptics might act to increase dopamine transmission. Thus one might postulate that neuroleptics improve schizophrenia by restoring dopaminergic activity, and thus adopt a dopaminergic deficiency hypothesis. The balance between autoreceptor and postsynaptic receptor blockade in producing neuroleptic effects has been further clarified by observations that mesocortical dopaminergic neurons lack autoreceptors. Thus the dopamine system anatomically most apparently relevant to explaining schizophrenic symptoms can only respond to neuroleptic by decreasing its activity. Thus, the conclusion that neuroleptics decrease dopaminergic activity in producing their effects upon schizophrenic symptoms appears the better of the two conceivable hypotheses, however, some doubts must await further data.

The neuroleptics have also been successfully used to produce anxiolysis in patients with anxiety not associated with schizophrenia. In demented patients, neuroleptics reduce the anxiety of catastrophic reactions without producing further deterioration of mental status. In borderline patients who don't also have attention deficit disorder, neuroleptics reduce anxiety associated with identity crisis, don't result in abuse, and are unlikely to be successfully used in a suicide attempt. In double-blind studies of mixed "neurotic" patients, neuroleptics are as effective as benzodiazepines in reducing anxiety. The doses used are much lower than (10-20% of) those used to treat schizophrenia. Autoreceptors have a higher affinity for neuroleptic than postsynaptic receptors do, and the effect of these doses upon dopaminergic activity may well be to increase it. This hypothesis receives support from the anxiolytic effects of dopamine agonists in these patients.

Dopamine neuron agonists have been successfully used as anxiolytics and antidepressants. Apomorphine is a popular drug in some European countries in the treatment of anxiolysis. Benztropine which blocks dopamine reuptake is advocated for social phobics. Buispirone is an anxiolytic equivalent in efficiency to diazepam which disinhibits dopamine neurons and acts primarily as an agonist. Bupropion is thought to act by selectively blocking dopamine reuptake and it is effective in major depression and dysthymic disorder.

The second major observation that has been used to support the dopaminergic hyperactivity hypothesis of schizophrenia is that chronic administration of amphetamines or cocaine causes a syndrome of paranoid fear and accusatory auditory hallucinations which is phenomenologically indistinguishable from paranoid schizophrenia. Acute administration of these same drugs results in catecholamine reuptake blockade and increased turnover and activity. Thus, perhaps dopaminergic (or adrenergic) potentiation causes paranoid schizophrenia. This hypothesis rests upon the assumption that chronic cocaine administration produces chronic potentiation of catecholamine neurotransmission, and that assumption has been questioned by recent experiments. Some experiments suggest that chronic cocaine produces a state of reduced catecholamine turnover secondary to depletion of neuronal stores. It is also associated with postsynaptic receptor supersensitivity. The resultant of these two forces is a state of catecholamine deficiency and reduced dopaminergic activity.

The data presented about the effects of neuroleptics and various dopamine agonists to lessen anxiety and probably guilt in various mental disorders support the hypothesis that modification of dopaminergic activity is often therapeutic in mental disorders. Future experiments measuring dopamine turnover and receptor densities in various stages of the different mental syndromes will further clarify the specific kinds of dopaminergic dysfunctions involved in them.

The evidence that associates adrenergic neurotransmission and emotional state is extensive.

In animals, studies in monkeys suggest that activation of the LC causes anxietylike behaviors. Low-intensity electrical pulse stimulation of the LC results in threat response behaviors. Piperoxane, which activates the LC by blocking the inhibitory alpha-1 autoreceptor, also increases threat response behaviors. Natural stressors such as pain activate the LC and produce threat response behaviors. Thus, increased adrenergic activity is associated with increased anxiety and stressful stimuli produce increased adrenergic activity and anxiety. Gold and coworkers suggested LC hyperactivity was the final common neuronal pathway for opiate withdrawal and opiate withdrawal-related panic and anxiety. Pharmacologic surgical treatments that inhibit LC would work in both drug withdrawal and naturally occurring panic.

In contrast, suppression of the LC reduces anxiety, and ablation of the LC decreases threat response behaviors. Suppression of the LC with morphine, clonidine, or diazepam reduces threat response behaviors. Finally, blockade of beta-adrenergic receptors with propranolol reduces threat response behaviors. Thus decreased adrenergic activity is associated with decreased anxiety.

Psychiatrists have studied adrenergic turnover, and response to adrenergic drugs in various mental syndromes. Early studies that examined affective disorders demonstrated altered adrenergic function. Some patients with major depression or bipolar depression have low daily excretion of the major brain adrenergic catabolite, 3-methoxy-4-hydroxyphenylglycol (MHPG). The finding of low daily MHPG excretion is highly correlated with that patient responding with several hours of euphoria after D-amphetamine 30 mg, the amphetamine challenge test. Low daily MHPG excretion, or a positive response to amphetamine challenge predicts ultimately a favorable response to adrenergic reuptake blocking antidepressants (e. g. , desipramine, nortriptyline, maprotiline). Recovery from depression in patients with initially reduced adrenergic turnover measured by daily MHPG is associated with normalization of MHPG excretion. Animal brain experiments show that the acute administration of tricyclics results in arrest of adrenergic neuron firing and decreased adrenergic turnover. Presumably this is the result of the stimulation of alpha-2 adrenergic autoreceptors caused by adrenergic reuptake blockade. Chronic desipramine causes increased turnover associated with downregulation of alpha-2 and beta-adrenergic receptors and no change in alpha-1 receptors. Chronic desipramine treatment is necessary to produce increased MHPG excretion and recovery from depressive symptoms. Thus, some major depressives and bipolar depressives have lowered adrenergic turnover and adrenergic reuptake blocking drugs ultimately normalize adrenergic turnover and relieve these depressions.

Mania in some bipolar subjects is associated with increased adrenergic turnover. This effect is still demonstrable when control of the diet and activity are included. Adrenergic but not serotonin reuptake blockers have been known to provoke mania with its increased energy, euphoria, and irritability. Thus increased adrenergic activity has been associated with mood states of euphoria and rage.

Studies of the relationship of adrenergic activity to anxiety and anxiety syndromes have recently received attention. Propranolol, a beta-adrenergic receptor blocker, is effective to lower anxiety in agoraphobia with panic attacks, in social phobia, in adjustment anxiety, and in posttraumatic stress disorder. It is partially effective in sedative withdrawal and in opiate withdrawal. Clonidine, an alpha-2 adrenergic agonist acutely decreases plasma MHPG, blocks the anxiety of opiate withdrawal, and blocks panic attacks and generalized anxiety in patients with agoraphobia with panic attacks. Unfortunately, tolerance develops to the effects of clonidine upon anxiety in agoraphobia with panic attacks. Agoraphobic panic patients subjected to a phobophobic stress increased their anxiety and plasma MHPG. Clonidine blocked both changes. Plasma MHPG is highly correlated with brain adrenergic turnover and with state anxiety level in agoraphobics. However, daily MHPG excretion is low in agoraphobia with panic patients and this predicts ultimate response to desipramine when the daily excretion normalizes. Finally, patients with Parkinson's disease who have LC lesions and presumably low adrenergic turnover have spontaneous anxiety attacks. A relationship of anxiety and adrenergic activity is uniformly supported. A relationship of adrenergic activity to anxiety in animal models appears to exist.

A relationship of adrenergic activity to anxiety in human

anxiety syndromes appears to exist. The precise nature of these relationships, whether hyper- or hypoactivity produces anxiety, remains to be clearly established.

A relationship of adrenergic activity to major depression and bipolar depression also appears to exist, and in this case support for a hypoadrenergic condition is clear. Conversely, a relationship of hyperadrenergic transmission and the euphoria/rage of mania is also reasonably clear, although increased dopaminergic activity may also play a role in this.

A relationship of increased catecholaminergic transmission (adrenergic and dopaminergic) to relief of attentional problems in attention deficit disorder is suggested by the widespread successful use of amphetaminelike drugs in the treatment of this condition.

Thus catecholaminergic activity seems to play an important role in the response to stress; in moods of fear, guilt, joy, anger, and interest. Catecholaminergic drugs now constitute the bulk of useful psychotropics, and they benefit many patients whose mental dysfunctions are associated with emotional disruption. The development of knowledge about catecholamine neurons and drugs is a prototype first step toward the development of a rational basis for psychopharmacology.

BIBLIOGRAPHY

Charney, O. , Menkes, D. , and Heninger, G. : Receptor sensitivity and the mechanism of action of antidepressant treatment. Arch Gen Psychiatry 38(10):1160, 1981.

Dahlstrom, A. , and Fuxe, K.: Evidence for the existence of monoamine containing neurons in the central nervous system: demonstration of monoamines in the cell bodies of brain stem neurons. Acta Physiol Scand 232:1, 1964.

Giannini, A. J. , Extein, I. , Gold, M. S. , Pottash, A. L. C. , and Castellani, S. : Clonidine in mania. Drug Dev Res 3:101, 1983.

Gold, M. , Redmond, D. , and Kleber, H. : Clonidine in opiate withdrawal. Lancet 1:929, 1978.

Kathol, R. , Noyes, R. , and Slyman, D. : Propranolol in chronic anxiety disorders: a controlled study. Lancet 1:788, 1966.

Langer, S.: Modern concepts of adrenergic transmission. In: Neurotransmitter Systems and Their Chemical Disorders (Edited by N. Legg). Academic Press, London, 1980, p. 29.

Maas, J., and Huang, Y.: Norepinephrine neuronal system functioning and depression. In: The Psychobiology of Affective Disorders. S. Karger, Basel, 1980, pp. 40-56.

Raymond, M., Lucan, C., Beasley, M., O'Connel, B., and Roberts, J.: A trial of five tranquilizing drugs in psychoneurosis. Br Med J 2:63, 1957.

Redmond, E.: Alterations in the function of the nucleus locus coeruleus: a possible model for studies of anxiety. In: Animal Models in Psychiatry and Neurology (Edited by I. Hanin, and E. Usdin). Pergamon Press, London, 1977, p. 295.

Sweeney, P., Maas, J., and Heninger, G.: State anxiety: physical activity and urinary MHPG excretion. Arch Gen Psychiatry 35:1418, 1978.

Ungerstedt, U.: Brain dopamine neurons and behavior. In: The Neurosciences: Third Study Program (Edited by F. Schmitt, and F. Worden). MIT Press, Cambridge, 1974, p. 695.

Chapter 5

INDOLEAMINES

Sam Castellani, M.D.

INTRODUCTION

Serotonin or 5-hydroxytryptamine (5HT) was discovered in the
1930s by two different groups of investigators who independently observed that a substance in the serum and gastrointestinal
mucosa caused powerful vasoconstriction and smooth muscle
contraction, respectively. Hence, the terms "serotonin" and
"enteramine." In 1951, this substance was synthesized and 1
year later it was found that "serotonin" and "enteramine" were
identical. Serotonin is present in many body cells, including
platelets, mast cells, enterochromaffin cells of the intestinal
mucosa, and central nervous system (CNS) neurons. The understanding of CNS 5HT functioning is crucial to biological
psychiatry since it is important in the mediation of basic life
processes such as sleep, food intake, sex, and pain, and has
been substantially implicated in the pathogenesis of affective
illness, hallucinogen-induced psychosis, and anxiety. The following review will deal with key aspects of 5HT neurobiology
with a brief mention of its relevance to psychiatric illness.

ANATOMY

The localization of 5HT in the CNS has been accomplished
with extreme precision due to the methodologic advances of
histochemical fluorescence, immunohistochemistry, and autoradiographic connection tracing. Serotonin structures delineated by these methods in the rat brain consist of nine discrete
cell clusters located in the midline of the midbrain, pons, and
medulla, termed raphe nuclei. Three caudal nuclear groups
send descending projections to the medulla and spinal cord.

The more rostral groups, termed median, dorsal, and central superior raphe nuclei give rise to six ascending projections which terminate in several areas of the forebrain: limbic system (amygdala, hippocampus, septum, hypothalamus), neostriatum, thalamus, sensory relay nuclei (lateral geniculate, superior colliculus), and cerebellar and cerebral cortices.

BIOSYNTHESIS AND CATABOLISM

Synthesis of 5HT in the brain is dependent on the essential amino acid, L-tryptophan. Tryptophan arises mainly from diet and is taken up from the plasma into brain cells by an active, high-affinity uptake process. Tryptophan uptake into brain cells is competitively inhibited by the uptake of large neutral amino acids (tyrosine, phenylalanine, leucine, isoleucine, valine). Intraneuronal tryptophan is converted to 5HT by two enzymes: tryptophan hydroxylase, which hydroxylates the amino acid at the 5 position; and aromatic-L-amino acid decarboxylase, which removes the carboxyl group to form 5HT. Tryptophan hydroxylase is found mainly in 5HT cells and is the rate-limiting step in 5HT formation. The activation of tryptophan hydroxylase requires molecular oxygen and pteridine cofactor. Sufficient data indicate that the availability of tryptophan is the major factor regulating the biosynthesis of 5HT. End product inhibition of synthesizing enzymes is of little physiologic significance.

Other factors that influence the brain synthesis of 5HT are dietary carbohydrate and to a lesser extent, protein. Ingestion of a carbohydrate meal in rats leads to rapid increase in blood and brain tryptophan and brain 5HT synthesis. This sequence of reactions occurs because insulin secretion produces a fall in competing amino acids by enhancing their uptake into muscle. Protein ingestion leads to increased blood levels of both tryptophan and competing amino acids, and thus increments in brain 5HT synthesis following dietary protein are small. In summary, a major factor influencing brain tryptophan levels and thus 5HT synthesis is the ratio of plasma tryptophan to competing amino acid concentration.

Plasma tryptophan exists in "free" and "bound" (to albumin) forms. However, tryptophan has a notably greater affinity for brain than serum albumin, and thus free versus bound tryptophan has little bearing on brain 5HT synthesis.

A dynamic relationship exists between brain tryptophan levels and intraneuronal tryptophan hydroxylase such that enhanced tryptophan uptake leading to increased 5HT synthesis causes a compensatory decrease in tryptophan hydroxylase and subsequent return of 5HT synthesis to normal levels.

Following hydroxylation of tryptophan, 5-hydroxytryptophan is rapidly decarboxylated to 5HT. Aromatic-L-amino acid decarboxylase, which catalyzes this reaction, is thought to be identical or very similar to the enzyme that decarboxylates dihydroxyphenylalanine in the synthesis of catecholamines.

Catabolism of 5HT takes place primarily by intraneuronal deamination by monoamine oxidase (MAO), which forms 5-hydroxyindoleacetaldehyde. The latter compound can be converted to either 5-hydroxyindoleacetic acid (5-HIAA) (by oxidation) or 5-hydroxytryptophol (reduction) depending on the ratio of NAD^+ to reduced nicotinamide adenine dinucleotide (NADH) in tissue. The usual end product is 5-HIAA, and the concentration of this compound in the cerebrospinal fluid is considered an index of central 5HT activity. Other possible catabolic pathways, which are not clearly established, are conjugation by a sulfotransferase and N-methylation. The latter reaction has been proposed as an abnormal pathway for the formation of an endogenous psychotogen in the pathogenesis of schizophrenia (see Chapter 15).

SYNAPTIC DYNAMICS

STORAGE AND RELEASE

There is ample evidence that 5HT is stored in synaptic vesicles which protect it from deamination by MAO, and is released in response to neural impulse into the synaptic cleft by exocytosis. Exocytotic release of 5HT is thought to be dependent on Ca^{2+}. In addition, there is evidence that there exist two intraneuronal 5HT pools: a large relatively stable pool resistant to release, and a small newly synthesized pool readily accessible to release. However, the relationship between these pools and the intraneuronal compartmentalization of 5HT in storage vesicles is not known. Release of 5HT is regulated by intraneuronal MAO activity and autoreceptors. Numerous studies demonstrate that 5HT receptors exist on 5HT raphe cell bodies and nerve terminals and in response to stimulation by 5HT inhibit the release of 5HT (see Chapter 3, Neuroreceptors). These receptors thus are termed "autoreceptors." Stimulation of raphe autoreceptors has been postulated as an important mechanism in the psychotomimetic effects of hallucinogens. Studies indicate that postsynaptic neuronal control

of raphe activity and subsequent 5HT release by feedback inhibition does not exist.

REUPTAKE

After release into the synaptic cleft, 5HT is rapidly taken
back up into the nerve terminal by an active, energy-dependent
process. Inhibition of this process is hypothesized to be an
important mechanism of action of tricyclic antidepressant
drugs (see Chapter 22).

POSTSYNAPTIC RECEPTORS

Radioreceptor binding methods have demonstrated high-affinity,
saturable, reversible, stereospecific binding of tritiated 5HT
and lysergic acid diethylamide (LSD) in brain regions that
have a high density of 5HT nerve terminals. The lack of changes in this binding following raphe lesions indicates it reflects
labeling of postsynaptic 5HT receptors.
    Several observations indicate that there are two types of
anatomically and functionally distinct brain 5HT receptors:
$5HT_1$, located in many brain regions, labeled by tritiated 5HT
and LSD, with LSD agonist actions, and showing drug potencies correlating with 5HT-stimulated adenylate cyclase; and
$5HT_2$, located predominately in cerebral cortex and caudate,
labeled by tritiated spiroperidol and LSD, with LSD antagonist
actions, and showing drug potencies correlating with blockade
of head twitch behaviors.

PHYSIOLOGY

CELLULAR

Electrophysiologic unit recording reveals that 5HT raphe neurons fire with a regular rhythm and slow rate (1-2 spikes/sec),
and between spikes (which are a sudden large depolarization)
there is hyperpolarization followed by gradual depolarization.
The interspike depolarization has been termed "pacemaker
potential." Systemic administration or direct application (microiontophoretic) of 5HT and LSD produces a profound inhibition of raphe neuronal firing. Intricate studies show that LSD
inhibits raphe firing presumably by causing a sustained hyperpolarization and elimination of the pacemaker potential.
    Studies of cats with chronically implanted electrodes al-
lowing free spontaneous activity demonstrate that raphe

electrical activity is correlated positively with arousal, showing highest firing rates during maximal arousal and electrical
silence during rapid eye movement (REM) sleep.

Postsynaptic CNS 5HT sites show predominately inhibitory, but also excitatory electrical activity upon direct application of 5HT. An interesting finding is that LSD and related
indoleamine hallucinogens (N, N-dimethyltryptamine, psilocin,
5-methoxydimethyltryptamine) show much greater inhibition of
raphe than postsynaptic firing in contrast to 5HT which inhibits
neuronal firing equally between pre- and postsynaptic sites.
This characteristic of the hallucinogens has been postulated to
be important in their hallucinogenic effects, presumably by
disinhibition of postsynaptic areas.

BEHAVIORAL

A large body of evidence indicates that CNS 5HT has a general
inhibitory function on several vital behaviors of the organism.
Thus, decreased brain 5HT by lesions or synthesis inhibition
results in enhancement of arousal, food intake, sexual behaviors, pain sensitivity, and blood pressure, while increased
brain 5HT by precursor administration or inhibition of catabolism causes a suppression of these behaviors. Elaborate
hypotheses have been put forth relating brain stem 5HT to the
production of slow-wave sleep, and catecholamines recipro-
cally to behavioral arousal and REM sleep. Studies of CNS
5HT in pain perception indicate the presence of a pain-suppress-
ing 5HT system originating in the nucleus raphe magnus of
the medulla which sends descending projections to pain-trans-
mitting afferents in the trigeminal nucleus and spinal cord. Although endocrine effects of central 5HT are not fully established, there is evidence that 5HT has important effects on anterior pituitary regulation of adrenocorticotropic hormone
(ACTH) (enhances secretion), prolactin (enhances secretion),
and growth hormone (enhances secretion).

PHARMACOLOGY

The clinically relevant drugs whose pharmacological actions
and mechanisms are presumably related to central 5HT are
illustrated in Table 5-1. Certain features of these drug effects
deserve mention. L-Tryptophan shows hypnotic effects and
equivocal but heuristically interesting antidepressant effects
in man. The therapeutic efficacy of tricyclic antidepressants
and trazodone has been presumed to result from a classical

Table 5-1 Clinically Relevant Drugs Affecting Central Nervous
System 5-Hydroxytryptamine

Drug	Pharmacologic Action	5HT Mechanism
L-Tryptophan	Hypnotic, antidepressant(?)	Increased synthesis
Tricyclic antidepressants Trazodone	Treatment of depression and panic disorders	Reuptake blockade Increased electrophysiologic response, decreased brain binding(?)
MAO inhibitors	Treatment of depression and panic disorders	MAO inhibition
Quipazine	Treatment of depression(?)	Postsynaptic receptor stimulation(?)
Reserpine	Sedation, depression	Depletion of intraneuronal storage
LSD and related hallucinogens	Visual hallucinations	Inhibition of raphe neuronal firing(?)
Methysergide	Treatment of vascular headaches	Peripheral, central(?) receptor blockade

reuptake blockade mechanism at central 5HT (and norepinephrine) nerve terminals. However, this mechanism has failed to fully explain the clinical actions of antidepressants (e.g., the long duration to onset of therapeutic effect) (see Chapter 22). The possibility that the increased electrophysiologic response and decreased binding of brain 5HT with chronic antidepressant administration are important mechanisms in the therapeutic effects of these agents is interesting but strictly hypothetical. Similarly, the assumed antidepressant mechanism of MAO inhibitors, i.e., enhanced central 5HT and catecholamines has not been fully established (see Chapter 23). Quipazine shows potential antidepressant effects in man and possible central 5HT receptor agonist actions but demands further study. Reserpine is of historical importance in that its depletion of central 5HT was initially thought to be a key mechanism causing sedation in animals and depression in man. However, later studies demonstrated that depletion of central catecholamines was more important in these effects of reserpine. As mentioned above, the 5HT actions of LSD and related hallucinogens on raphe neurons have been implicated in their hallucinogenic effects. Methysergide, which has peripheral 5HT receptor antagonist actions, is successful in treating vascular headaches. Although initially thought to possess central 5HT receptor blocking actions, data in support of this notion are not available.

RELEVANCE TO PSYCHIATRY

Several lines of evidence support the involvement of central 5HT in the pathogenesis of affective illness, suicide, anxiety, schizophrenia, and hallucinogen-induced psychosis.

The notable importance to biological psychiatry of gaining an understanding of underlying 5HT neurobiological mechanisms is emphasized by the intimate association of 5HT with the limbic system, coupled with the striking central 5HT physiologic effects as reviewed above.

BIBLIOGRAPHY

Aghajanian, G. K.: The modulatory role of serotonin at multiple receptors in brain. In: Serotonin Neurotransmission and Behavior (Edited by B. L. Jacobs and A. Gelperin). MIT Press, Cambridge, MA, 1981, pp. 156-185.

Aghajanian, G. K.: Influence of drugs on the firing of serotonin-containing neurons in brain. Fed Proc 31:91-95, 1972.

Aghajanian, G. K.: Regulation of serotonergic neuronal activity: autoreceptors and pacemaker potentials. In: Serotonin ir Biological Psychiatry (Edited by B. T. Ho, et al.). Raven Press, New York, 1982, pp. 173-181.

Aghajanian, G. K., Haigler, H. J., and Bennett, J. L.: Amine receptors in CNS. III. 5-hydroxytryptamine in brain. In: Biogenic Amine Receptors (Edited by L. L. Iverson, S. D. Iverson, and S. H. Snyder). Plenum Press, New York, 1975, pp. 63-96.

Aprison, M. H., and Hingtgen, J. N.: Serotonin and behavior: a brief summary. Fed Proc 31:121-128, 1972.

Azmitia, E. C.: The serotonin-producing neurons of the midbrain median and dorsal raphe nuclei. In: Chemical Pathways in the Brain (Edited by L. L. Iverson, S. D. Iverson, and S. H. Snyder). Plenum Press, New York, 1978, pp. 233-295.

Basbaum, A. I.: Descending control of pain transmission: possible serotonergic-enkephalinergic interactions. In: Serotonin-Current Aspects of Neurochemistry and Function (Edited by B. Haber, S. Gabay, M. R. Issidorides, and S. G. A. Alivisatos). Plenum Press, New York, 1981, pp. 177-189.

Brown, G. L., Goodwin, F. K., and Bunney, W. E.: Human aggression and suicide: their relationship to neuropsychiatric diagnoses and serotonin metabolism. In: Serotonin in Biological Psychiatry (Edited by B. T. Ho, et al.). Raven Press, New York, 1982, pp. 287-306.

Fernstrom, J. D.: Physiological control of brain serotonin synthesis: relevance to physiology and behavior. In: Serotonin Neurotransmission and Behavior (Edited by B. C. Jacobs and A. Gelperin). MIT Press, Cambridge, MA, 1981, pp. 75-102.

Garattini, S., and Samanin, R.: Drugs affecting serotonin: a survey. In: Serotonin in Health and Disease, Vol. 2. Physiological Regulation and Pharmacological Action (Edited by W. B. Essman). Spectrum Publications, Jamaica, NY, 1978, pp. 247-293.

Giannini, A. J., Castellani, S., and Dvoredsky, A. E.: The role of atmospheric actions in hyperserotonergic anxiety states. J Clin Psychiatry 7:262-264, 1983.

Haigler, H. J., and Aghajanian, G. K.: Serotonin receptors in the brain. Fed Proc 36:2159-2164, 1977.

Jacobs, B. C., and Trulson, M. E.: The role of serotonin in the action of hallucinogenic drugs. In: Serotonin Neurotransmission and Behavior (Edited by B. L. Jacobs and A. Gelperin). MIT Press, Cambridge, MA, 1981, pp. 366-400.

Krieger, D. T.: Endocrine processes and serotonin. In: Serotonin in Health and Disease, Vol. 3. The Central Nervous System (Edited by W. B. Essman). Spectrum Publications, Jamaica, NY, 1978, pp. 51-67.

Mandell, A. J., and Knapp, S.: Regulation of serotonin biosynthesis in brain: role of the high affinity uptake of tryptophan into serotonergic neurons. Fed Proc 36:2142-2148, 1977.

Morgane, P. J., and Stern, W. C.: Serotonin in the regulation of sleep. In: Serotonin in Health and Disease, Vol. 2. Physiological Regulation and Pharmacological Action (Edited by W. B. Essman). Spectrum Publications, Jamaica, NY, 1978, pp. 205-245.

Peroutka, S. J., and Snyder, S. H.: Recognition of multiple serotonin receptor binding sites. In: Serotonin in Biological Psychiatry (Edited by B. T. Ho, et al.). Raven Press, New York, 1982, pp. 155-172.

Sanders-Bush, E.: Regulation of serotonin storage and release. In: Serotonin in Biological Psychiatry (Edited by B. T. Ho, et al.). Raven Press, New York, 1982, pp. 17-34.

Trulson, M. E., and Jacobs, B. L.: Activity of serotonin-containing neurons in freely moving cats. In: Serotonin Neurotransmission and Behavior (Edited by B. L. Jacobs and A. Gelperin). MIT Press, Cambridge, MA, 1981, pp. 339-365.

Chapter 6

ACETYLCHOLINE

Robert L. Gilliland, M.D.

Acetylcholine is a neurotransmitter of great importance in
nervous system function. The chemical was first recognized
for its possible role as a neurotransmitter by Dale in 1914 and
on the basis of experimental evidence it was proposed by Dikshit
in 1934 as a transmitter of nervous system function. In recent
years the research on the function of this neurotransmitter has
rapidly increased and the roles of its associated enzymes,
choline acetyltransferase and acetylcholinesterase, which are
involved in its synthesis and hydrolysis have been greatly clarified. The molecular structure of the acetylcholine receptor has
also been clearly defined. The sequence of events involved in
the neurohumoral transmission of this particular chemical has
been defined. Defects in the transmission of acetylcholine
across the synaptic junction and the interference of its attachment to the receptor site have been clarified and the substances
that interfere with its attachment to the receptor site have produced an understanding of the disease myasthenia gravis.

CHOLINERGIC TRANSMISSION IN THE PERIPHERAL NERVOUS SYSTEM

Acetylcholine is synthesized by the acetylation of choline with
acetyl coenzyme A. This is accomplished by the enzyme choline
acetyltransferase which is a basic protein with a molecular
weight of approximately 65,000. Choline acetyltransferase is
synthesized within the neuron membrane and is transported
along the length of the axon to its terminal.
　　Acetylcholine is synthesized in the terminal portion of the
motor axon and is stored and released from the synaptic vesicles to traverse the small gap of the terminal portion of the

axon to the receptor site on the motor end-plate. The synaptic vesicle may contain several thousand molecules of acetylcholine and it has been calculated that a single motor nerve terminal may contain as much as 300, 000 or more vesicles. In the skeletal muscle the junctional site occupies a small portion of the surface of the individual fiber. It is at this site that the stimulation for contraction of the skeletal muscle cell occurs. The arrival of an action potential down the motor axon causes the release of the vesicles of acetylcholine and they traverse the gap to the receptor sites of the motor end-plate where the molecules of acetylcholine are inactivated with a "flashlike suddenness" by another enzyme, acetylcholinesterase. This allows the muscle membrane to become depolarized and then repolarized.

There is some random occurrence of spontaneous depolarization unrelated to the action potential stimulation. This is at a level much lower than required to stimulate the contraction of the muscle. These are miniature end-plate potentials (MEPPS). With the release of 100 or more quanta (vesicles) of acetylcholine, the depolarization of the muscle cell receptor site is accomplished, in the presence of calcium ions. The combination of acetylcholine with the receptor on the external surface of the muscle membrane induces an immediate, marked increase in permeability to sodium and potassium ions. This triggers the muscle action potential and results in the contraction of the muscle cell.

AUTONOMIC NERVOUS SYSTEM

The smooth muscle of the intestinal tract and the cardiac conduction system are influenced by acetylcholine in a different manner. The smooth muscles of the intestinal tract exhibit intrinsic activity which is modified but not initiated by nerve impulses. Acetylcholine will directly produce contraction of smooth muscles even when they are in the denervated state. In the cardiac conduction system, acetylcholine is released by the preganglionic fibers of the vagus nerve, and inhibits the action of the cardiac muscle by producing a state of hyperpolarization of the fiber membrane and a marked decrease in the rate of depolarization.

CHOLINERGIC SYSTEMS OF THE
CENTRAL NERVOUS SYSTEM

The cholinergic systems of the central nervous system are primarily involved in the arousal mechanisms of the cortex. These systems are located primarily within the midbrain and forebrain with projections to the cerebellum, tectum, thalamus, hypothalamus, striatum, lateral cortex, and olfactory bulb. One area of the forebrain, labeled the basal nucleus of Meynert, lying in the substantia innominata has neurons that are cholinergic. They constitute the major source of cholinergic input to the cortex. The studies on the nervous system have been determined by biochemical, enzyme histochemical, immunocytochemical, and ablation techniques. There is degeneration of the basal nucleus of Meynert and its cholinergic influence on the other cortex in such degenerative diseases as Alzheimer's disease. Studies currently show that choline acetyltransferase is diminished by 50-90% in the neocortex and the hippocampus of brains of patients with Alzheimer's disease. This results in a marked diminution of acetylcholine as a neurotransmitter of the brain.

THE RECEPTOR

Acetylcholine is the smallest of the neurotransmitters. Its receptor on the muscle cell membrane is more accessible for study than the receptors of the brain. Using the techniques of electron microscopy, x-ray diffraction, recombinant DNA, monoclonal antibodies, and the patch clamp membrane procedure, the chemical anatomy and function of the receptor has been established.

The acetylcholine receptor in the three-dimensional view has a funnel-shaped configuration with the wide end extending extracellularly above the membrane surface (synaptic side). The small end extends intracytoplasmically through the lipid bilayer of the cell membrane. This establishes a pore for the ion channel. The densely packed receptors may be single or may be found in groups of two or three in the cell membrane.

Each receptor is composed of subunits that are polypeptide chains. There are four different types of polypeptide chains in each receptor, which are arranged as pentamers. That means that each receptor will be composed of two identical and three unique chains. Each chain spans the membrane. They are labeled alpha, beta, gamma, and delta and are immunologically specific. In the receptor, there are 12 possible arrangements of these subunits of polypeptide chains in the plane of the cell membrane.

The presence of two acetylcholine molecules (agonist), affects the receptor site by producing a rapid transition of the subunits from a resting (closed) state, to the active (open) state thus allowing ion transport to occur. This is followed by a de-sensitized state where the binding of the acetylcholine molecule does not lead to opening of the channel. During the opened phase, an equal number of sodium and potassium ions flow through, causing a drop in the membrane voltage potential to near zero. This produces the excitatory state for the muscle membrane. In the nervous system, the acetylcholine transmission may be excitatory or inhibitory.

Sites on the receptor are effected in different ways by various chemicals. D-Tubocurarine and some snake venoms act primarily at the acetylcholine receptor. Other noncompetitive inhibitors such as certain local anesthetics, aromatic tertiary amines, antimuscarinic agents, antiarrhythmic agents, psychogenic agents, antiviral agents, alkaloid toxins, detergents, and alcohol act at some other unknown site on the receptor. Indications are that they bind within, blocking the channel for ion transport.

Neurotoxins from snake venom (D-bungarotoxin) has been the most important resource for the study of the receptor site. The affinity for this neurotoxin at the receptor site is equal to acetylcholine.

The development of techniques for producing monoclonal antibodies has made it possible to identify each subunit of the receptor immunologically. This has helped in understanding the autoimmune character of myasthenia gravis. Monoclonal antibodies have been developed that are specific for each subunit chain (or part of a chain) in the receptor.

The antireceptor site antibodies seen in myasthenia gravis not only bond to the receptors, but excite the production of complement, producing local lysis of the receptors. The resulting reduced number of receptors produces a functional denervation. These antibodies differ from patient to patient and may be specific for different regions of the receptor site. The stimulation and regulation of this autoimmune response is unknown.

The intensified study of the cholinergic system of neuro-muscular transmission is leading research in the direction of defining the nervous system in terms of its molecular anatomy.

BIBLIOGRAPHY

Aquilonius, S. M.: Role of acetylcholine in the central nervous system. Handbook Clin Neurol 29(22):435-458, 1977.

Corey, D. P.: Patch clamp: current excitement in membrane physiology. Neurosci Comment 1:99-110, 1983.

Dale, H. H.: The action of certain esters and ethers of choline, and their relation to muscarine. J Pharmacol Exp Ther 6:147-190, 1914.

Dikshit, B. B.: Action of acetylcholine on the brain and its occurrence therein. J Physiol 80:409-421, 1934.

Iversen, L. L.: The chemistry of the brain. Sci Am 241:134-149, 1979.

Karlin, A.: The anatomy of a receptor. Neurosci Comment 1: 111-123, 1983.

Lindstrom, J.: Using monoclonal antibodies to study acetylcholine receptors and myasthenia gravis. Neurosci Comment 1: 139-156, 1983.

Price, D. L., et al.: Alzheimer's disease and Down's syndrome. Ann NY Acad Sci 396:145-164, 1982.

Stevens, C. F.: The neuron. Sci Am 241:134-149, 1979.

Stroud, R. M.: Acetylcholine receptor structure. Neurosci Comment 1:124-138, 1983.

Terry, R. D., and Katzman, R.: Senile dementia of the Alzheimer type. Ann Neurol 14:497-506, 1983.

Chapter 7

OPIOIDS: THE ENDORPHINS AND ENKEPHALINS

A. James Giannini, M.D.

A. James Giannini, M.D.

It has always been a source of some academic curiosity that
the sap of an injured poppy could alleviate pain and produce a
euphoria. In the past decade it has been discovered that this
sap is effective because it resembles in both structure and
function mammalian peptides or opioids that act at specific receptor sites in the brain to produce similar results.

There are two types of opioids, the endorphins or "endogenous morphines" and the enkephalins. Both are fragments of
beta-lipotropin, a 91-amino-acid peptide probably manufactured
in the pituitary or, less likely, in the hypothalamus. This larger
unit is then subjected to cleavage by enzymes to produce the desired endorphin and enkephalin fragments as well as adrenocorticotropic hormone (ACTH). (An alternative hypothesis specu-
lates that pituitary and brain opioids are independently synthesized.) Distribution then occurs in those areas of the brain that
are associated with pain perception or mood. Such opioid-rich
areas would include:

Amygdala

Cingulate

Habenula

Hippocampus

Hypothalamus

Inferior frontal lobe

Interpeduncular nuclei

Locus coeruleus

Olfactory bulb

Periaqueductal gray area

Reticular formation

Septum

Striatum

Subcollosal striae

Substantia gelatinosa

Substantia nigra

Temporal lobe

Thalamus

Though both the enkephalins and endorphins both modulate analgesia and mood there are numerous differences. The enkephalins are all pentapeptides with identical sequences [tyrosine (tyr)-glycerine (gly)-gly-phenylalanine (phe)] for the first four amino acids. Endorphins are much larger and include the largest known opioid, a 31-amino acid fragment, beta-endorphin. In addition, there is no similarity among endorphin fragments. The smaller enkephalins act and are degraded more rapidly. Finally, enkephalins and endorphins are thought to act at different types of receptor sites. An interesting possibility has been raised that enkephalins are endorphin subfragments and possibly only artifacts.

All opioid receptors are probably protein-glycolipid complex located at both presynaptic and postsynaptic sites. Presynaptically they function regulate transmitter release in a fashion similar to alpha-2 noradrenergic receptor sites. Postsynaptically they can either excite or inhibit. Thus far excitatory activity has been found only at the hippocampal pyramids and the Renshaw cells. Inhibitor activity has been noted everywhere else. The highest proportion of such activity is seen in the caudate and thalamus. This inhibition is due to hyperpolarization and occurs with any type of neuron (e.g., adrenergic, cholinergic, dopaminergic, etc.). This is affected through overstimulation of guanylate cyclase, a cyclic nucleotide.

Two types of opioid receptors have been differentiated. Delta-receptors act to modulate emotional tone and accordingly are concentrated in those areas of the brain that are concerned with this function—amygdala, nucleus accumbens and pontine raphe nuclei, and locus coeruleus. Quite possibly delta-receptors have a lower addictive potential. They are rather specific to metkephamid, an experimental analgesic known to have little addicting activity. Leu-enkephalin [tyr-gly-gly-phe-leucine (leu)] has delta selectivity.

The second type of opioid receptor is the mu-receptor that is specific to met-enkephalin [tyr-gly-gly-methionyl (met)]. It is found in greatest amounts in tracts and nuclei regulating pain perception including the hippocampal pyramids, hypothalamus inferior colliculi, periaqueductal gray area, and the thalamus. Morphine is approximately 50 times more selective for mu- than delta-receptors. Both types of receptors are found in nucleus ambiguus, nucleus solitarius, substantia gelatinosa, and vagus cords.

An alternative classification system has been developed which is based on the interaction of cations with opioid receptors. Using this scheme, the receptors are divided into mu-, kappa-, and sigma-receptors. The mu-receptors in this system bear no relationship to the previous one. This type of mu-receptor has a high affinity to dihydromorphine, and is most sensitive to regulation by guanosyl triphosphate and sodium ion. Kappa-receptors are highly agonized by ethylketocyclazocine but have low affinities for dihydromorphine, ala-enkephalin, and leu-enkephalin. Sigma receptors have high affinity to leu-enkephalin and ala-enkephalin and a lesser sensitivity to dihydromorphine, but are quite sensitive.

A number of endorphins have been differentiated that are important in psychiatry. Alpha-endorphin regulates analgesia about the head and face. Adding a leu residue produces gamma-endorphin which produces convulsions, hyperthermia, and stimulation. Beta-endorphin modulates total body analgesia and is also a potent euphoriant. Leu-endorphin has been implicated in schizophrenia.

From a psychiatric perspective, the most important site of extraneuronal opioids is in the adrenal medulla. Leu- and met-enkephalin are found in specific organelles within the chromaffin cells. They are stored within specific organelles whose buoyant density approximates that of the catecholamines. Overall opioid release is quantitatively proportional to the amount of combined epinephrine-norepinephrine release.

This association with ACTH and opioids is also seen in the central nervous system. Beta-endorphin and ACTH have been found to coexist in at least some cell bodies of the mediobasal hypothalamus of the rat. Work in progress shows a similar relationship in dog and cat hypothalami. Thus there appears to be an intimate relationship between opioids, catecholamines, and at least one pituitary hormone.

Opioids are situated where they can act as welding devices to interconnect pain, stress, and affect. Their intimate association with the peripheral and decreased central catecholamines and the peripheral catecholamine regulator, ACTH, places them in a unique position to mediate mood and stress responses. Their propinquity to sensory and pain centers assures their ability to regulate the perception of these sensations. Since they interact with pain, stress, and mood areas, they are able to define a sensory sensation in terms of emotional response and to give an "affective coloration" to all sensory input including pain.

BIBLIOGRAPHY

Agnati, L. F., Fuxe, K., Locatelli, V., Benfanaty, F., and Zini, I.: Neuroanatomical methods for the quantitative evaluation of transmitters in nerve cells. J Neurosci Methods 5:203, 1982.

Bergstrom, L., and Terenius, L.: Enkephalin levels decrease in rat striatum during morphine abstinence. Eur J Pharmacol 60:349, 1979.

Childers, S. R., and Snyder, S. H.: Differential regulation by guanine nucleotides of opiate agonist and antagonist interactions. J Neurochem 34:583, 1980.

Chung, K. J., and Cuatrecasas, P.: Multiple opiate receptors. J Biol Chem 254:2610, 1979.

Clement-Jones, V., Lowry, P. J., Rees, L. H., and Besser, G. M.: Met-enkephalin circulates in human plasma. Nature 283: 295, 1980.

Constanti, A., and Nistri, R.: Presynaptic opioid receptor sites. Br J Pharmacol 57:347, 1976.

Frederickson, R. C. A., Southwick, E. L., and Shuman, R.: Methkephamid. Science 211:603, 1981.

Fuxe, K., Andersson, K., and Locatelli, V.: Neuropeptides and central catecholamine systems. In: Neural Peptides and Neuronal Communications (Edited by E. Costa and M. Trabucchi). Raven Press, New York, 1980, pp. 37-50.

Fuxe, K., Agnati, L. F., Hokfelt, T., Anderson, K., Culza, L., Bernardi, P., and Locatelli, V.: Possible functional meaning of coexistence of amine and peptides in the same neuron. Neurosci Suppl 7:544, 1981.

Goldstein, A.: Opioid peptides in pituitary and brain. Science 193:1081, 1976.

King, A. C., and Cuatrecassas, P.: Peptide induced receptor mobility, aggregation and internalization. N Engl J Med 305(2): 77, 1981.

Kline, N. S.: Beta-endorphin induced changes in schizophrenic and depressed patients. Arch Gen Psychiat 34:1111, 1977.

LaMotta, C. C., Snowman, A., Pert, C. P., and Snyder, S. H.: Opiate receptor binding activity: association with limbic systems. Brain Res 155:374, 1978.

Leinen, R., and Giannini, A. J.: Effect of eyestalk removal on glucagon-induced hyperglycemia in crayfish. J Neurosci Abstr 9:604, 1983.

Lord, J., Waterfield, A., and Hughes, J.: Endogenous opioid peptides: multiple agonists and receptors. Nature 267:495, 1977.

Pasternak, G. W., Childers, S. R., and Snyder, S. H.: Naloxone, a long-acting opioid antagonist. J Pharmacol Exp Ther 214: 455, 1980.

Pert, C. B., Kuhar, M. J., and Snyder, S. H.: Opiate receptor. Proc Natl Acad Sci USA 73:3729, 1976.

Pfeiffer, A., Sadee, W., and Herz, A.: Differential regulation of gamma, delta and kappa opiate receptor subtypes by guanyl nucleotides and metal ions. J Neurosci 2:912, 1982.

Sicuteri, F.: Exorcizing migraine through the magic of opioids. In: Headache (Edited by M. Critchley, A. Friedman, and S. Curini). Raven Press, New York, 1980, pp. 7-96.

Snyder, S. H.: Opiate receptors in the brain. N Engl J Med 5: 266, 1977.

Snyder, S. H.: Opiate receptors and internal opiates. Science 236:44, 1977.

Snyder, S. H.: The opiate receptor and morphine-like peptides in the brain. Am J Psychiatry 135:645, 1978.

Terenius, L., Wahlstrom, A., and Lindstrom, L.: Increased CSF levels of endorphins in chronic psychosis. Neuroscience 3:157, 1976.

Watson, S. J., Akil, H., Richard, C. W., and Barchas, J. D.: Evidence for two separate opiate peptide neuronal systems. Nature 275:226, 1978.

Chapter 8

GAMMA-AMINOBUTYRIC ACID (GABA)

David E. Sternberg, M.D.

In recent years several amino acids have gained recognition as major neurotransmitter candidates in the mammalian central nervous system (CNS). Since these substances are also involved in intermediary metabolism, it has been difficult to fulfill all the required criteria that would give these substances legitimate status as neurotransmitters in the mammalian CNS. These amino acids can be divided into two general classes based on their neurophysiologic action—excitatory amino acids which depolarize neurons, and inhibitory amino acids which hyperpolarize neurons and prevent an action potential. Gamma-aminobutyric acid (GABA) appears to be an inhibitory neurotransmitter and is one of the most widely distributed substances in the brain, with 30% of all synapses believed to be GABAergic. The finding that brain concentrations of GABA are 15 times higher than those for catecholamines or serotonin and that GABA was markedly localized, implicates a major physiologic role for GABA in the CNS.

HISTORY

Synthesized in 1883, GABA was known for many years as a product of microbial and plant metabolism. It is formed largely from glutamic acid, which is a shunt of the Krebs' cycle of carbohydrate metabolism. Not until 1950, however, did investigators identify GABA as a normal constituent of the mammalian CNS and find that no other mammalian tissue, with the exception of the retina, contains more than a mere trace of this material. Almost 35 years later we still have no conclusive proof as to the precise role this compound plays in the mammalian CNS, although much evidence has accumulated supporting the hypothesis that GABA functions as an inhibitory transmitter.

Figure 8-1   Metabolism of GABA

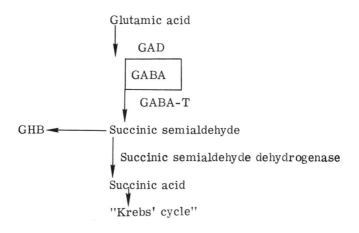

Figure 8-1   Metabolism of GABA

METABOLISM (Fig. 8-1).

GABA is synthesized from the amino acid glutamic acid, by
the enzyme glutamic acid decarboxylase (GAD). The localization of GAD in the brain correlates quite well with GABA content
and thus can be used to localize GABA synthesis to specific neurons.
    GABA transaminase (GABA-T) degrades GABA by transfer-
ring its amino group thereby generating succinic semialdehyde,
which when oxidized enters the Krebs' cycle as succinic acid.
Thus, GABA has an integral connection to general metabolic
functioning in addition to a presumed neurotransmitter action.
In addition, GABA can undergo other metabolic transformations
in the brain, producing active substances such as gamma-
hydroxybutyrate (GHB).

DISTRIBUTION

GABA appears to have a discrete distribution within the CNS. In
the mammalian brain, the highest levels of GABA are found in
the substantia nigra, limbic region, globus pallidus, and hypothalamus. A relationship between GABAergic and dopaminergic

neurons involving GABA-modulated feedback systems has been proven and has possible relevance to schizophrenia (see below).

NEUROTRANSMITTER ROLE

The identification of a compound as a neurotransmitter requires that it be neuronally produced, stored, released, bind to a specific receptor, exert a specific action, and then be rapidly removed from its site of action. Most of the criteria necessary for GABA to be called a neurotransmitter have been identified: the precursor glutamic acid, the synthesizing enzyme (GAD), GABA-receptors, the catabolizing enzymes (GABA-T), and succinic semialdehyde dehydrogenase. There seem to be two types of GABA-receptors: one that binds to tritiated muscimol and tritiated GABA (high-affinity sites) and one that corresponds to the allosteric site which is under modulatory control of a benzodiazepine (BZ) binding site (low-affinity sites). GABA acts postsynaptically by increasing membrane conductance to chloride ions. The net effect of this "hyperpolarization" is to inhibit the generation of an action potential in the postsynaptic neuron. Thus, application of GABA, or of GABA agonists, inhibits neuronal firing.

PATHOPHYSIOLOGY IN DISEASE

GABA deficiencies have been implicated in the pathogenesis of Huntington's disease, epilepsy, schizophrenia, dementia, and normal aging. GABA-mediated inhibition of neuronal firing has been clinically harnessed via the use of valproic acid, a GABA-T inhibitor which increases central GABA, for the treatment of seizure disorders. Research has led to major hypotheses of GABA involvement in schizophrenia and anxiety disorders.

SCHIZOPHRENIA

A GABA disturbance in schizophrenia was first suggested by Roberts (1975). He hypothesized that low levels of GABA in the brain might lead to a state of disinhibition which, in turn, could produce the symptoms seen in schizophrenia. By infusing a GABA antagonist into the area of the nucleus accumbens, Stevens and colleagues induced "paranoid, psychosis-like" behavior in rats. Given the knowledge that GABA and dopamine activity interact, changes in dopamine sensitivity in schizophrenia might be the result of alterations in GABA activity or vice versa. However, clinical trials with GABAergic agents or assays of GABAergic function in schizophrenic patients have failed to show major clinical improvement or to prove consistent GABA abnormalities, respectively.

ANXIETY

In 1967, Schmidt and coworkers reported that diazepam potentiated neuronal inhibition in the spinal cord. Subsequent studies indicated that GABA was the neurotransmitter mediating this so-called presynaptic inhibition—i.e., GABA acts on the presynaptic nerve terminal to inhibit release of an excitatory neurotransmitter. Electrophysiologic experiments have shown that BZs enhance not only presynaptic but also postsynaptic GABAergic inhibition at various sites throughout the CNS. This action does not involve changes in the synthesis, release, or inactivation of GABA, nor is there a direct effect of BZs as GABA agonists on the recognition site of the receptor. A further advance in the understanding of the mechanism of action of BZs and in the understanding of anxiety was the discovery, in 1977, of BZ receptors. Different BZs offer a wide range of pharmacologic potencies, and it was demonstrated that these potencies correlate well with the strength with which the BZ binds to the binding protein. Such a correlation suggests that binding has functional relevance and indicates that the binding protein is a receptor for BZs. In 1978, Tallman and colleagues observed that stimulation of GABA receptors by GABA enhanced the affinity of BZ receptors for BZs. This raised the possibility that the two receptors were close together in neuronal membranes. The BZ receptor seems to be coupled to both the GABA receptor and the chloride channel in a GABA/BZ-receptor/chloride channel complex. Remarkably little happens to chloride or to GABA-receptors when BZs occupy BZ-receptors—i.e., BZs by themselves do not open chloride channels or inhibit neurons. However, when GABA is added to a neuron in addition to a BZ, it produces a greater chloride flux through the neuronal membrane than before the BZ was added. Thus, when a BZ is present on the BZ-receptor, GABA has greater success in opening chloride channels and thereby in inhibiting the neuron's firing. GABA and BZs appear to derive their antianxiety synergism in this manner.

BIBLIOGRAPHY

Cooper, J.R., Bloom, F.E., and Roth, R.H.: Gamma-amino-butyric acid, glycine, glutamic acid, and taurine. In: The Biochemical Basis of Neuropharmacology. Oxford University Press, New York, 1978, pp. 223-258.

Fuxe, K., Perez de la Mora, M., Hokfelt, T.: GABA-DA interactions and their possible relation to schizophrenia. In: Psychopathology and Brain Dysfunction (Edited by G. Shagass, S. Gershon, and A. J. Friedhoff). Raven Press, New York, 1977, pp. 97-111.

Haefely, W., Role, P., Schaffner, R., et al.: Facilitation of GABAergic transmission by drugs. In: GABA Neurotransmitters (Edited by P. Krogsgaard-Larsen, J. Scheel-Kruger, and H. Kofod). Munksgaard, Copenhagen, 1979, pp. 357-375.

Perry, T. L., Buchanan, J., Kish, S. J., et al.: Gamma-aminobutyric acid deficiency in brain of schizophrenic patients. Lancet 1:237-239, 1979.

Roberts, E.: GABA in nervous system function—an overview. In: The Nervous System, Vol. 1: The Basic Neurosciences (Edited by R. O. Brady). Raven Press, New York, 1975, pp. 541-552.

Stevens, S. T., Daris, R. L.: GABA concentrations in a population of schizophrenics. Lancet 231:1173, 1972.

Tallman, J. F., Paul, S. M., Skolnick, P., et al.: Receptors for the age of anxiety: pharmacology of the benzodiazepines. Science 207:274-281, 1980.

Van Kammen, D. P., Sternberg, D. E., Hare, T., et al.: CSF levels of gamma-aminobutyric acid in schizophrenia. Arch Gen Psychiatry 39:91-97, 1982.

Chapter 9

PROSTAGLANDINS

Julian Lieb, M.D.

INTRODUCTION

Close to 60 years ago, Raphael Kurzrock and Charles Lieb made the observation that when artificial insemination was attempted in the treatment of sterility, the injected semen often was promptly expelled. Thus prompted, they devised a series of experiments to investigate the actions of semen on uterine muscle. In some patients uterine muscle contracted while in others it relaxed. These contradictory responses can today be explained by the nature of dose-response curves and by tachyphylaxis.

In 1934, Von Euler observed that human semen and extracts of sheep vesicular glands lower arterial blood pressure on intravenous injection and stimulate isolated intestinal and uterine smooth muscle preparations. He showed that the active principle, which he termed prostaglandin (PG), was a lipid soluble acid and thus different chemically from all other known substances with similar biological activity. Prostaglandins were isolated by Samuelsson in 1960. For a long time it was believed that PGs exist only in semen, but they now are known to be synthesized by every cell in the body, with the possible exception of the mature red blood cell.

The discovery that aspirin and other anti-inflammatory drugs such as indomethacin inhibit cyclooxygenase, an important enzyme in the PG pathway, stimulated intensive research in the involvement of PGs in drug action and disease. As a consequence, conclusive evidence has emerged that PGs and their counterparts, the leukotrienes (LTs) are important in the pathogenesis of many medical, surgical, and reproductive disorders. Demonstrated involvement of PGs in causing patent ductus arteriosus and other congenital heart defects presages the demonstration of PG involvement in many disorders of organogenesis.

Physiologic activity of the PGs in the central nervous system was first demonstrated in 1965 when Horton published a report on the sedative-tranquilizer properties of prostaglandin E1 (PGE1), prostaglandin E2 (PGE2), and prostaglandin E3 (PGE3) in chicks. These findings were subsequently confirmed in mice. Anticonvulsive and analgesic effects of PGE1 in animals were also demonstrated.

Interest in the actions of lithium on the adenyl cyclase-cyclic AMP system led to the demonstration that lithium significantly reduces PGE1-induced stimulation of adenyl cyclase in vivo and in vitro. Subsequent investigation demonstrated excessive synthesis of PGE1 in platelets of manic patients and reduced synthesis of this PG in platelets of depressives. This discovery has been complemented by the observations that lithium selectively inhibits PGE1 synthesis, that monoamine oxidase (MAO) inhibitors (MAOI) inhibit PGE2 synthesis and that tricyclic antidepressants (TCAs) antagonize the actions of PGs, particularly PGE2.

BASIC CHEMISTRY

PROSTAGLANDINS

Prostaglandins are products of fatty acids that are released from membrane phospholipids. A fatty acid cyclooxygenase catalyzes the fatty acids, mainly arachidonic acid, to PG endoperoxides prostaglandin G2 (PGG2) and prostaglandin H2 (PGH2). The endoperoxides are then converted to compounds such as prostacyclin (PGI2), PGE2, thromboxane B2 (TXB2), and prostaglandin D2 (PGD2). PGD2 appears to be particularly important in the central nervous system.

The dietary essential fatty acid linoleic acid is converted by chain elongation and desaturation reactions into dihomo-gammalinolenic acid (DGLA). DGLA is converted into endoperoxides from which PGE1, prostaglandin F1 alpha, and thromboxane B1 are formed.

The release of arachidonic acid may be governed by the enzyme phospholipase A2, although other enzymes such as phospholipase C may also be involved. Glucocorticoids inhibit arachidonic acid release, while aspirin and nonsteroidal anti-inflammatory drugs (NSAID) inhibit cyclooxygenase. MAOIs inhibit arachidonic acid release, but may act at other loci in the PG pathway. Lithium selectively inhibits the formation of PGE1 by inhibiting the mobilization of DGLA. Prostaglandins undergo enzymatic degradation in the lungs or other organs, and excretion is mainly in the urine.

Prostaglandins are not stored in tissues and they usually produce their actions in tissues in which they are synthesized or in adjacent tissues. They are rapidly metabolized to biologically inactive forms. Prostaglandins are categorized on the basis of the number of double bonds present. Thus, PGs may contain one, two, or three double bonds and thus earn the appellation of 1-, 2-, and 3-series PGs, respectively.

LEUKOTRIENES

Leukotrienes were isolated by Samuelsson and colleagues while studying arachidonic acid metabolism in white blood cells. They were named leukotrienes because they are manufactured by leukocytes and have three conjugated double bonds.

Leukotrienes are formed by transformation of arachidonic acid into an unstable epoxide intermediate, leukotriene A4 (LTA4), which can be converted enzymatically by hydration to leukotriene B4 (LTB4), and by addition of glutathione to leukotriene C4 (LTC4). LTC4 is metabolized to leukotrienes D4 (LTD4) and E4 (LTE4) by successive elimination of an alpha-glutanyl residue and glycine.

Cysteinyl-containing LTs are potent bronchoconstrictors, increase vascular permeability, and stimulate mucus secretion. LTB4 causes adhesion and chemotactic movement of leukocytes. Leukotrienes C4, D4, and E4 are released from the lungs of asthmatic subjects exposed to specific allergens and seem to play a role in immediate hypersensitivity reactions. The slow-reacting substance of anaphylaxis consists of LTs C4, D4, and E4.

INTERACTIONS OF PROSTAGLANDINS

Prostaglandins interact with many other compounds. Some of their most important interactions are:

CYCLIC NUCLEOTIDES

In human platelets, PGs sequentially activate adenylate cyclase and cyclic AMP (cAMP) phosphodiesterase. Cyclic AMP appears to be the second messenger for PGs in lymphocytes and in many other systems.

OPIOIDS

There is a growing volume of evidence that PGs and cAMP are involved in the actions of morphine and of endorphins.

CALCIUM

Calcium appears to be necessary for phospholipase activity, and hence PG synthesis could depend on local concentrations of calcium. Prostaglandin effects cannot occur in the absence of calcium and many calcium effects cannot occur in the absence of PGs. Prostaglandins may be involved in facilitating calcium entry into and exit from mitochondria, and stimulation of sodium transport caused by calcium ionophores is secondary to the release of PGs.

CATECHOLAMINES

Prostaglandins appear to be modulators of biogenic amines, both in peripheral organs as well as in the central nervous system. Prostaglandins modulate noradrenergic, dopaminergic, and serotoninergic transmission. Serotoninergic neurons mediate the depressive behavioral effects of PGE2 and PGF2 alpha and the hyperthermic and hypertensive actions of PGF2 alpha.

HORMONES

Prostaglandins modulate the interactions between the sympathetic nervous system and the pineal enzymes that are involved in melatonin synthesis. Prostaglandins also modulate the release of hypothalamic peptide hormones. Prostaglandins, therefore, appear to be modulators of the neuroendocrine junction. Prostaglandins and LTs also play an important role in the synthesis of endocrine and exocrine secretions. Both PGs and LTs have important functions as secretagogue in insulin production.

PROSTAGLANDINS AND PSYCHIATRY

AFFECTIVE DISORDERS

Abdullah and Hamadah demonstrated that platelet formation of PGE1 is elevated in patients with mania and lowered in those with depression when the platelets are stimulated with half-maximal levels of ADP. The discovery that lithium selectively inhibits PGE1 formation and that alcohol, which can induce identical symptoms to mania, selectively enhances PGE1 production complement this finding.

MAOIs are effective inhibitors of PGE2 synthesis, and at clinically relevant concentrations TCAs antagonize PG actions. PGE1 inhibits the mobilization of arachidonic acid, the precursor of PGE2 and TXA2, so that reduced production of PGE1 in depression should be associated with enhanced PGE2 production. These data lead us to suspect that increased PGE2 synthesis could play a role in depression.

We measured plasma PGE2 and TXB2 levels in 30 depressed outpatients (17 unipolars and 13 bipolars) who qualified for a diagnosis of depression by achieving a score of 18 or more on the Hamilton rating scale. We also measured PGE2 and TXB2 in the plasma of 5 healthy nondepressed subjects and in 10 patients suffering from conditions such as hypomania, allergic rhinitis, and psoriasis who were not depressed.

When compared to the normal control values, 29 of the 30 depressed patients had significantly elevated levels of PGE2, and all 30 patients had significantly elevated plasma levels of TXB2. The 10 patients who were not depressed all had PGE2 levels within the range found in the 5 healthy control subjects.

Linnoila and colleagues measured PGE2 levels in the spinal fluid of small samples of unipolar and bipolar depressives and schizophrenics. When compared to schizophrenics, the unipolar depressives were found to have significantly elevated levels of PGE2.

The current theoretical basis for the therapeutic action of MAOIs and TCAs is the catecholamine concept of depression in which depression is associated with deficient formation or action of catecholamines and mania with the converse. However, in addition to the studies cited above, there is both in vitro evidence that MAOIs are effective inhibitors of PG synthesis and in vivo evidence that MAOIs lower brain PG levels, as well as evidence that at clinically relevant concentrations TCAs antagonize PG actions. It can thus be concluded that PGs should be integrated into contemporary concepts of depression.

SUBSTANCE ABUSE

Until recently, it was assumed that any factor that modified conversion of free arachidonic acid to 2-series PGs would affect conversion of the PGE1 precursor DGLA in the same way. However, evidence has emerged that the two pathways can be selectively regulated.

In human platelets, ethyl alcohol has no effect on the conversion of AA to 2-series PGs, but over a range relevant to human intoxication of 30-300 mg/100 ml (7-65 mmol/liter) it greatly enhances the formation of PGE1 from DGLA. These observations are supported by the observation that ethanol enhances the effect of PGE1 on cAMP formation.

Based on these data, it has been argued that ethanol consumption leads to the following reactions:

1. An initial increase in PGE1 synthesis which may be a factor in causing euphoria. However, as PGE1 inhibits PGE2 synthesis euphoria could result from the reduction of PGE2.
2. With continued drinking of alcohol, prolonged mobilization of DGLA occurs; when drinking ceases DGLA stores are relatively depleted.
3. Reduced availability of DGLA would result in reduced levels of PGE1, in turn leading to increased production of PGE2. This mechanism could account for alcohol withdrawal symptoms. When PGE1 is administered to mice following chronic exposure to alcohol, the intensity of the withdrawal syndrome is significantly reduced.

Based on these considerations, raising the intake of the DGLA precursors gammalinoleic and gammalinolenic acids should reduce withdrawal symptoms. This effect has been observed in a few patients.

Ethanol also directly inhibits the formation of 2-series PGs in human platelets. As 2-series PGs are increased in depression, an attractive hypothesis concerning the etiology of alcoholism emerges. Added to these speculations concerning PGs in the etiology of alcoholism is the copious evidence of PG involvement in the chronic effects of alcohol.

There is also a growing volume of evidence concerning the involvement of PGs in mediating the effects of amphetamines, opiates, cannabinoids, and nicotine.

ANXIETY, PHOBIA, AND COMPULSION

1. Drugs that are known to be effective for these disorders include lithium, MAOIs, TCAs, amphetamines, benzodiazepines, beta-adrenergic blockers, and phenothiazines. All have inhibitory actions on PG synthesis.
2. PG synthesis inhibitors such as ibuprofen and naproxen are effective in treating phobias and obsession-compulsion in some patients.
3. Aspirin, commonly used for the relief of mild anxiety and tension, is capable of producing electroencephalographic (EEG) changes consistent with a mild antianxiety property.

STRESS

Recently, "stress" has become the province of the laiety, particularly the media. All kinds of benefits are assured those who commit themselves to control it. Stress reduction can be "taught" and "learnt."

Sufferers from "psychosomatic" disorders are frequently subjected to moralizing speculations regarding their handling of stress. Such value judging should decrease when it is more widely understood that the asthmatic probably can no more control his mobilization of arachidonic acid than can a patient with cholecystitis, appendicitis, or herpes.

Prostaglandins may be involved in mediating stress, either through their increased production or through enhanced tissue sensitivity to them. These speculations are supported by a study in which lymphocytes from subjects undergoing either of two stressful events, cardiac surgery or childbirth, were shown to have an enhanced sensitivity to PGE2. Patients who are sensitive to stress may either increase their production of PGE2 when stressed or become more sensitive to existing levels of PGE2. Increased production of or sensitivity to PGE2 would further increase sensitivity to stress, thus establishing a vicious cycle.

This model holds well for depression. Depressives are often excessively sensitive to stress, and stress tends to intensify their symptoms. Remission of depression with mood-regulating drugs is often followed by an enhanced capacity to handle stress, along with reduction in stress perception.

PSYCHOSOMATIC DISORDERS

Nowhere has the involvement of PGs and LTs in causing illness been more dramatically demonstrated than in those disorders which have earned for themselves the appellation "psychosomatic. " In the section that follows, some of the studies that have established the importance of PGs and/or LTs in these disorders will be summarized.

Irritable Bowel Syndrome

Recently, specific foods were shown to provoke symptoms of irritable bowel syndrome in 14 of 21 patients suffering from this condition. In these patients, challenge with the offending food (e. g. , wheat, corn, dairy products, coffee, citrus) caused pronounced increases in rectal PGE2.

Significant elevations of serum PGE2 and PGF2 alpha occur after challenging food-intolerant individuals with offending foods such as lactose and shellfish. When PG inhibitors such as aspirin or ibuprofen are administered prior to repeat challenge an increase in PGs does not occur and the subjects do not experience their characteristic symptoms.

Asthma

Prostaglandins have marked effects on airway smooth muscle, and asthmatics often respond to steroids, which block PG synthesis.

Although there is evidence implicating 2-series PGs in asthma, LTs may play even a more important role in causing this disorder. Not only are LTs potent bronchoconstrictors, but they also play a role in mucus secretion, edema, and pulmonary vasoconstriction. Allergen challenge of lung tissue from asthmatics elicits bronchial constriction that correlates with the release of LTs C4, D4, and E4.

Rheumatoid Arthritis

Prostaglandins act as mediators of inflammation and it is not surprising that human rheumatoid synovial tissue explants and derived synovial cells in vitro produce large amounts of PGs, primarily PGE2, which probably participate in the pathogenesis of rheumatoid inflammation and promote the osteoclastic resorption of juxtaarticular bone. Furthermore, PG synthesis inhibitors inhibit PGE2 synthesis by rheumatoid synovial organ cultures at concentrations similar to those achieved in plasma during therapy.

The group of drugs, alternately referred to as NSAIDs or PG synthesis inhibitors, all have in common the ability to alleviate the symptoms of rheumatoid arthritis, and all inhibit PG synthesis. MAOIs, which can alleviate or remit the symptoms of rheumatoid arthritis, also have the ability to inhibit PG synthesis.

Migraine

Injection of PGE1 or PGE2 into humans often induces a throbbing headache. Lithium, TCAs, MAOIs, NSAIDs, ergotamine, steroids, and beta-adrenergic blockers are all effective in the treatment and/or prophylaxis of migraine in selected patients and all have inhibitory actions on PG synthesis.

Dysmenorrhea

The investigations that ultimately led to the isolation of PGs were stimulated by the observation that semen appeared to stimulate uterine contractions.

Dysmenorrheic women have more PGs in their menstrual blood than women who have painless periods. It is, therefore, not surprising that NSAIDs can remit dysmenorrhea as well as other premenstrual symptoms such as vomiting and diarrhea.

Duodenal Ulcer

PGE2 and certain methyl analogs of PGE2 inhibit gastric acid secretion in animals and humans, and they prevent the formation of experimental gastric and duodenal ulcers.

Although it is widely accepted that these PGs have a peripheral site of action, PGE2 strongly inhibits gastric acid secretion induced by insulin, electrical vagal stimulation, or acetylcholine in anesthetized rats when administered into the cerebral ventricle.

15(R)-15-Methyl prostaglandin E2, a potent analog of PGE2, increases the incidence of duodenal ulcer healing to approximately the same degree as has been reported in most extensive studies with cimetidine.

Psoriasis

The pathogenesis of psoriasis is marked by infiltration of polymorphonuclear leukocytes into the epidermis, frequently with the formation of microabscesses.

LTB4 and LTB5 are highly potent stereospecific factors which stimulate the migration and degranulation of polymorphonuclear leukocytes and enhance vascular permeability. LTB4 has been found in significant quantities in psoriatic skin, but not in uninvolved skin or in the skin of healthy volunteers.

A strong correlation has been found between the antipsoriatic activity of various drugs and their lipoxygenase inhibition. Benoxaprofen, a 5-lipoxygenase inhibitor, is capable of producing dramatic improvement in the skin of psoriatic patients.

Hypertension

Prostaglandins and LTs appear to be involved in the regulation of blood pressure, probably through both central and peripheral mechanisms. Antihypertensive drugs have important actions on PG synthesis, and PGs are involved in causing renal hypertension. PGE2 has hypertensive and cardiac accelerating effects when injected into the lateral ventricle and discrete hypothalamic nuclei in rats, and a significant increase of plasma PGE2 has been identified in borderline hypertensive patients.

Thyroid Disease

The thyroid contains high concentrations of PG-like substances, and both PGE1 and PGE2 are released in culture media of medullary carcinoma cells. Furthermore, PGE1 mimics the action of thyroid-stimulating hormone on the thyroid by increasing cAMP formation, and lithium, which inhibits PGE1 synthesis, is capable of inducing hypothyroidism. Therefore, it is likely that PGs are involved in the secretion of thyroid hormone.

Anorexia Nervosa and Bulimia

Anorexia nervosa is generally considered to be a psychiatric disorder, and is often classified as psychosomatic.

The primary symptoms of anorexia nervosa are a compulsive desire for thinness accompanied by a delusional self-image, hyperactivity, disordered food intake, compulsive behavior aimed at maintaining thinness, and amenorrhea. Other features include hypothermia, leukopenia, lanugo hair growth, and bradycardia.

Prostaglandins are involved in regulating food intake, and in thermoregulation, ovulation, menstruation, hair growth, hematopoiesis, and depression, and they may be involved in obsession-compulsion. Supporting a possible role of PGs in anorexia/bulimia is the finding that genetically obese mice show large reductions of excessive body weight and excessive food intake when treated with polymeric prostaglandin PGB2.

Lithium, TCAs, and MAOIs can all be effective in treating anorexia and bulimia. All can influence appetite, weight, ovulation-menstruation, and thermoregulation, and all have potent effects on PG synthesis.

SCHIZOPHRENIA

Abdulla and Hamadah demonstrated that adenosine diphosphate (ADP) stimulates the synthesis of PGE1 in platelets from normal subjects and patients with affective disorders, but not in platelets from patients with schizophrenia. Subsequently, Rotrosen and colleagues found that accumulation of PGE1-stimulated [3H cAMP] was reduced in patients with schizophrenia compared with control subjects. Supporting the hypothesis that schizophrenia is a PG deficiency disease are the following data:

1. High doses of PGs antagonists can cause schizophrenia-like syndromes.

2. Penicillin, which enhances PG synthesis, has been reported to be beneficial in a group of patients with chronic schizophrenia.

3. Improvement has been reported in chronic schizophrenics treated with a combination of evening primrose oil, which is rich in the PGE1 precursor gamma-linolenic acid, and penicillin.

In contrast, an excess of PG synthesis has also been proposed as a cause of schizophrenia. The basis of this hypothesis is as follows:

1. There are high cerebrospinal fluid (CSF) PGE levels during fevers, and a temporal relationship between febrile episodes and clinical exacerbations of catatonic states has been reported to occur in some schizophrenics.

2. PGE concentrations have been measured in the CSF of a group of schizophrenics and were found to be higher than in CSF from several nonschizophrenic groups.

Increasingly, doubts are being raised about the validity of various diagnostic schemata for schizophrenia, and even about the validity of schizophrenia itself as a disease entity. Many subjects entered into studies as "schizophrenic" may well be suffering from paranoid mania or hypomania or from delusional depression.

The data cited here concerning schizophrenia are tentative and, to an extent, contradictory, and it may be more productive to integrate them into concepts of psychosis rather than into schizophrenia per se.

EFFECTS OF PSYCHOTROPIC DRUGS
ON PROSTAGLANDIN SYNTHESIS

A considerable number of studies have shown that both TCAs and MAOIs are potent inhibitors of PG synthesis in vitro. In one study, phenelzine was found to be a more potent PG inhibitor than indomethacin. The inhibitory action of MAOIs on PG synthesis is caused, at least partially, by inhibition of arachidonic acid release. TCAs, such as clomipramine, are potent PG antagonists and weak agonists. The action of TCAs on PG synthesis and metabolism appears to be highly selective; clomipramine appears to selectively inhibit PGE2 activity, while imipramine may increase PGF2 alpha synthesis. There are conflicting data concerning possible neuroleptic inhibition of PG synthesis.

In the early 1970s, lithium was shown to inhibit

PGE1-induced cAMP formation by human platelets. The discovery that platelets from manics make excessive PGE1 enhanced these findings. Subsequently, lithium was found to selectively inhibit PGE1 synthesis while not inhibiting PGE2 formation. Recent work has shown that lithium enhances 2-series PG production.

The significance of these findings pertains not only to the therapeutic actions of lithium, but also the mechanisms involved in lithium's side effects. Inhibition of PGE1 synthesis could be an important step in lithium's actions on mania, cluster headache, herpes, thyrotoxicosis, abnormal thermoregulation, leukopenia, and in enhancing immune function. In contrast, the increase in 2-series PG formation could explain many of lithium's side effects, such as hypothyroidism, tremor, diabetes insipidus, and exacerbation of rheumatoid arthritis, psoriasis, and acne.

The promotion of an increase in 2-series PG production by lithium may be a direct effect or could indirectly follow initial inhibition of PGE1. PGE1 inhibits arachidonic acid mobilization, and reducing PGE1 below a critical level would release this inhibition and lead to increased production of 2-series PGs.

IMPLICATIONS OF ACTIONS OF MOOD-REGULATING DRUGS ON PROSTAGLANDIN SYNTHESIS

Mood-regulating drugs are effective in treating a wide range of nonpsychiatric illnesses in which a disturbance of PG synthesis is either known to be or is strongly suspected of being pathogenetically important. TCAs can be effective in managing migraine, colitis, peptic ulcer, asthma, and pain, while MAOIs are capable of remitting hypertension and migraine. Lithium can be effective in treating leukopenia, chronic cluster headache, thyrotoxicosis, hypothermia, familial Mediterranean fever, viral infections, and asthma.

Demonstration of PG involvement in the pathogenesis of a major psychiatric disorder such as affective illness and in a host of medical illnesses suggests that the therapeutic action of these drugs in both affective disorders and these medical illnesses is mediated by a common mechanism: the inhibition of PG synthesis.

CONCLUSIONS

Prostaglandins are involved in the pathogenesis of a plethora of medical illnesses, and there is increasing evidence of their involvement in psychiatric illness. Drugs that inhibit PG synthesis are effective in both psychiatric and medical illness as well as in those diseases termed "psychosomatic."

Advances in our knowledge of PG physiology and pharmacology threaten to weaken, if not obliterate, the traditional divisions between "medical" and "psychiatric," and portend a drastic revision of the concept of "psychosomatic."

So many novel insights into pathogenesis have been provided by PG research that there can be little doubt that this area holds extraordinary promise for the pharmacologic prevention and treatment of disease.

BIBLIOGRAPHY

Abdulla, Y. H., and Hamadah, K.: Effect of ADP on PGE1 formation in blood platelets from patients with depression, mania and schizophrenia. Br J Psychiatry 127:591-595, 1975.

Alvarez, R., Taylor, A., Fazzari, J. J., and Jacobs, J. R.: Regulation of cyclic AMP metabolism in human platelets. Mol Pharmacol 20:302-309, 1981.

Barchfield, C. C., Maasen, Z. F., and Medzihradsky, F.: Receptor-related interactions of opiates with PGE-induced adneylate cyclase in brain. Life Sci 31:1661-1665, 1982.

Bartmann, W., Beck, G., Lerch, U., Teufel, H., and Scholkens, B.: Luteolytic prostaglandin synthesis and biological activity. Prostaglandins 17(2):301-311, 1979.

Brain, S. D., Camp, R. D. R., Dowd, P. M., Black, A. K., Woollard, P. M., Mallet, A. I., and Greaves, M. W.: Psoriasis and leukotriene B4. Lancet 216:762-763, 1982.

Brus, R., Herman, Z. S., Szkilnik, R., and Zabawska, J.: Mediation of central prostaglandin effects by serotoninergic neurons. Psychopharmacology 64:113-120, 1979.

Buisseret, P. D., Heinzelmann, D. I., Youlten, L. J. F., and Lessof, M. H.: Prostaglandin-synthesis inhibitors in prophylaxis of food intolerance. Lancet 1:906-908, 1978.

Burstein, S., Hunter, S. A., Sedor, C., and Shulman, S.: Prostaglandins and cannabis-IX. Biochem Pharmacol 31(14): 2361-2365, 1982.

Caldwell, J., and Putman, J. L.: The potentiation of certain effects of amphetamine by inhibitors of prostaglandin synthesis. Proc Br Paedodont Soc 8:249-250, 1975.

Cardinali, D. P., Ritta, M. N., Speziale, N. S., and Gimeno, M. F.: Release and specific binding of prostaglandins in bovine pineal gland. Prostaglandins 18(4):577-589, 1979.

Chan, W. Y., and Hill, J. C.: Determination of menstrual prostaglandin levels in non-dysmenorrheic and dysmenorrheic subjects. Prostaglandins 15(2):365-375, 1978.

Collier, H. O. J., and Roy, A. C.: Morphine-like drugs inhibit the stimulation by E prostaglandins of cyclic AMP formation by rat brain homogenate. Nature 248:24-27, 1974.

Cubitt, T.: Lithium and thyrotoxicosis. Lancet 1:1247, 1976.

Dahlen, S. E., Hansson, G., Hedqvist, P., Bjorck, T., Granstrom, E., and Dahlen, B.: Allergen challenge of lung tissue from asthmatics elicits bronchial contraction that correlates with the release of leukotrienes C4, D4, and E4. Proc Natl Acad Sci USA 80:1712-1716, 1983.

Ellis, F., Rosenblum, W. I., Birkle, D. L., Traweek, D. L., and Cockrell, C. S.: Lowering of brain levels of the depressant prostaglandin D2 by the antidepressant tranylcypromine. Biochem Pharmacol 31(9):1783-1784, 1982.

Erlij, D., Gersten, L., and Sterba, G.: Calcium, prostaglandin and transepithelial sodium transport. J Physiol 320: 136, 1981.

Feuerstein, G., Adelberg, S. A., Kopin, I. J., and Jacobowitz, D. M.: Hypothalmic sites for cardiovascular and sympathetic modulation by prostaglandin E2. Brain Res 231: 335-342, 1982.

Frolich, J. C., Leftwich, R., Ragheb, M., Oates, J. A., Reimann, I., and Buchanan, D.: Indomethacin increases plasma lithium. Br Med J 1:1115-1116, 1979.

George, F. R., and Collins, A. C.: Prostaglandin synthetase inhibitors antagonize the depressant effects of ethanol. Pharmacol Biochem Behav 10:865-869, 1978.

Godard, P., Chantreuil, J., Clauzel, A. M., Crastes de Paulet, A., and Michel, F. B.: Plasma concentrations of prostaglandins E2 and F2a in asthmatic patients. Respiration 42:43-51, 1981.

Goodwin, J. S., Bromberg, S., and Messner, R. P.: Studies on the cyclic AMP response to prostaglandin in human lymphocytes. Cell Immunol 60:298-307, 1981.

Goodwin, J. S., Bromberg, S., Staszak, C., Kaszubowski, P. A., Messner, R. P., and Neal, J. F.: Effect of physical stress on sensitivity of lymphocytes to inhibition by prostaglandin E2. J Immunol 127(2):518-522, 1981.

Griffin, M. W., Weiss, A. G., Leitch, E. R., McFadden, E. J., Corey, K. F., Austen, J. M., and Drazen, T. S.: Effects of leukotriene D on the airways in asthma. N Engl J Med 308(8): 436-439, 1983

Hanukoglu, I.: Prostaglandins as first mediators of stress. N Engl J Med 296(24):1414, 1977.

Holroyde, M. C., Altounyan, R., Cole, M., Dixon, M., and Elliot, E. V.: Bronchoconstriction produced in man by leukotrienes C and D. Lancet 2:17-18, 1981.

Hong, S. L., Carty, T., and Deykin, D.: Tranylcypromine and 15-hydroperoxyarachidonate affect arachidonic acid release in addition to inhibition of prostacyclin synthesis in calf aortic endothelial cells. J Biol Chem 255(20):9538-9540, 1980.

Hornych, A., Safar, M., Bariety, J., Simon, A., London, G., and Levenson, J.: Thromboxane B2 in borderline and essential hypertensive patients. Prostaglandins Leukotrienes Med 10:145-155, 1983.

Horrobin, D. F.: Schizophrenia as a prostaglandin deficiency disease. Lancet 1:936-937, 1977.

Horrobin, D. F., and Manku, M. S.: Possible role of prostaglandin E1 in the affective disorders and in alcoholism. Br Med J 1:1363-1366, 1980.

Horrobin, D. F., Manku, M. S., and Mtabaji, J. P.: A new mechanism of tricyclic antidepressant action. Blockade of prostaglandin-dependent calcium movements. Postgrad Med J 53(4):19-23, 1977.

Horrobin, D. F., Mtabaji, J. P., Manku, M. S., and Karmazyn, M. : Lithium as a regulator of hormone-stimulated prostaglandin synthesis. In: Lithium in Medical Practice (Edited by F. N. Johnson and F. Johnson). University Park Press, Baltimore, 1978, pp. 243-263.

Horton, E. W. : Prostaglandins. Springer-Verlag, New York, 1972.

Hwang, D. H. : Ethanol inhibits the formation of endoperoxide metabolites in human platelets. Prostaglandins 7:511-513, 1981.

Hwang, D. H., LeBlanc, P., and Chanmugan, P. : In vitro and in vivo effects of ethanol on the formation of endoperoxide metabolites in rat platelets. Lipids 16(8):583-588, 1981.

Hwang, E. C., and Van Woert, M. H. : Role of prostaglandins in the antimyoclonic action of clonazepam. Eur J Pharmacol 71: 161-164, 1981.

Janicke, U., and Forster, W. : Effects of imipramine, chlorpromazine and promazine pretreatment on the in vitro prostaglandin biosynthesis of rabbit brain and renal medulla. Pharmacol Res Commun 9(5):501-507, 1977.

Jones, V. A., McLaughlan, P., Shorthouse, M., Workman, E., and Hunter, J. O. : Food intolerance: a major factor in the pathogenesis of irritable bowel. Lancet 2:1115-1117, 1982.

Kapadia, L., and Elder, M. G. : Flufenamic acid in treatment of primary spasmodic dysmenorrhea. Lancet 2:348-350, 1978.

Komlos, M., Seregi, A., and Schaffer, A. : The role of monoamine oxidase in catecholamine-stimulated prostaglandin biosynthesis of rat brain homogenates. J Pharm Pharmacol 32:592-593, 1980.

Kragballe, K., and Herlin, T. : Benoxaprofen improves psoriasis. Arch Dermatol 119:548-552, 1983.

Laborit, H., Thuret, F., and Laurent, J. : The action of arachidonic acid on the locomotive activity of mice. Chemico-Biol Interact 10:309-312, 1975.

Lazarus, J. H., Richards, A. R., Addison, G. M., and Owen, G. M.: Treatment of thyrotoxicosis with lithium carbonate. Lancet 2:1160-1163, 1974.

Lee, R. E.: The influence of psychotropic drugs on prostaglandin biosynthesis. Prostaglandins 5(1):63-68, 1974.

Levine, A. S., and Morley, J. E.: The effect of prostaglandins (PGE2 and PGF2 alpha) on food intake in rats. Pharmacol Biochem Behav 15:735-738, 1982.

Lieb, J.: Remission of recurrent herpes infection during therapy with lithium. N Engl J Med 301(17):942, 1979.

Lieb, J.: Prostaglandin E1 in affective disorders and alcoholism. Br Med J 1:453, 1980.

Lieb, J.: Immunopotentiation and inhibition of herpes virus activation during therapy with lithium carbonate. Med Hypotheses 7:885-890, 1981.

Lieb, J.: Remission of herpes virus infection and immunopotentiation with lithium carbonate: inhibition of prostaglandin E1 synthesis by lithium may explain its antiviral, immunopotentiating, and antimanic properties. Biol Psychiatry 27:695-698, 1981.

Lieb, J.: Treatment of phobic-anxiety, obsession-compulsion, and excessive drinking with prostaglandin-synthesis inhibitors. J Psychiatric Treat Eval 3:95-97, 1981.

Lieb, J.: Lithium carbonate in vasopastic disorders. Med Hypotheses 9:179-181, 1982.

Lieb, J.: Remission of rheumatoid arthritis and other disorders of immunity in patients taking monoamine oxidase inhibitors. Int J Immunopharmacol 5(4):353-357, 1983.

Lieb, J., and Horrobin, D. F.: Treatment of lithium-induced tremor and familial essential tremor with essential fatty acids. Prog Lipid Res 20:535-537, 1981.

Lieb, J.: Linoleic acid in the treatment of lithium toxicity and familial tremor. Prostaglandins Med 4:275-279, 1983.

Lieb, J., and Karmali, R.: Elevated levels of prostaglandin E2 and thromboxane B2 in depression. Prostaglandins Leukotrienes Med 10:361-367, 1983.

Lieb, J., and Zeff, A.: Lithium treatment of chronic cluster headaches. Br J Psychiatry 133:556-558, 1978.

Lieb, J., Lombard, D., and Nazzaro, A.: Lithium treatment of hypothermia caused by electric shock. Med Hypotheses 6: 769-772, 1980.

Linnoila, M., Whorton, A. R., Rubinow, D. R., Cowdry, R. W., Ninan, P. T., and Waters, R. N.: CSF prostaglandin levels in depressed and schizophrenic patients. Arch Gen Psychiatry 40:405-406, 1983.

Manku, M. S., and Horrobin, D. F.: Chloroquine, quinine, tricyclic antidepressants, and methylxanthines as prostaglandin agonists and antagonists. Lancet 2:1115-1117, 1976.

Manku, M. S., Oka, M., and Horrobin, D. F.: Differential regulation of the formation of prostaglandins and related substances from arachidonic acid and from dihomogammalinolenic acid. 1. Effects of ethanol. Prostaglandins Med 3:119-128, 1979.

Mathe, A. A., Sedvall, G., Wiesel, F. A., and Nyback, H.: Increased content of immunoreactive prostaglandin E in cerebrospinal fluid of patients with schizophrenia. Lancet 2:16-17, 1980.

Michibayashi, T.: Prostaglandins A and E levels in human essential hypertension. Adv Prostaglandin Thromboxane Res 7: 791-796, 1980.

Moore, T. J., et al.: Contribution of prostaglandins to the antihypertensive action of captopril in essential hypertension. Hypertension 3(2):168-173, 1981.

Mtabaji, J. P., Manku, M. S., and Horrobin, D. F.: Actions of the tricyclic antidepressant clomipramine on responses to pressor agents. Interactions with prostaglandin E2. Prostaglandins 14(1):125-132, 1977.

Murphy, D. L., Donnelly, C., and Moskowitz, J.: Inhibition by lithium of prostaglandin E1 and norepinephrine effects on cyclic adenosine monophosphate production in human platelets. Clin Pharmacol Ther 14(5):810-814, 1973.

Nasr, S. J., and Atkins, R. W.: Coincidental improvement in asthma during lithium treatment. Am J Psychiatry 134(9):1942-2043, 1977.

Pennington, S. N., Smith, C. P., Jr., and Strider, J. B.: Alterations in prostaglandin catabolism in rats chronically dosed with ethanol. Biochem Med 21:246-252, 1977.

Persaud, T. V. N.: Prostaglandins and organogenesis. Adv Prostaglandin Thromboxane Res 4:139-156, 1978.

Pickles, V. R.: Prostaglandins in the human endometrium. Int J Fertil 12(3):335-338, 1967.

Pickles, V. R.: Indomethacin, prostaglandins, dysmenorrhea. Br Med J 285:49, 1981.

Polis, E., and Cope, F. W.: Dose-dependent reduction of hereditary obesity in the non-diabetic mouse by polymeric prostaglandin PGBx. Physiol Chem Phys 12:564-568, 1980.

Puurunen, J.: Inhibition of gastric acid secretion by intracerebroventricularly administered prostaglandin E2 in anaesthetized rats. Br J Pharmacol 78:131-135, 1983.

Raab, W. P.: Cyclic nucleotides and prostaglandins in psoriasis. Int J Clin Pharmacol Ther Toxicol 18(5):212-224, 1980.

Rathaus, M., and Bernheim, J.: Effect of propranolol treatment on urinary excretion of prostaglandins E2 and F2-alpha in patients with essential hypertension. Isr J Med Sci 18:231-234, 1982.

Robinson, D. R., Dayer, J. M., and Krane, S. M.: Prostaglandins and their regulation in rheumatoid inflammation. Ann NY Acad Sci 279-294, 1979.

Rotrosen, J., Miller, A. D., Mandio, D., Traficante, L. J., and Gershon, S.: Prostaglandins, platelets, and schizophrenia. Arch Gen Psychiatry 37:1047-1054, 1980.

Rotrosen, J., Mandio, D., Segarnick, D., Traficante, L. J., and Gershon, S.: Ethanol and prostaglandin E1: biochemical and behavioral interactions. Life Sci 26:1867-1876, 1980.

Ruilope, L., Robles, R. G., Brnis, C., Barrientos, A., Alcazar, J., Tresguerres, J. A. F., Sancho, J., and Rodicio, J. L.: Role of renal prostaglandin E2 in chronic renal disease hypertension. Nephron 32:202-206, 1982.

Safar, M. E., Hornych, A. F., Levenson, J. A., Simon, A. C., London, G. M., Bariety, J. L., and Milliez, P. L.: Central haemodynamics and plasma prostaglandin E2 in borderline and sustained essential hypertensive patients before and after indomethacin. Clin Sci 61:323S-325S, 1981.

Samuelsson, B.: Leukotrienes: mediators of immediate hypersensitivity reactions and inflammation. Science 220:568-575, 1983.

Samuelsson, B., Borgeat, P., Hammarstrom, S., and Murphy, R. C.: Leukotrienes: a new group of biologically active compounds. Adv Prostaglandin Thromboxane Res 6:1-18, 1980.

Sircar, J. C., and Schwender, C. F.: Antipsoriatic drugs as inhibitors of soybean lipoxygenase. A possible mode of action. Prostaglandins Leukotrienes Med 11:373-380, 1983.

Taube, C., Block, H. U., and Forster, W.: Antihypertensive drugs alter the production and ratio of prostaglandins E and F in the organs of spontaneously hypertensive rats. Acta Biol Med Germ 41:477-485, 1982.

Vantrappen, G., Janssens, J., Popiela, T., Kulig, J., Tytgat, G. N. J., Huibregtse, K., Lambert, R., Pauchard, J. P., and Robert, A.: Effect of 15(R)-15-methyl prostaglandin E2 (arbaprostil) on the healing of duodenal ulcer. Gastroenterology 83:357-363, 1982.

Wang, Y. C., Pandey, G. N., Mendels, J., and Frazer, A.: Effect of lithium on prostaglandin E1-stimulated adenylate cyclase activity of human platelets. Biochem Pharmacol 23:845-855, 1973.

Weiss, J. W., Drazen, J. M., Coles, N., McFadden, E. R., Weller, P. F., Corey, E. J., Lewis, R. A., and Aarten, K. E.: Bronchoconstrictor effects of leukotriene C in humans. Science 216:196-198, 1982.

Chapter 10

SUBSTANCE P

A. James Giannini, M.D.

Nociception is mediated by a neurotransmitter with the intriguing name of substance P. This is a undecapeptide with the
sequence Arg-pro-lys-pro-glu-phe-phe-gly-leu-met. It is found
in the brain, spinal cord, throughout the intestinal wall, and in
the peripheral nervous system. Peripherally it tends to cause,
at least in vitro, smooth muscle contractility and vasodilatation.
   In neuronal tissue it acts as an excitatory transmitter. In
fact, it was the first peptide considered to act as a neurotransmitter. Its release is dependent upon calcium ion and postsynaptically causes a depolarization. Its slow onset of action has
caused some researchers to consider it a neuromodulator rather than a true neurotransmitter. It appears to share a common
axon with acetylcholine, at least in the avian preciliary ganglia
and the habenulointerpeduncular pathway. Two distinct types of
vesicles, each containing either substance P or acetylcholine,
have been noted. Two separate types of synaptic systems exist
to accommodate the shared heritage in the axoplasm. Immuno-
histochemical investigations have shown that substance P is
manufactured in the perikaryon and is not a synaptosomal artifact. Studies of the substantia nigra have demonstrated that this
peptide is subject to gamma-aminobutyric acid (GABA)nergic
inhibition by quantitative reduction of presynaptic release.
   Substance P is localized in the small unmyelinated neurons
of the dorsal horns of the spinal cord. It is also known to be
produced in the habenular cells and substantia nigra as well as
being found in the fourth ventricular floor, mesencephalon, diencephalon, and caudate nuclei. As a quick rule of thumb, it
may be remembered that brain substance P is found in the gray
matter and spinal substance P in the dorsal horns.
   Several interesting but isolated properties have been noted
for this transmitter. It can stimulate prolactin release though

95

this action is blocked by dephenhydramine, an H histamine antagonist. It also blocks the symptoms of opiate withdrawal.
During Wallerian degeneration its concentration increases prox-
imally but decreases distally.

BIBLIOGRAPHY

Chang, M. M., and Leeman, S. E.: Isolation of a sialogogic
peptide from Abvine Hypothalamus tissue and its characterization as Substance P. J Biol Chem 245:4784, 1970.

Costa, E., and Trubucchi, M. (Editors): Neural Peptides and
Neuronal Communications. Raven Press, New York, 1980, pp.
1-23.

Cuello, A. C., Galfri, G., and Milstein, C.: Detection of substance P in the central nervous system by monoclonal antibody.
Proc Natl Acad Sci USA 76:3532, 1979.

Erichsen, J. T., Kurten, H. J., Eldred, W. D., and Brecha,
N. C.: Localization of substance P-like and enkephalin-like im-
munoreactivity within preganglionic terminals of the avian ciliary ganglion. J Neurosci 2:994, 1982.

Haefely, W., and Hurlimann, A.: Substance P a highly active
naturally occurring polypeptide. Experientia 18:297, 1962.

Terzuolo, C. A.: Research in the ciliary ganglion of birds. Z
Zellforsch Mikrosk Anat 36:255, 1951.

Wilson, W. S. R., Schulz, R. A., and Cooper, J. R.: The
isolation of cholinergic synaptic vesicles from bovine superior
cervical ganglion. J Neurochem 20:659, 1973.

Part II

PATHOPSYCHOPHYSIOLOGY

Chapter 11

THE BIOLOGICAL BASIS OF DEPRESSION

Irl Extein, M.D., A. L. C. Pottash, M.D., and
Mark S. Gold, M.D.

A number of avenues of research over the past three decades
have given credibility to the working assumption that neurobiological abnormalities underlie the major affective illnesses—
major unipolar depressive disorders and manic-depressive
disorders. This research has included identification of a strong
genetic component in the etiology of affective disorders; documentation of a variety of biochemical, neuroendocrinologic,
and electrophysiologic abnormalities in depression; and perhaps
most important of all, development of effective and specific
pharmacotherapies for major depression and manic-depression,
including tricyclics, monoamine oxidase inhibitors (MAOI), and
lithium. The psychopharmacologic revolution has not only
brought effective treatment, but studies of the mechanisms of
action of psychotropic medications have sparked hypotheses
about the pathophysiology of depression.

THE CLINICAL SPECTRUM OF DEPRESSION

When one mentions biological factors in affective disorders, it
is useful to conceptualize this in terms of a spectrum. The
word depression is used to describe a spectrum of conditions
ranging from an ordinary human emotion to a full-blown medical syndrome with fixed depressed mood and physiologic symptoms. These conditions differ phenomenologically and have different causes and treatments. In general, one would emphasize
psychosocial variables such as character structure and environment stresses as causal at the end of the spectrum that refers
to the ordinary human emotion of depression. Biological predisposition receives more causal emphasis at the end that refers
to the medical syndrome of depression.

Let us define the kind of depression to which we will be referring when discussing biological findings. We refer to patients who meet the criteria of the American Psychiatric Association Diagnostic and Statistical Manual of Mental Disorders, 3d ed. , for major depressive disorder and bipolar disorder, depressed. This kind of depression represents a clearly altered mental state compared to the patient's usual self. The depression has a definite onset, clear impairment of functioning, and definite duration. The important point is that patients with this kind of depression manifest not only a relatively fixed, autonomous depressed mood, but also a cluster of symptoms involving multiple body systems, such as those regulating sleep, appetite, sexual drives, and gastrointestinal and other visceral functions. This kind of depression is not part of another psychiatric diagnosis, but stands as an illness by itself. These are the clinical markers for the kind of depression that is likely to have a biological component, reflected both in drug responsiveness and in the evidence for a genetic contribution. There are many depressions secondary to medical conditions or drug abuse. These needed to be carefully considered by clinicians, but will not be focused on in this chapter.

THE MONOAMINE HYPOTHESIS OF DEPRESSION

Three basic monoamine neutrotransmitter systems are of interest in relation to depression. Each of these neuronal systems is defined by the neurotransmitter utilized: the catecholamines dopamine (DA) and norepinephrine (NE) and the indoleamine serotonin [5-hydroxytryptamine (5HT)]. These systems, although neuroanatomically distinct from each other, are intimately interrelated. These important monoamine systems contain relatively few neurons. However, the tiny clusters of neuronal cell bodies called nuclei, in the brain stem and midbrain, project diffusely up toward critical brain regions, including the cerebellum, cortex, limbic system, striatum, and hypothalamus. The NE system, for example, contains less than one-tenth of 1% of the total neuron count in the brain, yet despite its small number of neurons its projections are widely distributed. The neurons that utilize norepinephrine as a neurotransmitter are very long neurons, they have very long axonal processes, and they make many connections. Each norepinephrine neuron can synapse with up to 75, 000 other neurons. In searching for the neuronal substrate of the complex affective disorder syndromes, one would start looking in systems that are widely distributed and that have projections to many crucial areas of the central nervous system. This description fits the NE, serotonin, and DA systems well.

In order to understand the mechanisms of action of drugs used to treat affective disorder, it is important to be familiar with the monoaminergic neuron, with special emphasis on synaptic transmission (Fig. 11-1). The neurotransmitter is released into the synapse from an outpouching of the nerve ending, called a vericosity. The synapse is the very narrow (100 A or less) gap between neurons across which the neurotransmitter must move in order to interact with its receptors on the postsynaptic neuron and exert its effect. In addition to interacting with its receptors, the neurotransmitter can be metabolized or taken back up into the neuron that released it. The synapse is, in effect, the neurochemical transducer of the central nervous system. It is at the synapse that multiple key processes take place, and that the predominant regulatory effects and drug effects occur. We are learning about the many feedback systems whereby synaptic and postsynaptic events influence events in the cell body through feedback neuronal circuits.

The NE system is one in which the neurochemistry and physiology have been extensively described. Synthesis of NE begins from the dietary amino acid tyrosine, which is hydroxylated to dopa by the enzyme tyrosine hydroxylase. This step is rate-limiting in the synthesis of NE. Dopa is decarboxylated to DA, which is hydroxylated to NE, which is then stored in vesicles. When the electrical event (nerve impulse) arrives, shifts in calcium and magnesium occur by an incompletely understood process, with a resultant migration of the NE storage vesicle to the inner wall of the nerve terminal. There is a fusion of the vesicle wall and neuronal membrane and then a release of the NE into the synapse where it can interact with the postsynaptic receptor. In interacting with its receptor, NE exerts control over the enzyme adenyl cyclase, which is associated with the receptors and can influence chemical and electrical events in the next neuron, be it cortical, limbic, or hypothalamic. Again, a number of other things can happen to the NE before or after it reaches the receptor. It can be metabolized extraneuronally [catechol-O-methyl transferase (COMT)] or it can be actively taken up into the neuron, where it can be metabolized by oxidative deamination with monoamine oxidase (MAO) or can be taken back into the storage vesicle.

How were monoamines first associated with affective disorder? It had to do with a series of accidental observations and some alert connections being made by people who were aware of what was happening clinically and also were aware of recent advances in neuropharmacology. For example, almost 20 years

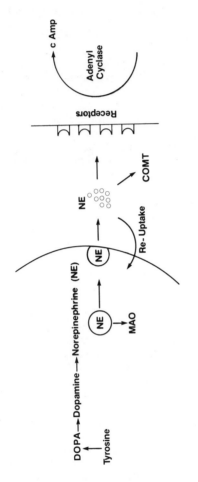

Fig. 11-1.   The noradrenergic synapse

ago reserpine was being used as an antihypertensive. Reserpine would precipitate depression in some individuals. At about this same time it was noted independently, by people who originally knew nothing about what was going on in the clinical sphere, that reserpine could deplete brain monoamines in animals. People began to wonder whether the depletion of monoamines had something to do with the precipitation of depression. Also, at about the same time, in the late 1950s, the MAO inhibitors were found to be antidepressants. Actually, a drug called isoniazid, which was not known to be a MAO inhibitor, used at the time as an antitubercular drug, was found to have mood-elevating properties. It increased activation and alleviated depression in some tubercular patients. Again, quite accidentally, isoniazid was found to inhibit MAO, limiting its availability to metabolize brain monoamines and hence increasing their level at the synapse. Tricyclic antidepressants were also accidentally discovered by researchers. Eventually, it was found that these drugs increased the functional level of monoamines by inhibiting their reuptake. Gradually a coherent story emerged—possibly the lowering of brain amine levels had something to do with depression, and elevation of these levels had something to do with antidepressant effects.

CEREBROSPINAL FLUID AND URINARY METABOLITES AND ANTIDEPRESSANT RESPONSES

One approach to the study of brain monoaminergic functioning in patients which has played an important role in biological psychiatry has been the measurement of metabolites of NE, 5HT, and DA in cerebrospinal fluid (CSF) and urine. There have been many methodologic problems and controversies in this area. However, these studies have suggested that there is a subgroup of major depressives with a "serotonin deficiency" marked by low CSF 5-hydroxy-indoleacetic acid (5HIAA), and a subgroup with a "norepinephrine deficiency" marked by low urinary levels of 3-methoxy-4-hydroxyphenylglycol (MHPG), the end metabolite of NE in brain. Low urinary MHPG tends to be associated with bipolar depression. There was initial excitement concerning these subgroups because of reports that the low serotonin depressives tended to respond preferentially to tricyclics that preferentially block reuptake of 5HT, such as amitriptyline, and that the low-norepinephrine depressives tended to respond preferentially to tricyclics which were thought to preferentially block reuptake of NE, such as imipramine. However, this clean distinction has not held up. One problem is that the above tricyclics are not completely selective, and along with their metabolites affect 5HT and NE. However, some of the drug-response prediction has been replicated, particularly low MHPG-predicting response to NE—potentiating antidepressants such as desipramine and maprotiline. The National Institute of Mental Health Collaborative Program on the Psychobiology of Depression has attempted to study more definitively these correlates of metabolite subgroups. One interesting and potentially useful association reported in Denmark has been the higher incidence of suicide in patients with low CSF 5HIAA. The concept of low 5HT depression has continued to be of value, as in the recent example of lithium's hypothesized potentiation of 5HT neurotransmission leading to the successful use of lithium to potentiate tricyclics in nonresponders.

LONG-TERM RECEPTOR CHANGES AND ANTIDEPRESSANT RESPONSES

New research has cast doubt on the importance of increased availability of synaptic NE and 5HT as the mechanism for antidepressant effect. Some newer nontricyclic antidepressants such as iprindole and mianserin fail to inhibit neuronal uptake of 5HT and NE. In addition, the time course of drug effects on amine availability and clinical improvement are not consistent. While tricyclic blockade of amine reuptake occurs within hours, clinical antidepressant responses take 2-3 weeks at least. Long-term treatment with tricyclics, MAOI, newer nontricyclic antidepressants, and electroconvulsive therapy (ECT) has been shown to reduce postsynaptic beta-adrenergic receptor sensitivity as measured by decreased cyclic AMP (cAMP) accumulation in response to beta-agonists, as well as by decreased binding of labeled beta-agonists. This suggests a common mechanism of antidepressant action. Certainly future research must take into account long-term receptor changes both pre- and postsynaptically.

NEUROENDOCRINE MARKERS FOR DEPRESSION

An approach to biological markers for major depression that has shown much promise for clinical use is the so-called "neuroendocrine strategy. "

The vegetative symptoms of depression, including disturbances of sleep, appetite, weight, and libido-the hypothalamic symptoms of depression-long have suggested neuroendocrine abnormalities in depression. A variety of abnormalities in neu-roendocrine function and response to provocative stimulation have been reported in patients with major depression (Table 11-1). Two tests that have been extensively studied and show relia-ble or reproducible changes in patients with affective disorders are the dexamethasone suppression test (DST) and the thyrotropin-releasing hormone (TRH) tests. Both are standard endocrine tests which have been used for years in the diagnosis of diseases of the hypothalamic-pituitary-adrenal (HPA) axis and hypothalamic-pituitary-thyroid (HPT) axis, respectively. Only more recently have these tests been applied to psychiatry. These tests can confirm clinical diagnoses of major depression and help monitor response to treatment.

The DST begins with administration of 1 mg dexamethasone orally at midnight. Small samples of blood are obtained by veni-puncture at the time of dexamethasone administration and then at two to six time points the next day for determination of serum cortisol in duplicate by radioimmunoassay (RIA). The test is abnormal (i.e., shows failure to suppress cortisol production) if the cortisol level is $\geqslant 5.0$ μg/dl at any of the time points after dexamethasone administration. Approximately 50% of all pa-tients with a clinical diagnosis of major depression fail to sup-press on a standard DST. In addition, many of these patients have hypercortisol secretion and some have a loss of the normal diurnal pattern of cortisol secretion. Thus, we see that while most patients with major depression do not have true Cushing's syndrome, about half of them have a Cushing's-like biochemical profile.

The TRH test consists of measurement of the thyroid stim-ulating hormone (TSH) response to intravenous infusion of 500 μg of the hypothalamic tripeptide TRH. Patients with major uni-polar depressions tend to have a blunted TSH response to TRH, compared to patients with nonmajor depressions of the kind seen in adjustment reactions, grief reactions, or personality disorders, who tend to have normal TSH response to TRH. Sev-eral factors can decrease the TSH response to TRH and they must be taken into account in interpreting TRH test results in depression. These include hyperthyroidism, corticosteroids, alcoholism, some drugs, and age over 60 in males. Factors that can augment the TSH response to TRH include hypothyroid-ism and lithium therapy. The mean Δ TSH in 20 normal volunteer subjects tested by our laboratory was 13.4 ± 1.0 IU/ml. We have found the definition of Δ TSH $\leqslant 7.0$ μIU/ml as a blunted TSH response to TRH useful in discriminating subgroups of depres-sion. In a study of 50 consecutive euthyroid, nonalcoholic pa-tients who had both a DST and a TRH test, 50% failed to suppress

Table 11-1 Summary of Neuroendocrine and Metabolite
Abnormalities in Major Depression

Hormone	Basal	Challenged
GH	−	Insulin, L-dopa, amphetamine, and clonidine stimulation
PRL		Opioid stimulation
LH		LHRH stimulation
TSH	−	TRH stimulation (unipolar)
ACTH/cortisol		Dexamethasone nonsuppression

Metabolite		
Urinary MHPG		(Bipolars)
CSF 5HIAA		Bimodal

Abbreviations: GH, growth hormone; LH; luteinizing hormone; LHRH; luteinizing hormone releasing hormone; PRL, prolactin; other abbreviations as in text.

on the DST and 64% had a blunted TSH response to TRH. There was no relationship between these two abnormalities by chi-square test. Thirty-four percent of patients had an abnormality on the TRH test only, 20% on the DST only, 30% on both, and 16% on neither. Thus each of the two tests identifies patients not recognized by the other, and the two tests seem necessary and complementary in the neuroendocrine evaluation of the depressed patient. The abnormalities in these two tests in patients with affective disorder probably reflect changes in the central neurotransmitters NE, 5HT, and DA which regulate both mood and hypothalamic function. In a sense the DST and the TRH tests are "windows into the brain" which enable us to see neurobiological changes in the brain in patients with affective illness that otherwise could not be detected safely and easily. For example, a failure to suppress on the DST may reflect low central noradrenergic activity, overactivity in serotonergic activity in brain, as well as possible primary alterations in the HPA axis. Recent advances allowing assay of adrenocorticotropic hormone (ACTH) and corticotropic releasing hormone (CRH) will help elucidate the mechanism of nonsuppression in the DST.

Dexamethasone suppression test and TRH test abnormalities tend to normalize with successful antidepressant treatment. Patients who have the persistence of DST or TRH test abnormalities after treatment have a much higher probability of relapse, regardless of clinical appearance or outcome up to that time. The prognostic value of the DST and TRH test in depression is an exciting area for further research.

OTHER BIOLOGICAL ABNORMALITIES IN DEPRESSION

One well-studied biological marker for depression that does not involve biochemical testing is the shortened latency for the onset of rapid eye movement (REM) sleep as measured electrophysiologically in a sleep laboratory. Another interesting approach to the biology of depression involves measurement of circadian rhythms in depressed patients. Alterations in these rhythms may play a role in the pathophysiology of depression, and interventions such as sleep deprivation have led to transient antidepressant responses.

Recent studies have shown that major depressives have decreased urinary levels of phenylacetic acid (PAA), the metabolite of the sympathomimetic phenylethylamine (PEA). These new findings are consistent with the monoamine hypothesis of depression.

The identification of endogenous opioid peptides (endorphins) in the brain sparked interest in the possible role of endorphins in depression. Clinical work with addicts before and after detoxification, anecdotal reports of antidepressant responses to beta-endorphin and exogenous opioids, and reports of decreased prolactin response to opioids all support this notion. Improved techniques for assay of endorphin in humans will help provide more direct information. As more psychoactive neuropeptides are identified, roles for these substances in mood regulation are being explored.

CONCLUSIONS

It is clear that neurobiological abnormalities play a predominant role in the etiology of major depression and manic depression. Despite its flaws, the monoamine deficiency hypothesis still is the central hypothesis concerning the biology of depression. Focus has shifted from turnover studies to studies of long-term receptor adaptations in depression and in pharmacologic response to antidepressants. Neuroendocrine challenge tests have become useful as clinically practical markers for major depression and treatment response, and as "windows into the brain" to elucidate pathophysiology. Studies of the mechanism of action of the increasing array of specific antidepressants continue to be crucial to our understanding of the biology of depression.

BIBLIOGRAPHY

Asberg, M., Thoren, P., Traskman, L., Bertilsson, L., and Rinberger, V.: "Serotonin depression"—a biochemical subgroup with the affective disorders? Science 191:478-480, 1976.

Ayd, F. K., Jr., and Blackwell, B. (Editors): Discoveries in Biological Psychiatry. J. B. Lippincott, Philadelphia and Toronto, 1970.

Bunney, W. E., Jr., Davis, J. M.: Norepinephrine in depressive reactions. Arch Gen Psychiatry 13:483-494, 1965.

Carroll, B. J., Feinberg, M., Greden, J. F., et al.: A specific laboratory test for the diagnosis of melancholia. Arch Gen Psychiatry 38:15-22, 1981.

Charney, D. S., Menkes, D. B., and Heninger, G. R.: Receptor sensitivity and the mechanism of action of antidepressant treatment. Arch Gen Psychiatry 38:1160-1180, 1983.

Cooper, J. R., Bloom, F. E., and Roth, R. H.: The Biochemical Basis of Neuropharmacology. Oxford University Press, New York, 1982.

Extein, I., Pottash, A. L. C., and Gold, M. S.: The thyrotropin-releasing hormone test in the diagnosis of unipolar depression. Psychiatry Res 5:311-316, 1981.

Gold, M. S., Pottash, A. L. C., and Extein, I.: Diagnosis of depression in the 1980's. JAMA 245:1562-1564, 1981.

Goodwin, F. K., and Extein, I.: The biological basis of affective disorders. In: Progress in the Functional Psychoses (Edited by R. Cancro, L. Shapiro, and M. Kesselman). Spectrum Publications, Jamaica, NY, 1979, pp. 129-152.

Goodwin, F. K., Cowdry, R. W., and Webster, M. H.: Predictors of drug response in the affective disorders: toward an integrated approach. In: Psychopharmacology: A Generation of Progress (Edited by M. A. Lipton, A. DiMascio, and K. F. Killam). Raven Press, New York, 1978, pp. 1277-1288.

Greden, J. F., Albala, A. A., Hasket, R. F., et al.: Normalization of dexamethasone suppression test: a laboratory index of recovery from endogenous depression. Biol Psychiatry 15:449-458, 1980.

Heninger, G. R., Charney, D. S., and Sternberg, D. E.: Lithium carbonate augmentation of antidepressant treatment. Arch Gen Psychiatry 40:1327-1334, 1982.

Kirkegaard, C., Bjorum, N., Cohn, D., et al.: Studies on the influence of biogenic amines and psychoactive drugs on the prognostic value of the TRH stimulation test in endogenous depression. Psychoneuroendocrinology 2:131-136, 1977.

Klein, D. F.: Endogenomorphic depression. Arch Gen Psychiatry 31:447-454, 1974.

Koslow, S. H., Maas, J. W., Bowden, C. L., et al.: CF and urinary biogenic amines and metabolites in depression and mania. Arch Gen Psychiatry 40:999-1010, 1983.

Kupfer, D. J.: REM latency: a psychobiologic marker for primary depressive disease. Biol Psychiatry 11:159-174, 1976.

Maas, J. W.: Biogenic amines and depression. Arch Gen Psychiatry 32:1357-1361, 1975.

Martin, J. P., Reichlin, S., and Brown, G. M.: Clinical Neuroendocrinology. F. A. Davis, Philadelphia, 1977.

Pickar, D., Extein, I., Gold, P. W., Summers, R., Naber, D., and Goodwin, F. K.: Endorphins and affective illness. In: Endorphins and Opiate Agonists in Psychiatric Research: Clinical Implications (Edited by N. S. Shah and A. G. Donald). Plenum, Press, New York, 1982, pp. 375-397.

Sachar, E. J., Hellman, L., Roffwang, H. F., Halpern, F. S., Fukushima, D. K., and Gallagher, T. F.: Disrupted 24 hour patterns of cortisol secretion in psychotic depression. Arch Gen Psychiatry 28:19-24, 1973.

Schildkraut, J. J.: The catecholamine hypothesis of affective disorders: a review of supporting evidence. Am J Psychiatry 122:509-522, 1965.

Schildkraut, J. J.: Norepinephrine metabolites as biochemical criteria for classifying depressive disorders and predicting responses to treatment: preliminary findings. Am J Psychiatry 130:695-698, 1973.

Shore, P. A., and Brodie, B.: Influence of various drugs on serotonin and norepinephreine in the brain. In: Psychotropic Drugs (Edited by S. Garrattini,and S. Ghetti). Elsevier, Amsterdam, 1957, pp. 423-427.

Ungerstedt, U.: Sterotaxic mapping of the monoamine pathways in the rat brain. Acta Physiol Scand suppl 367:1-48, 1971.

Wehr, T. R.: Phase and biorhythm studies of affective illness. In: The switch process in manic depressive psychosis (Moderated by W. E. Bunney, Jr.). Ann Intern Med 87:319-335, 1977.

Chapter 12

THE BIOLOGICAL BASIS OF DELUSIONAL DEPRESSION

Duane G. Spiker, M.D.

This chapter will briefly review some of the known differences between delusional and nondelusional depressives including new data regarding treatment of these patients, and discuss one of the more promising current hypotheses regarding the biological basis of this illness. At least three recent articles have reviewed the similarities and differences between delusional and nondelusional depressives and the results will only be summarized here. Although there are some exceptions, most investigators find no differences between delusional and nondelusional depressives with respect to current age, age at first depressive episode, number of prior episodes, duration of current episode, and sex ratio. There is some disparity with respect to current symptomatology with some investigators finding differences and others not finding differences between delusional and nondelusional depressives.

Some of the more consistent findings comparing delusional to nondelusional depressives concerns their response to treatment. Delusional depressives do not respond to placebo while nondelusional depressives have a placebo response rate of approximately 30%. Several authors have also reported that delusional depressives have a much lower response rate to tricyclic antidepressants than nondelusional depressives. Other authors have reported that delusional depressives respond well to the combination of a tricyclic antidepressant and an antipsychotic, while others have reported a favorable response to antipsychotics alone. However, these studies can be criticized because they were either retrospective surveys or used nonrandom assignment of patients to treatment. This led to a large prospective double-blind study in which patients with a delusional depression were randomly assigned to amitriptyline (AT) alone, perphenazine (PER) alone, or the combination of AT + PER for 35 days.

Details of this recently completed study have been presented elsewhere. Fourteen (77.8%) of the 18 patients assigned to AT + PER were responders compared to 7 (41.2%) of the 17 patients treated with AT alone and 3 (18.8%) of the 16 patients on PER alone (p < 0.01). This alone is certainly important information for clinicians. However, some insight into possible biological mechanisms can be gained by combining the plasma level data and analyzing the response rates of the AT alone group and the AT + PER group. By using an analysis of variance to control for the plasma levels of AT and its biological active metabolite nortriptyline (NT), several aspects of the relationship between the AT + NT plasma levels, the presence of PER, and clinical response can be evaluated. Such an analysis shows that there is a positive relationship between the log of AT + NT plasma levels and clinical response (F = 4.29, p < 0.05). However, AT + PER is still a superior treatment to AT alone even when the AT + NT plasma levels are controlled for (F = 4.58, p < 0.05). Even more important to understanding the biological basis of delusional depression, there is virtually no interaction between AT + NT plasma levels and the presence of PER [F = 0.05, p = not significant (NS)]. In other words, no matter what the AT + NT plasma level, the addition of PER increases the response rate. These observations suggest that there is a threshold beyond which antidepressants are not effective and the presence of a phenothiazine is needed. As one of the more prominent effects of phenothiazines is on the dopaminergic system, this seems to suggest some role of that system in the etiology of delusional depression.

Some of the earliest work looking at the dopaminergic system in delusional depression was done by Meltzer and associates. In 1976 they reported that delusional unipolar and to a lesser extent bipolar depressives have decreased levels of dopamine-beta-hydroxylase (DBH) in their plasma compared to nondelusional depressives. Thus delusional depressives might have elevated dopamine levels from decreased metabolism of dopamine secondary to decreased DBH activity. There is some support for the role of increased dopamine levels causing psychosis in depressed patients based on cerebral spinal fluid (CSF) studies. Homovanillic acid (HVA) is the metabolite of dopamine. In 1978, Sweeney and associates reported that CSF HVA levels were significantly higher in delusional than in nondelusional depressives (see Bibliography at end of chapter). Although this is certainly encouraging, another study did not find this when they examined the CSF of delusional and nondelusional depressives. However, in both of these studies, the sample sizes are small and there was wide variation in HVA in both delusional and nondelusional depressives.

Probably the most consistently found biological difference between delusional and nondelusional depressives concern the secretion of cortisol and the failure of dexamethasone to sustain the suppression of the endogenous production of this hormone. In the studies that have reported on the results of the dexamethasone suppression test (DST) in these two groups of depressed patients, the delusional patients almost uniformly have elevated baseline cortisol levels and/or an increased incidence of failure to suppress cortisol secretion using the DST.

Rothschild and associates recently reported on a series of experiments in which they produced data to support a hypothesis relating the elevated cortisol levels and the development of psychosis. They first measured dopamine levels in normal volunteers before and after the administration of dexamethasone. Prior to the dexamethasone, dopamine levels were either below levels of detection or very low. Afterward, they uniformly found higher levels of dopamine. Rothschild and coworkers conducted an experiment in rats to demonstrate that exogenous dexamethasone not only led to measurable plasma levels of dopamine but also to increased dopamine levels in the brain. They gave one group of rats $20 \mu g$ dexamethasone intraperitoneally, sacrificed them after 1 or 4 hours, immediately froze their brains, and measured dopamine levels in several areas of the brain. They compared these findings to those from a control group of rats given intraperitoneal injections of water. The rats given dexamethasone had statistically significant higher levels of dopamine than the control group in the hypothalamus and nucleus accumbens but no difference in the frontal or striatal areas. Thus, their basic hypothesis is that the markedly increased cortisol levels seen in delusional depressives is associated with an increased central nervous system dopamine level that produces the psychosis.

There is little question that there are differences between delusional and nondelusional depressives. Whether these differences are simply expressions of differential severity or whether they represent the end result of a biological divergence is simply not known at this time. In any case, the most promising area currently being investigated regarding the biological basis of delusional depression is the dopamine hypothesis. Experiments currently in progress should answer these questions.

BIBLIOGRAPHY

Caroff, S., Winokur, A., Rieger, W., et al.: Response to dexamethasone in psychotic depression. Psychiatry Res 8:59-64, 1983.

Carroll, B. L., Greden, J. F., Feinberg, M., et al.: Neuroendocrine dysfunction in genetic subtypes of primary unipolar
depression. Psychiatry Res 2:251-258, 1980.

Charney, D. S., and Nelson, J. C.: Delusional and nondelusional unipolar depression: further evidence for distinct subtypes. Am J Psychiatry 138:328-333, 1981.

Coryell, W., Gaffney, G., and Burkhardt, P. E.: The dexamethasone suppression test and familial subtypes of depression
—a naturalistic replication. Biol Psychiatry 17:33-39, 1982.

Frances, A., Brown, R. P., Kocsis, J. H., et al.: Psychotic
depression: a separate entity? Am J Psychiatry 138:831-833,
1981.

Glassman, A. H., and Roose, S. P.: Delusional depression.
A distinct clinical entity? Arch Gen Psychiatry 38:424-427,
1981.

Kaskey, G. B., Nasr, S., and Meltzer, H. Y.: Drug treatment
in delusional depression. Psychiatry Res 1:267-277, 1980.

Meltzer, H. Y., Cho, H. W., Carroll, B. J., et al.: Serum
dopamine-beta-hydroxylase activity in the affective psychoses
and schizophrenia. Decreased activity in unipolar psychotically
depressed patients. Arch Gen Psychiatry 33:585-591, 1976.

Mendels, J., Frazer, A., Fitzgerald, R. G., et al.: Biogenic
amine metabolites in cerebrospinal fluid of depressed and manic
patients. Science 175:1380-1381, 1972.

Minter, R. E., and Mandel, M. R.: The treatment of psychotic
major depressive disorder with drugs and electroconvulsive
therapy. J Nerv Ment Dis 167:726-733, 1979.

Moradi, S. R., Muniz, C. E., and Belar, C. D.: Male delusional depressed patients: response to treatment. Br J Psychiatry 135:136-138, 1979.

Nelson, J. C., and Bowers, M. B.: Delusional unipolar depression: description and drug response. Arch Gen Psychiatry
35:1321-1328, 1978.

Rothschild, A. J., Schatzberg, A. F., Langlais, P. J., et al.: Dexamethasone elevates dopamine in human plasma and rat brain. Abstracts of Panels and Posters presented at the Annual Meeting of the American College of Neuropsychopharmacology, San Francisco, December 12-16, 1983, p. 16.

Rudorfer, M. V., Hwu, H. G., and Clayton, P. J.: Dexamethasone suppression test in primary depression: significance of family history and psychosis. Biol Psychiatry 17:41-48, 1982.

Spiker, D. G., Hanin, I., Perel, J. M., et al.: Pharmacological treatment of delusional depressives: a summary of protocol results. Abstracts of the American College of Neuropsychopharmacology, San Francisco, December 12-16, 1983, p. 16.

Sweeney, D., Nelson, C., Bowers, M., et al.: Delusional versus nondelusional depression: neurochemical differences. Lancet 2:100-101, 1978.

Chapter 13

MANIA: THE DUAL NATURE OF ELATION

Jonathan M. Himmelhoch, M.D.

> In 1665 and 1666 a large proportion of the members of
> the world Jewish communities acknowledged the ar-
> rival of a "messiah" in the person of a Turkish Jew,
> Shabbatai Zvi. . . . The biographical details. . . leave
> little doubt that he suffered manic-depressive illness
> . . . but it was Nathan of Gaza rather than
> Shabbatai who instigated diffusion of the messianic
> claim. . . [and] Nathan's was what we have been call-
> ing a "hypomanic personality."
>
> Mortimer Ostow

THE NATURE AND SOURCES OF ELATION

The relationship between Nathan of Gaza and Shabbatai Zvi
catches the dual, paradoxical nature of elation nicely. On the
one hand, elation is a consummation devoutly to be wished—a
source of joy, of energy, of creative genius, even of sainthood.
Unlike syphilis which is always blamed on the other guy (the
French call it the Italian disease; the Spanish, the French disease, and so forth), people are happy to be labeled manic or
hypomanic. Indeed, they will frequently call themselves manic-
depressive as an explanation for any sort of queer or aberrated
behavior for which they have a particular fondness. No one ever
caught mania from a toilet seat. Morris Fishbein describes it
as the illness of geniuses. Mabel Baker-Cohen claims it for up-
ward striving, intellectually oriented, middle-European Jews.
Americans honor it as the essence of entrepreneurship. The
Scandinavians feel they have prior claim to it, and the Russians
hallow manics to the same degree they do epileptic vurodivies.
It cannot be said that mania has the royal lineage of hemophilia
or porphyria, but then again it is not so decadent.

116

On the other hand, elation can represent a failing organism's last gasp attempt at adaptation and survival. The assault may take the form of creeping senescence, of implacable medical disease, or of overwhelming environmental stress. Conversely, the organism may be constitutionally unable to stand up to even the most trivial threat. Whichever the case, all that is left to it is a frail tissue composed of absolute denial, cheerful delusion, exaggerated religiosity, and desperate driveness. Sometimes the masque succeeds: Solshenitzen's notes in The Gulag Archipelago that any given Zek's (shortened Russian form of zaklyuchennye, meaning prisoner) survival depended directly on his abilities to mobilize hypomanic denial; and no wise physician would interfere with this survival maneuver in cancer patients undergoing chemotherapy. But just as often it fails. The psychotic and delusional nature of the organism's denial becomes readily apparent, and worse yet, underlying protest, depression, and despair well up through the cracks and crazes of imperfect denial. It is in this situation that we see the young male patient with a fresh coronary doing pushups at the side of his bed, monitor leads still on his chest, proving to the coronary care unit personnel, brought running by his monitor's alarm, that he is perfectly healthy, nay, even better, immortal; and it is also in this situation that the worst forms of manic-depressive illness—rapid cycling, psychotic, or chronically manic ¬occur. This form of elation can be viewed as the organism's ultimate emergency response, mobilized when there is a perceived threat to survival that is both serious and prolonged (acute, short-term threats to existence mobilize those well-known fight-flight responses originally described by Cannon). A similar ethologic hypothesis has been made to explain the evolutionary role of the naturally occurring, polypeptide opiates and the systems of central receptors which they modulate. If both these hypotheses have any ethologic validity, the mobilization of such emergency responses by an organism should be extremely difficult, restricted either to the occurrence of serious subacute threats to existence, or to those situations where the organism's access to such dire behavioral patterns (response threshold) is set low because of constitutional predisposition. Mandell has neatly described the formidable neurobiologic barriers to euphoria that exist just at the locus of the synaptic cleft (Table 13-1). It is inevitable that the central nervous system props up these barriers with broader homeorhetic influences. In Mandell's own words:

> From both the neurobiological and clinical points of
> view it is clear that the extension of central euphorigenic
> action over time has reached a technical barrier, the

Table 13-1   Neurologic Barriers to Elation

The amount of neurotransmitter released into the synapse.

The state of the mechanism for reuptake of neurotransmitter into the presynaptic nerve ending.

The amount, availability, and affinity for substrate of the enzymes that metabolized neurotransmitters.

The amount and proximity to the rate-limiting enzyme of a product that can inhibit enzymatic function.

The supply and transport into the cell of the precursors of neurotransmitters.

The physical state and/or conformation of the enzyme as a regulator of activity or of affinity for substrate.

existence of acute and chronic mechanisms of adaptation. . . . I recall a statement Heinz Lehmann made to
me recently. . . . It seems to me that puritanical attitudes toward pleasure must have as part of their sub-
stantive grounds these neurobiological mechanisms of
adaptation.

It may be legitimately asked that if these intense, ecstatic,
often psychotic, and more rarely occurring elations represent
ethologically derived patterns of emergency response, what does
hypomanic behavior, which Ostow states is "often not only not
pathologic, but in many instances. . .seems to confer an advantage, " represent? Ostow believes hypomania is the same psychic
process as psychotic elation, but limited in degree. It is the
basic contention of this chapter, however, that it represents an
entirely different process, connected with different ethologic
and developmental issues, and even in those instances when it
forms a part of a "manic-depressive illness, " this illness is not
only descriptively different from classical bipolar illness (often
known as bipolar I) but has a different course and treatment response. Kurt Goldstein, in attempting to explain the difference
between the neurologically normal and the neurologically abnormal organism, concluded:

Whenever anxiety, as the mainspring of an organism,
comes into the foreground, we find that something is
awry in the nature of that organism. To put it conversely, an organism is normal and healthy when its tendency toward self-actualization issues from within, and
when it overcomes the disturbance arising from its
clash with the world, not by virtue of anxiety but
through the joy of coming to terms with the world.

The experience of fulfillment contingent upon self-actualization
therefore, serves as the model for "hypomania. " The evolutionary advantage of such contingent reinforcement as part of the
everyday armamentarium that the organism uses to come to
terms with the problems of quotidian existence is self-evident.
Margaret Mahler in her article "Notes on the Development of
Basic Moods" attaches this hypomanic mood state to that phase
of individuation and separation she calls "the practicing period
par excellence" - the period where the 14- or 15-month-old
toddler has developed enough locomotor skills to, in Piaget's
terms, run "physics" experiments with every object within his
reach. Mahler states: "These functions, during the practicing
period, attract so much libido that the junior toddler is emotion-
ally relatively independent of [mother] and absorbed in his own
narcissistic pleasures. " Seen in this light, hypomania; even

when it is a marker to a form of manic-depressive illness (in some cases called bipolar II illness; where the patient functions well in his hypomanic phase, but only comes for treatment in his depressed phase) represents an entirely different adaptive position from that desperate emergency mobilization that is usually part of any intense euphoria, but is the very essence of psychotic elation. An argument may be erected against the dual nature of elation, and the clear distinction between hypomania and mania, based on the correct observation that severely ill, primary and secondary manic-depressives often pass through a nonpsychotic, pleasantly hypomanic period as they escalate into full-blown mania. However, it is just this relative absence of those "neurobiological barriers" against euphoria that justifies the separation, whether the defective barrier arises from constitutional factors, from frank neurologic illness, or from an overwhelming, clear, and present danger.

THE CLINICAL PRESENTATION OF HYPOMANIA AND MANIA

Although the nature of elation is obscure, its meaning is hard to decipher, and its differential diagnosis diverse and complex, hypomania and mania are far and away the easiest psychopathologic syndromes for the clinician to recognize. The patient's motor behavior is markedly accelerated, although not as much as his thinking. In elated episodes secondary to complex partial epilepsy or subictal cerebral dysrhythmias, motor acceleration is muted and hypomania/mania can be expressed as an elation of pure thought, usually involving religious themes or, more rarely, sexual ones. In most circumstances, however, motor behavior is frenetic, but purposive, which helps distinguish it from the aimless motor patterns of the excited catatonic or acutely schizophrenic patient. When a severely hypomanic/manic is restrained from carrying out his plans, he can become assaultive and extremely dangerous. If, on the other hand, there are no environmental obstacles to his schemes, the patient is often infectiously jovial. He frequently will develop six or seven business deals simultaneously, while heading up charity drives and other civic-minded endeavors. He becomes extremely social and gregarious as his mood elevates, and joins numerous clubs and organizations. The patient will talk long hours on the telephone, frequently long distance. He will spend outrageous sums of money, on occasion bankrupting himself and his family. Finally, the subject suffers from major vegetative changes; sleeping less and less as his illness gets worse. Sex drive is usually elevated, sometimes leading to "promiscuous" behavior prodigal in proportion. Appetite is effected, but just as often decreased as increased, because sometimes the patient becomes so enmeshed in the Byzantine matrix of his own schemes that there is no time left for eating in the daily schedule.

However, elation is an essentially cognitive experience. Almost every well-known observer of manic-depressive illness has commented on the "role of the word" in hypomania and mania. The patient's thinking and logic seems rational but extremely quick. One can follow his thinking as it expands to encompass every tangential concept and percept. This process in its purest form is known as "flight of ideas" and is distinguished from the fragmented cognitive structure or schizophrenia by the fact that the logic of associations is still retained and the chain of associations can be followed by the listener. An excerpt from the letter of a very creative patient, which she posted during a hypomanic episode demonstrates this almost pathognomonic cognitive pattern:

Dear Doctor,
Would you like to hear my theory regarding your recent illness? Hah! This is a letter, so you have no choice, unless you decide not to read it which is almost as impossible as not eating the last piece of candy in a bag of M&M's (unless you don't go for M&M's in the first place – in which case you wouldn't have opened the bag, which just goes to prove my point because you've already opened the letter, which does not necessarily mean you like M&M's. I happen not to like them myself, having proven (contrary to popular opinion) that with patience and enough time they do melt in your hand . . . which just goes to show that the peanut [candy] people are not all they are cracked up to be (there's a pun in there somewhere. . .); to make a long parenthesis short − I guess it's already too late for that − I shall get back to the letter.

The integral part played by "word-play" in the nature of wit is evident here, and has been well described by both Freud and Henri Bergson. But mania and hypomania are intrinsically hypersocial behaviors, particularly when compared to those socially isolating maneuvers that almost define schizophrenia. Katan has observed that: "In schizophrenia the external world is restored by means of the word; in mania, contact with the outside world is maintained by means of the word."

This difference becomes important in distinguishing intensely psychotic manic episodes from schizophrenic ones. Manic cognition can range from the pufferies of the gregarious, high-pressure automobile salesman, to paranoia and grandiose delusions that are bizarre enough to often be mislabeled schizophrenic. However, the concept of intensity weighs heavily on the interpretation of any behavioral symptom. It is often impossible to interpret a behavioral syndrome at the height of its intensity. Manic patients at the extreme end of their episode can be dissociated, paranoid, and riddled with Schneiderian first-rank symptoms, including specific auditory and visual hallucinations. Occasionally elements of confusion and disorientation will also appear — usually associated with extreme sleep depri vation and fatigue — injecting the differential diagnosis of delirium into the clinician's thinking. It is, therefore, often wise to wait for intensely psychotic and/or confusional episodes to cool off so that both final diagnosis and maintenance treatment plans are made interepisodically, instead of at the height of an episode. The psychotic manic's ability to maintain social contact during his episode, plus his more complete adaptive recovery at its end should usually resolve any confusion that has developed around the issues of schizophrenia and of organic brain disease.

A NOSOLOGY OF ELATION

Whenever a bipolar patient presents with severe psychotic symptomatology during a manic episode the question of the so-called "third psychosis," schizoaffective illness, arises, Himmelhoch and colleagues have demonstrated that this diagnosis cannot be made during an acute episode. However, the presence of a formal or an informal thought disorder between affective episodes does indicate that the patient suffers from an illness more closely akin to schizophrenia than to even the more severe, pure bipolar syndromes. Subjects with interepisodic thought disorders have much higher relapse rates, tend to deteriorate into sheltered care situations, and are more likely to commit suicide even than rapid-cycling bipolars. Nevertheless, investigators such as Carpenter have hypothesized that bipolar illness and schizophrenia are on a dimensional continuum of psychotic illnesses where mild bipolar states are at one end, pure, but psychotic bipolar illness and schizoaffective illness represent successive steps along the continuum, and schizophrenia is at the other end. Such a hypothesis is a sophisticated reiteration of Ostow's conceptualization that hypomania is a milder form of mania, in which adaptive capabilities are preserved, or even enhanced. Psychiatry as a discipline has always had a predilection for dimensional concepts of illness, as is well demonstrated by the ill-fated conceptualization of reactive versus endogenous depression. This dimensional hypothesis has enamored nosologists for years, but in the end has had no value for predicting which depressive responds to which treatment, be that treatment electroconvulsive therapy, drugs, or psychotherapy. It has been the consistent experience of the Affective Disorders Clinic at the University of Pittsburgh that bipolar illness is heterogenous in the categorical statistical sense that the anemias and dementias are, not in the dimensional sense described above. At present one can only use clinical variables − initial presentation, course, and outcome − that tap into this categorical heterogeneity. Nevertheless useful, if crude, nosologies can be developed in regard to the differential diagnosis and treatment of elation. The critical clinical variables in any given patient consist of: (1) the above-described differentiation between mania and hypomania, (2) the relative degree of disability produced by elated episodes in the same patient, (3) cycle frequency or, conversely, the length of symptom-free, normal intervals, and (4) the presence or absence of chronic hypomania or mania.

Patients who develop hypomanic episodes, become disabled exclusively in their depressed phases, and have substantial symptom-free intervals have far better prognoses, respond more definitively to lithium salts, and need fewer adjunctive pharmacologic treatments than patients who cycle rapidly or who present chronic mania. As cycle frequency increases, patients respond less and less well to lithium, are more subject to mixed dysphoric, manic episodes (episodes where manic and depressive symptomatology are simultaneously present), and are more likely to have other neuropsychopathology, such as sedative habituation or cerebral dysrhythmias, confounding their clinical presentation. Finally, when patients present with chronic hypomania or mania, they almost invariably are also afflicted with some form of central nervous system deterioration, usually either an early, mild dementia or a primary or secondary Parkinsonian motor syndrome.

Dunner was the first to suggest a nondimensional typology for manic syndromes when he differentiated bipolar I illness from bipolar II (mentioned earlier in this chapter). He was also the first to produce systematic data demonstrating the negative effect on outcome of rapid cycling (greater than four manic or depressed episodes per year). Angst arrived at a categorization similar to the one described in this chapter when he demonstrated in a group of 95 manic-depressive patients:

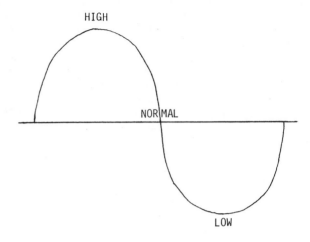

Fig. 13-1A   Conflicting models of manic-depressive illness bipolar model.

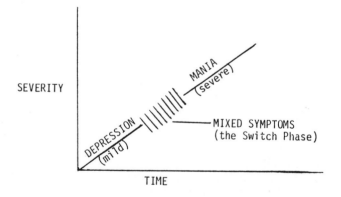

Fig. 13-1B   Conflicting models of manic-depressive illness continuum model (adapted from Court, 1968).

1. that "the preponderantly depressed sub-group of bipolar patients differ considerably in the course of the disorder from the other two groups" (severely manic and depressive patients and preponderantly manic patients).

2. that the better-prognosis subgroup (preponderantly depressed) had a heavier loading of psychiatric morbidity in their families, precisely the opposite of what would be expected, and highly suggestive that this "good prognosis bipolar illness" is a separate constitutional illness from the other forms.

CONCEPTUAL MODELS FOR THE DIFFERENTIAL DIAGNOSIS AND TREATMENT OF ELATION (Fig. 13-1)

The notion that elation is psychologically and physiologically opposite to depression forms the so-called "bipolar model" of manic-depressive illness. However, a large body of clinical, physiologic, biochemical, and pharmacologic evidence has been developed that suggests that many manic-depressive patients, particularly those with severe illness, do not conform to this model. Kraepelin observed early that mania as opposed to hypomania is almost always ushered in by brief periods of dysphoria and depression, and often presents with a continuing mixture of significant depressive symptoms. This state of affairs would be a logical impossibility if elation were truly the opposite to depression. As a result, a number of different models have been suggested to describe these more severe forms of manic-depressive illness. Court has suggested a continuum hypothesis (see Fig. 13-1B) where depression represents a mild deviation from normal mood and mania a severe deviation. Therefore, any given patient, as he gets more severely ill passes from depression, through a mixed state into mania. Bunney and colleagues, in their important article "The 'Switch Process' in Manic-Depressive Illness, " feel that the rapid switch from depression to mania usually includes a brief "normal period, " often overlooked because there is usually no opportunity to continuously observe such patients. They offer a third model, an extension of Prange's "serotonin-permissive" hypothesis, "which includes both an underlying dysfunction and a superimposed dysfunction. The underlying dysfunction, present during both depressive and manic phases, may not be related to catecholamine function. " Court's hypothesis, however, seems preferable because it explains both mixed states and rapid cycling, where the latter model seems preoccupied with rapid cycling. However, either model can be

Table 13-2 Differential Diagnosis and Treatment of Elation

Clinical Presentation	Model	Treatment
Hypomania/retarded depression; substantial normal intervals; mixed states — rare, usually associated with alcohol or sedative abuse	Bipolar	Low-dose lithium salts + adjunctive, alerting antidepressants
Mania/mixed states and agitated dysphorias/severe retarded depression; increasing cycle frequency; psychotic and schizoaffective markers can be present in any phase	Continuum Syndromes secondary to subictal seizure disorders	High-dose lithium salts + adjunctive thiazides; low-dose neuroleptic adjuncts and/or maintenance antidepressants sometimes necessary Carbamazepine in combination with lithium or less often alone; effective in either continuum or secondary model illness
Chronic hypomania/mania		Very difficult — lithium neurotoxicity can occur at low doses; severe dyskinesias likely from low-dose lithium-neuroleptic combination

evinced to describe severe, psychotic, and rapid cycling, manic-depressive illness. The traditional bipolar model, on the other hand, can be invoked as the constitutional anlage for those patients with hypomanic episodes, long symptom-free intervals, and excellent lithium responses. The differential diagnosis and treatment of elation can now be summarized (Table 13-2):

BIPOLAR MODEL ILLNESS

Bipolar model illness is found where retarded depression proves more disabling than does hypomania, which is often productive and highly adaptive. There are usually substantial normal intervals between episodes of hypomania and/or depression. Mixed states are only seen when a second neuropsychiatric factor is present, usually substance abuse. Treatment of choice is lithium salts, often at doses and blood levels lower than traditionally suggested (450-900 mg daily, blood levels at 0.35-0.60 mEq/liter). Antidepressants must sometimes be used adjunctively, and alerting varieties such as desmethylimipramine, or monoamine oxidase inhibitors (in compliant patients) are preferable. Neuroleptics tend to make these patients worse, often inducing depression, complicated by pseudoparkinsonism. For the most part they should be avoided.

CONTINUUM MODEL ILLNESS

Where severe hypomania and mania dominate the picture, mixed states are relatively common, and rapid cycling complicates treatment. Patients with rapid cycling do poorly on lithium and often need treatment with the limbic anticonvulsant, carbamazepine. Some of these patients probably represent subictal presentation of complex partial seizure disorders, others may be "true" manic-depressives, whose illness is best explained by Ballenger and coworkers' kindling hypothesis, where: "increasingly severe and rapid mood swings in manic-depressive illness also relate to the progressive dysregulation of transmitter-receptor feedback systems in a different biochemical anatomical substrates [than Parkinsonism with on-off oscillating dyskinesia, or complex partial seizure patients with interictal rapid cycling]." Even those continuum model patients who respond to lithium need higher doses and blood levels. As a result, such patients often develop renal concentrating defects and benefit from thiazide supplementation of their lithium treatment. These patients are also more likely to need neuroleptics and/or maintenance antidepressants as adjunctive therapy.

CHRONIC MANIA OR HYPOMANIA

Chronic mania is found where either of the above models of manic-depressive illness becomes complicated by encroaching senescence, other forms of dementia, or degenerative motor disease. It is almost impossible to manage these patients pharmacologically. They readily develop lithium neurotoxicity. Adjunctive neuroleptics produce severe dyskinesias, which are magnified by even low doses of lithium. Chronic hypomania can be understood as a bipolar patient's last gasp response to a deteriorating central nervous system and as such is related to those hypomanic reactions seen in normal subjects confronted with supreme and prolonged threats to their survival.

BIBLIOGRAPHY

Angst, J.: Clinical typology of bipolar illness. In: Mania, An Evolving Concept (Edited by R. H. Belmaker, and H. M. van Praag). Spectrum Publications, Jamaica, NY, 1980, pp. 61-76.

Bunney, W. E., Murphy, D. L., Goodwin, F. K., and Borge, G. F.: The "Switch Process" in manic-depressive illness, I., II., III. Arch Gen Psychiatry 27:295-317, 1972.

Carpenter, W. T., Jr., and Stephens, J. H.: The diagnosis of mania. In: Mania, an Evolving Concept (Edited by R. H. Belmaker, and H. M. van Praag). Spectrum Publications, Jamaica, NY, 1980, pp. 7-24.

Court, J.: Manic-depressive psychosis: an alternative conceptual model. Br J Psychiatry 114:1523-1530, 1968.

Dunner, D., Cohn, C., Gershon, E., et al.: Differential catechol-o-methyltransferase activity in unipolar and bipolar illness. Arch Gen Psychiatry 25:348-353, 1971.

Dunner, D. L., Fleiss, J. L., and Fieve, R. R.: The course of development of mania in patients with recurrent depression. Am J Psychiatry 133:905-908, 1976.

Goldstein, K.: Human Nature in the Light of Psychopathology. Schocken, New York, 1971, pp. 112-113.

Himmelhoch, J. M.: Mixed states, manic-depressive illness, and the nature of mood. Psychiatr Clin N Am 2:449-459, 1979.

Himmelhoch, J. M., Mulla, D., Neil, J. F., Detre, T. P., and Kupfer, D. J.: Incidence and significance of mixed affective states in a bipolar population. Arch Gen Psychiatry 33:1062-1066, 1976.

Himmelhoch, J. M., Forrest, J., Neil, J. F., and Detre, T. P.: Thiazide-lithium synergy in refractory mood swings. Am J Psychiatry 134:149-152, 1977.

Himmelhoch, J. M., Neil, J. F., May, S. J., Fuchs, C. Z., and Licata, S. M.: Age, dementia, dyskinesias, and lithium response. Am J Psychiatry 137:941-945, 1980.

Himmelhoch, J. M., Fuchs, C. Z., May, S. J., Symons, B. J., and Neil, J. F.: When a schizoaffective diagnosis has meaning. J Nerv Men Dis 169:277-282, 1981.

Katan, M.: The role of the word in mania. In: Manic-Depressive Illness, History of a Syndrome (Edited by E. A. Wolpert). International Universities Press, New York, 1977, pp. 209-235.

Klein, D. F.: Endogenomorphic depression: a conceptual and terminological revision. Arch Gen Psychiatry 31:447-454, 1974.

Kraepelin, E.: Lectures on Clinical Psychiatry (a facsimile of the 1904 edition). Hafner Publishing, New York, 1968.

Mahler, M. S.: Notes on the development of basic moods. In: Psychoanalysis − A General Psychology (Edited by R. M. Loewenstein, L. M. Newman, M. Schur, and A. J. Solnit). International Universities Press, New York, 1966, pp. 152-168.

Mandell, A. J.: Neurobiological barriers to euphoria. Am Scientist 61:565-573, 1973.

Ostow, M.: The hypomanic personality in history. In: Mania, an Evolving Concept (Edited by R. H. Belmaker, and H. M. van Praag). Spectrum Publications, Jamaica, NY, 1980, pp. 387-393.

Post, R. M.: Biochemical theories of mania. In: Mania, an Evolving Concept (Edited by R. H. Belmaker and H. M. van Praag). Spectrum Publications, Jamaica, NY, 1980, pp. 217-265.

Prange, A., Jr.: The use of drugs in depression: its theoretical and practical basis. Psychiatr Ann 3:2, 1973.

Solzhenitsyn, A.: Gulag Archipelago. Time-Life, New York, 1976.

Vaillart, G. E.: Adaptation to Life. Little Brown, New York, 1977.

Chapter 14

ANXIETY AND PANIC DISORDERS

Richard S. Goldberg, M.D.

MEDICAL DISORDERS MASQUERADING
AS ANXIETY AND PANIC

Anxiety is a nonspecific symptom whose appearance should always prompt the clinician to consider a variety of possible underlying medical causes. Anxiety, which is often ascribed to some nonspecific psychological or social problem, often represents the first and occasionally the only sign of undetected physical illness. The need for medical evaluation is not eliminated simply because social stresses and psychological conflicts can be identified. Table 14-1 lists a number of medical disorders that produce anxiety.

NEUROTRANSMITTERS AND ANXIETY

This section reviews some of the current speculations regarding the relationship of several neurotransmitter systems to anxiety.

Recently, the locus coeruleus (LC) has gained attention as a crucial factor in the central regulation of anxiety. The LC, as the name implies, is a small bluish area visible to the naked eye in the dorsal lateral tegmentum of the pons. It is thought to be a unique intergrative position due to its diverse neuroanatomic connections which include the principal noradrenergic innervations of the cerebral cortex and a major portion of the limbic system along with hypothalamic, medullary, and spinal areas. It has been estimated that this small nucleus supplies up to 70% of the noradrenergic neurons in the central nervous system (CNS).

Data are now available to support a hypothesis that changes in central norepinephrine (NE) are related to anxiety, and that

Table 14-1   Common Medical Disorders and Drugs
              Producing Anxiety

Cardiovascular disorders
  Angina pectoris
  Arrhythmias
  Mitral valve prolapse
  Congestive heart failure

Metabolic
  Carcinoid syndrome
  Cushing's syndrome
  Hypercalcemia
  Hyperkalemia
  Hyperthyroidism
  Hypoglycemia
  Hyponatremia
  Hypoxia
  Pheochromocytoma
  Porphyria

Neurologic
  Encephalopathies
  Essential tremor
  Postconcussion syndrome
  Temporal lobe seizures

Drug-related
  CNS sedative withdrawal
    (e.g., alcohol, benzodiazepines)
  Diuretics
  Hallucinogens
  L-Dopa
  Neuroleptics (akathisia may simulate anxiety)
  Opiate withdrawal
  Propranolol
  Stimulants (e.g., amphetamine, cocaine)
  Sympathomimetics (e.g., isoetharine, isoproterenol,
    terbutaline)
  Tricyclic antidepressants
  Xanthines (e.g., caffeine, theophylline)

the LC controls central noradrenergic function. Early studies of
LC function by electrical stimulation revealed increases in noradrenergic activity as reflected in increases in MHPG (3-
methoxy-4-hydroxyphenethyleneglycol), the major brain

metabolite of NE. One clinical study of psychiatric patients demonstrated a positive correlation of urinary MHPG with changes in rated anxiety. Since correlating changes of NE with changes in anxiety does not establish causality, it has been important to test more directly whether changes in NE (e. g. , by infusion) can induce changes in anxiety.

NOREPINEPHRINE

Norepinephrine (an alpha-1- and alpha-2-adrenergic agonist) was first reported to be the peripheral sympathetic neurotransmitter in 1946. It turns out, however, that infusions of NE cause a significant elevation of blood pressure only without producing anxiety. However, since NE does not cross the blood-brain barrier its effects on the CNS cannot be assessed by peripheral infusion studies. Furthermore, since adrenal stimulation produces approximately 80% epinephrine, NE infusions are probably not a physiologic event.

Yohimbine and piperoxan which do cross the blood-brain barrier and stimulate noradrenergic (NA) activity (as alpha-2-antagonists) have been used to investigate properties of brain NA systems including the LC. Piperoxan has been used in the past to help diagnose pheochromocytoma, however, the consistent emergence of panic and severe anxiety led to the discontinuation of its use in the early 1950s. Infusions of yohimbine consistently induce a subjective experience of anxiety. Therefore, consistent with the hypothesis in question, it appears that central NA activation indeed produces the experience of anxiety.

If anxiety is directly related to increased activity of the LC NA system, then one would expect that clonidine, a drug that inhibits the LC and lowers the NE output, should also decrease anxiety. The most outstanding effect of clonidine was a decrease in "anxiety attacks" rather than a decrease in generally experienced somatic symptoms. The results of these studies suggest that the NA system plays a role in anxiety but does not account exclusively for its manifestation.

EPINEPHRINE

Interest in the relationship between epinephrine and anxiety dates back to experiments reviewed by Walter Cannon in the 1920s. Cannon pointed out that epinephrine infusions do not invariably produce anxiety. Epinephrine was used in early psychophysiologic studies because of the observed relationship between adrenal function and fear. It is now recognized that epinephrine, which is both an alpha- and beta-adrenergic agonist, does not produce

anxiety per se, but rather a state of arousal which may be interpreted by the individual in a variety of ways depending on psychologic set and social setting. Nevertheless, the failure of epinephrine infusions to invariably produce anxiety is not inconsist-
ent with the LC model of anxiety since epinephrine in fact activates alpha-adrenergic receptors which actually inhibit LC firing, while at the same time activating peripheral adrenergic receptor function.

Given the relationship of NA systems to anxiety and the regulation of brain NA systems by the LC, the LC may function as
a central "anxiostat" by supplying ongoing modifications to the
limbic system, hypothalamus, cortex, and brain stem. This
anxiostat may set out tonic "trait" level of anxiety and also may
be responsible for the bursts of anxiety experienced by some
patients as panic attacks.

GAMMA-AMINOBUTYRIC ACID

The gamma-aminobutyric acid (GABA) system may be the neurotransmitter system most directly involved with the regulation of
anxiety and appears to be closely associated with the anxiolytic
mechanism of benzodiazepines (BZs). Receptors for BZs were
discovered in 1977. Naturally, the discovery of such receptors
initiated the search for endogenous BZ ligands, which have not
yet been identified. However, there has been progress in understanding the relationship of BZ activity and GABA. Apparently,
BZ receptors are functionally linked to GABA receptors to form
a GABA-BZ-chloride ionophore complex. GABA is the most
prevalent inhibitory neurotransmitter in the brain. Benzodiazepines are not direct GABA agonists but potentiate effects of
GABA on the influx of chloride into neurons, which then leads to
altered neuronal polarization and make selves less responsive
to other stimuli. Other sedatives with anxiolytic properties such
as barbituates and alcohol may also exert some of their pharmacologic properties by affecting the GABA-BZ-chloride complex.

Many questions remain in this area of neuroscience. The
reader should be cautioned that much information in this area
remains hypothetical, even regarding the relationship of BZ receptors to anxiety. It is also unclear to what extent the GABA-BZ
complex affects anxiety directly or indirectly through alterations
of the NE or serotonin systems that this complex affects.

CARDIOVASCULAR CAUSES

In the most extreme cardiovascular cause of anxiety, psychiatric
consultants may be called to see a hospitalized medical patient

whose sudden feelings of extreme anxiety and fearfulness are the first symptoms of impending shock. Patients who develop bradyarrhythmias or tachyarrhythmias (such as paroxysmal atrial tachycardia or atrial flutter) may have intermittent episodes of anxiety associated with palpitations or low cardiac output. Therefore, Holter monitoring occasionally plays a role in the evaluation of episodic anxiety. While there is no problem in recognizing severe congestive heart failure, borderline congestive failure in early stages of decompensation may present only with mild delirium and anxiety.

There appears to be an increased association of anxiety episodes in patients who have mitral valve prolapse. Mitral valve prolapse syndrome (MVPS) is due to an anatomic defect with redundancy of myxomatous connective tissue of the mitral valve (principally the posterior leaflet) and is most often idiopathic. Auscultatory findings typical of MVPS include a midsystolic click and a blowing apical late systolic murmur varying with position change. Patients with this syndrome are prone to episodes of anxiety associated with extrasystoles, palpitations, dyspnea, fatigue, and atypical chest pain. Symptoms associated with MVPS are indistinguishable from anxiety episodes due to a number of other causes. MVPS and anxiety/panic attacks both occur more often in females, begin before age 35, and tend to be familial. Furthermore, there have been a number of reports of increased incidence of mitral valve prolapse among patients with panic disorder and agoraphobia. Because patients with MVPS may be mislabeled as "anxiety neurotics," patients with panic attacks should have careful cardiac auscultation. If atypical findings are present, an echocardiogram may confirm the diagnosis.

DRUG-RELATED ANXIETY DISORDERS

Withdrawal from CNS sedatives or narcotics is a frequent cause of anxiety. The clinician should always take a very careful history of alcohol, other CNS sedatives, or opiate use in patients where the cause of anxiety episodes seems unclear. Occasionally toxicology screening will show the presence of some substance which the patient has not admitted to.

Diuretics, by altering electrolytes or neurotransmitters, can result in symptoms of anxiety. L-Dopa psychiatric side effects include severe anxiety along with depression or psychosis. Patients on neuroleptics may develop "akathisia" which may simulate anxiety. Akathisia is a sense of internal restlessness which the patient feels in the legs and often reports as an inner sense of anxiety. If this is not recognized as a side effect of the neuroleptic, the unwary clinician may often increase the dose of neuroleptic when in fact the appropriate treatment would be to either decrease the dose or to add an anticholinergic agent.

Stimulants can of course produce anxiety. Cocaine is being utilized by an increasing number of people. Symptoms of anxiety, irritability, tremulousness, fatigue, or depression may appear soon after use or following initial euphoriant effects. Caffeine is one of the most widely used psychotropic drugs in the United States. The approximate amount of caffeine in a cup of brewed coffee is 150 mg. While individual sensitivity varies, anxiety symptoms may occur at doses of 200 mg. The symptoms of caffeinism are identical to the classical description of an anxiety episode. Taking a thorough history of caffeine ingestion is crucial to every evaluation of anxiety. Caffeine abstinence as well as caffeine intoxication should be considered a source of intermittent anxiety. Other stimulant drugs that produce anxiety are the amphetamines as well as many of the agents used in the treatment of chronic obstructive pulmonary disease such as theophylline or the sympathomimetics. When symptoms of anxiety appear in any patient with asthma or emphysema who is on such agents, plasma levels of these drugs should be obtained and every effort should be made to lower their levels.

METABOLIC CAUSES

While there are some rather rare disorders such as pheochromocytoma, porphyria, or carcinoid syndrome which cause episodic anxiety, many more common metabolic disorders should be considered on a regular basis. Cerebral hypoxia should be considered as an etiology of anxiety in patients with asthma, chronic obstructive pulmonary disease (COPD), pneumonia, congestive heart failure, or surgery predisposing to pulmonary embolism. Electrolyte imbalance such as hyponatremia or hypokalemia can lead to symptoms of anxiety. Hyperthyroidism can produce symptoms of anxiety. Hypercalcemia is a cause of anxiety which should be considered especially in cancer patients with breast cancer, bronchogenic carcinoma, or multiple myeloma. Hypercalcemia is one of the most common metabolic abnormalities associated with being host to a malignant disease and patients with this condition can present with symptoms that include anxiety or psychosis.

Finally, hypoglycemia is one of the most controversial metabolic causes of anxiety. With fasting hypoglycemia, striking subjective symptoms of anxiety are most commonly absent and instead the patient reports mild impairment of motor performance, social judgment, or dull sensorium with mild confusion or apathy along with headaches and fatigue. Such symptoms typically occur in the morning following the overnight fast. With insulinoma, side and abrupt fluctuations in plasma insulin levels may lead to anxiety and panic states, including symptoms of depersonalization and sympathetic autonomic discharge. With insulinomas, unlike other fasting hypoglycemias, relief by eating is not regularly reported by patients. Between attacks, the patient feels well and functions in a normal manner.

Reactive (postprandial) hypoglycemia, in contrast, usually occurs 3-4 hours after eating, and results from an exaggerated and asynchronous physiologic response to carbohydrate ingestion. When the hypoglycemia is clinically significant it is associated with increased serum cortisol along with symptoms such as sympathetic autonomic arousal and anxiety. Episodes do not show the progression of frequency or severity that is characteristic of insulinoma. When reactive hypoglycemia is suspected on the basis of characteristic episodic symptoms, the appropriate diagnostic evaluation is a properly performed 5-hour glucose tolerance test (GTT).

NEUROLOGIC CAUSES OF ANXIETY

Subjective emotional symptoms of temporal lobe epilepsy (TLE) include feelings of intense depression, euphoria, paranoia, or severe anxiety with a sense of impending doom. Anxiety is the most common ictal emotional state associated with temporal lobe epilepsy. The characteristic abnormality in temporal lobe seizure disorder is the anterior temporal spike focus; however, in the waking state at least one-half of the patients have normal electroencephalograms (EEGs). A sleep record does increase the percentage of abnormal EEGs obtained in epileptic patients, although the percentage of false-negatives remains between 30 and 40%. Therefore, while the occurrence of an abnormal EEG may be diagnostic, a normal EEG finding does not rule out the presence of temporal lobe seizure disorder. Other neurologic causes of anxiety include nonbacterial meningoencephalitis which can present as an insidious chronic disorder with waxing and waning symptoms of anxiety. Encephalitis should be considered in any patient with a new psychiatric symptom who is an immune-compromised host.

Anxiety disorders also follow concussion. Cerebral concussion is classically regarded as a disorder which produces no irreversible anatomic lesions. However, it has been estimated that 20% of head injuries involving no demonstrable damage lead to a syndrome involving medically unexplained symptoms. Anxiety is one of the most frequent disabling symptoms for such patients. The postconcussion syndrome typically consists of anxiety, impairment of sleep and appetite, irritability, lightheadedness, headaches, and poor concentration. There are data to suggest that the symptoms that follow concussion are a direct result of neurobiological changes including direct neuronal damage and alteration of cerebral blood flow resulting in regional and generalized abnormalities correlating with the presence of psychological symptoms. In summary, the presentation of symptoms of anxiety require the psychiatrist to be a physician who supplements a meticulous history with selected physical and laboratory examinations. The multiplicity of possible underlying medical causes should be reviewed before triaging the patient into a purely psychosocial treatment modality. Naturally, the identification of such biomedical causes does not exclude the need to address concomitant psychological or social adjustment issues.

DRUG TREATMENT OF ANXIETY

BENZODIAZEPINES

The ubiquity of antianxiety drug prescribing is a well documented phenomenon. According to the Food and Drug Administration (FDA), about 10 million Americans take BZs yearly.

Since the introduction of chlordiazepoxide (Librium) in 1960, over a dozen BZs have been introduced. Some of the differences among available BZs are esoteric while others are clinically relevant, reflecting differences in pharmacokinetic properties. All the BZs are well absorbed orally and reach peak blood levels after a single dose, in times varying from 2 to 6 hours.

The bewildering metabolic fate of various BZs may be simplified by classifying these agents into two groups (Table 14-2). One group includes drugs that have no active metabolites, do not depend on the liver for metabolism, and are quickly inactivated by conjugative transformation. With relatively short lives, these drugs are most suited for use when prolonged sedation is undesirable. Because there are no active metabolites, these drugs will not tend to accumulate with repeated administration and require bid or tid administration if used as a maintenance medication. Drug accumulation is a special risk to be kept in mind with all other BZs, especially for older patients and those with liver impairment.

The second group of BZs includes those with long

Table 14-2 Pharmacokinetic Summary Comparison of Benzodiazepines

Drug Given	Peak Blood Level (hr)	Half-Life (hr)	Active Metabolites	Half-Life (hr)
		Short-acting		
Alprazolam (Xanax)	1-2	12-15	—	—
Lorazepam (Ativan)	2	12	None	—
Oxazepam (Serax)	2	6-8	None	—
Temazepam (Restoril)	2.5	9.5-12.4	None	—
Triazolam (Halcion)	1-1.5	2.3	Alpha-hydroxy-triazolam	3.9
			4-Hydroxytri-azolam	3.8
		Long-acting		
Chlordiazepoxide (Librium)	2-6	12 (7-28)	Desmethylchlor-diazepoxide	8-24
			Demoxepam	14-95
			Desmethyldiazepam	48-96
Chlorazepate dipotassium (Tranxene)	*	—	Oxazepam	6-8
			Desmethyldiazepam	48-96

Table 14-2 (Continued)

Drug Given	Peak Blood Level (hr)	Half-Life (hr)	Active Metabolites	Half-Life (hr)
Diazepam (Valium)	2	36 (20–50)	Desmethyldiazepam Oxazepam	48–96 6–8
Flurazepam (Dalmane)	2	—	N–Desalkylflurazepam	47–100
Prazepam (Verstran)	6	63 (43–78)	Desmethyldiazepam Oxazepam	48–96 6–8

* No known peak level.

half-lives. They share common oxidative metabolic pathways in the liver. On the basis of their pharmacokinetics, these medications may be prescribed on a once per day schedule. Nevertheless, most patients feel more comfortable psychologically with divided daily doses. Despite the long half-lives and accumulation of active substances, chronic use of these drugs usually does not lead to oversedation. The sedative and anti-anxiety effects of BZs appear to be distinct. As a steady state is reached, the CNS seems to adapt to the nonspecific sedative effects of the medication.

Drug Interactions

The major drug interaction involving BZs is augmentation of other CNS depressants. There are a few reports of BZs increasing diphenylhydantoin and digoxin levels and decreasing prothrombin times for patients on coumadin. Concomitant use of cimetidine can lead to increases in plasma diazepam levels.

Side Effects

The most common adverse effects of BZs involve CNS depression. There is some question as to whether or not BZs, in some people, release hostility and rage reactions.

Studies in humans reveal that BZs are quite innocuous to the cardiovascular systems even in patients with underlying cardiac disease. The respiratory depressant effects of BZs appear to be most marked in patients with CO_2 retention or who are on narcotics.

Toxicity

Benzodiazepines are the most benign of all psychoactive drugs with respect to the danger of overdose. In the medical literature there have been fewer than a dozen suicides with diazepam ingestion alone. However, BZs are often used in combination with other drugs in fatal overdoses.

Benzodiazepine Withdrawal and Addiction

Withdrawal from large doses of BZs resembles barbiturate withdrawal. Higher doses taken over longer durations create a greater risk of moderate to severe withdrawal. It may be that the short-acting BZs are associated with a greater prevalence and severity of withdrawal reactions because their plasma concentrations decline more rapidly following discontinuation.

Practically speaking, patients should be gradually tapered from BZs even though the likelihood of significant withdrawal is minimal. Rapid discontinuation may lead to some withdrawal which can be misinterpreted as a recrudescence of the underlying disorder and, therefore, lead to patient demands for restarting the medication. Most investigators feel that the addiction cannot occur at ordinary therapeutic doses of BZs, but require 10-20 times the usual dose for a period of months. Some investigators maintain that humans do not develop overt tolerance to the anxiolytic effects of BZs, although this point is controversial. However, it is widely recognized that a large number of patients appear psychologically dependent on BZs.

BETA-ADRENERGIC BLOCKING AGENTS

The cluster of autonomic symptoms associated with anxiety (such as palpitations and tremulousness) are peripheral symptoms mediated by beta-adrenergic sympathetic activity. Because beta-adrenergic blocking agents can antagonize these symptoms at the target organ, there has been considerable interest in the anxiolytic use of these agents.

It has also been suggested that propranolol has a unique role for patients in situations of acute situational distress, such as public performance anxiety, in which the psychomotor intellectual impairment produced by BZs is not desirable. Evaluation of the effectiveness of beta-blockers on anxiety has become more complex with the recognition that these agents enter the CNS and may produce direct neurologic and behavioral effects, including side effects such as insomnia, hallucinations, and depression.

Issues in Prescribing

Propranolol is almost completely absorbed following oral administration. It undergoes extensive first-pass metabolism in the liver. The half-life is initially about 3 hours and it may increase to 4 hours during chronic use. Propranolol is almost completely metabolized in the liver before urinary excretion.

Because of its effects on bronchial smooth muscle and interference with glycogenolysis during hypoglycemia, propranolol is contraindicated in patients with asthma and should be used cautiously in diabetics. Beta-receptor blockade has little effect on the normal heart at rest though there is some decrease in heart rate, cardiac output, and blood pressure. However, during exercise and anxiety, sympathetic responses may be significantly blocked. Therefore, maximum exercise

tolerance may be decreased in otherwise normal patients.
Serious cardiac depression is uncommon, but heart failure
may develop slowly or suddenly especially if the heart is com-
promised by intrinsic disease or by other drugs (such as digi-
talis).

Beta-adrenergic blockers such as propranolol are defin-
itely effective in the treatment of some anxiety disorders.
They appear especially useful when somatic, especially cardiovascular, symptoms are prominent. It is too early to make
any definitive statements on the comparative efficacy of beta-
blockers versus other antianxiety agents.

IMIPRAMINE

The identification of panic attacks has special implications for
drug selection. Spontaneous panic attacks are episodes of fearfulness and terror occurring acutely and often accompanied by
some cardiorespiratory distress. They typically emerge in an
apparently unthreatening setting in which the person reports
feeling entirely calm. A "panic attack" does not represent a
crescendo of gradually worsening anxiety and should be thought
of as a unique disorder rather than as fitting along a spectrum
of increasing anxiety. Although BZs are often used to treat
panic attacks, there is little evidence to support their efficiency in these situations, though there has been recent evidence
suggestive of special efficacy for alprozolan (Xanax).

Imipramine is the medication first shown to be effective in
abolishing spontaneous panic attacks in patients for whom BZs
and other sedatives were previously ineffective. However, imipramine is not a panacea since patients who have experienced
panic attacks become so fearful of their recurrence that they
often remain expectantly anxious even after the core disorder
is eliminated. More recent studies have confirmed the clinical
usefulness of imipramine in panic attacks as an important element of a comprehensive therapeutic program which includes
behavioral and psychologic approaches.

While some anxious patients are exquisitely sensitive to
imipramine side effects and report marked jitteriness and
overstimulation with small doses, patients on tricyclics for
panic attacks generally require similar dose ranges to patients
treated for depression.

MONOAMINE OXIDASE INHIBITORS

Although first introduced for the treatment of depression,
monoamine oxidase inhibitors (MAOIs) were noted quite early

to be effective for treatment of anxiety states including severe phobic-anxiety symptoms, phobias, and combined symptoms of anxiety with depression. It is important to identify when the anxious patient actually has an atypical depression for which MAOIs appear to be significantly more useful than tricyclic antidepressants or other agents. Some effectiveness of MAOIs in the treatment of phobia has been demonstrated. While an overview of these studies shows some superiority of MAOIs over placebos, the lack of overall strikingly positive findings may be due to the generally low doses used as well as the diagnostic heterogeneity of the patients sampled.

BIBLIOGRAPHY

Castillo-Ferrando, J. R., Garci, M., and Carmona, J.: Digoxin levels and diazepam. Lancet 2:368, 1980.

Goldberg, R.: Anxiety Biobehavioral Diagnosis and Therapy. Medical Examination Publishing, New Hyde Park, NY, 1982.

Hoehn-Saric, R.: Neurotransmitters in anxiety. Arch Gen Psychiatry 39:735-742, 1982.

Gronwall, D., and Wrightson, P.: Delayed recovery of intellectual function after minor head injury. Lancet 2:605-609, 1974.

Hoyumpa, A. M.: Disposition and elimination of minor tranquilizers in the aged and in patients with liver disease. South Med J 71:23-28, 1978.

James, I.M., Pearson, R. M., Griffith, D.N.W., et al.: Reducing the somatic manifestations of anxiety by beta-blockage - a study of stage fright. J Psychosom Res 22:327-337, 1978.

Kantor, J. S., Zitrin, C. M., and Zelis, S. M.: Mitral valve syndrome in agoraphobic patients. Am J Psychiatry 137:467-469, 1980.

Karch, F. E.: Rage reaction associated with clorazepate dipotassium. Ann Intern Med 91:61-62, 1979.

Kathol, R. G., Noyes, R., Slymen, D. J., et al.: Propranolol in chronic anxiety disorders—a controlled study. Arch Gen Psychiatry 37:1361-1376, 1980.

Klein, D., and Fink, M.: Psychiatric reaction patterns to imipramine. Am J Psychiatry 119:432-438, 1962.

Klotz, U., Anttila, V. J., and Reimann, I.: Cimetidine/diazepam interaction. Lancet 2:699, 1979.

Koranyi, E. K.: Morbidity and rate of undiagnosed physical illness in a psychiatric clinic population. Arch Gen Psychiatry 36:414-419, 1979.

Leigh, D.: Psychiatric aspects of head injury. Psychiatry Dig 40:21-32, 1979.

Mavissakalian, M.: Pharmacologic treatment of anxiety disorders. J Clin Psychiatry 43:487-491, 1982.

Mitchells-Heggs, P., Murphy, K., Minty, K., et al.: Diazepam in the treatment of dyspnea in the "pink puffer" syndrome. Q J Med 49:9-20, 1980.

Noyes, R., Jr., Clancy, J., Hoenk, P. R., et al.: Physical illness in anxiety neurosis. Comp Psychiatry 19:407, 413, 1978.

Pariser, S. F., Jones, B. A., Pinta, E. R., et al.: Panic attacks: diagnostic evaluations of 17 patients. Am J Psychiatry 136:105-106, 1970.

Paul, S. M., Maranges, P. J., and Skolnick, P.: The benzodiazepine-GABA-chloride ionophore receptor complex: common site of minor tranquilizer action. Biol Psychiatry 16:213-229, 1981.

Permutt, M. A.: Postprandial hypoglycemia. Diabetes 25:719-736, 1976.

Ravaris, C. L., Nies, A., Robinson, D. S., et al.: A multiple-dose, controlled study of pheneizine in depression-anxiety states. Arch Gen Psychiatry 33:347-350, 1976.

Shader, R. I., Greenblatt, D. J., Goodman, M., and Gever, J.: Panic disorders: current perspectives. J Clin Psychopharmacol 2 (suppl):2S-26S, 1982.

Sheehan, D. V.: Panic attacks and phobias. N Engl J Med 307: 156-158, 1982.

Taylor, A. R., and Bell, T. K.: Slowing of cerebral circulation after concussional head injury. A controlled trial. Lancet 2:178-180, 1966.

Vajda, F. J. E., Prineas, R. J., and Lovell, R. P. H.: Interaction between phenytoin and the benzodiazepines. Br Med J 1: 346, 1971.

Victor, B. S., Lubetsky, M., and Greden, J. F.: Somatic manifestations of caffeinism. J Clin Psychiatry 42:185-188, 1981.

Von Eules, U. S.: Catecholamines and stress. Acta Physiol Scand 12:73-97, 1946.

Weil, A. A.: Ictal emotions occurring in temporal lobe dysfunction. Arch Neurol 1:87-97, 1959.

White, B. C., et al.: Anxiety and muscle tension as consequences of caffeine withdrawal. Science 209:1547-1548, 1980.

Winokur, A., Rickels, K., Greenblatt, D. J., et al.: Withdrawal reaction from long-term, low-dosage administration of diazepam. Arch Gen Psychiatry 37:101-105, 1980.

Yager, J., and Young, R. T.: Non-hypoglycemia as an epidemic condition. N Engl J Med 291:907-908, 1974.

Chapter 15

SCHIZOPHRENIA

David E. Sternberg, M.D.

INTRODUCTION

The group of disorders known collectively as schizophrenia
continues to be a critical problem for modern psychiatry and
accounts for large expenditures for modern psychiatry and
tragedy for many families. Today an estimated ten million people worldwide suffer from schizophrenia. Schizophrenics account for 20% of those treated for mental disorders, and 35% of
psychiatric hospitalizations in the United States. More than half
of the beds in psychiatric hospitals are occupied by schizophrenics. And there is a one in a hundred chance that a person living
in the United States will be diagnosed as schizophrenic in his
lifetime.

Many different patterns of behavior, connected by some
commonly shared features, have come to be recognized and diagnosed as schizophrenia. It remains uncertain whether these
are varieties of one illness or are, in fact, several different
illnesses. This group of disorders is characterized by the disorganization of a previous level of functioning, by the presence
of specific psychotic features during the "active" phase of the
illness, by the absence of a full affective disorder, and by a
tendency toward chronicity. Schizophrenic symptoms have been
classified as being "positive" or "negative." Positive symptoms
are those whose presence reflects pathology—delusions, hallucinations, and thought disorder. Negative symptoms are defined
by the absence of affect, the lack of goal-directed behavior,
poverty of speech, deteriorated functioning, and the lack of
close personal ties.

Although research clearly indicates a major genetic contribution to the etiology of these disruptions of cognition, perception and, presumably, brain function, the pathophysiology

147

has nevertheless remained obscure. The heterogeneity of symptomatology and clinical course makes the goal of finding a single biochemical etiologic factor in this group of disorders suspect and suggests, rather, an underlying biochemical heterogeneity. It should also be noted that most current research on schizophrenia is done with heterogeneous groups of patients; therefore, significant factors which are characteristic of only a small percentage of the whole patient group will tend to disappear in studies of large groups of patients or will fail to be replicated when small groups of patients are studied.

To indicate that some aspect of schizophrenia is genetically transmitted is, de facto, to assert a biochemical component. Much research effort has been made to identify physiologic and biochemical factors associated with schizophrenia. Thus, much work has been done to identify ways in which the physiology and biochemistry of schizophrenic patients differ from that of "normal" individuals and nonschizophrenic patients. The findings thus far have failed to indicate a single etiologic source of the widespread pathology of schizophrenia. As various aspects of bodily function in schizophrenic patients have been studied, it has become evident that little of their physiologic functioning is normal. To what extent this indicates overall failure of physical function in schizophrenia and to what extent it is an artifact of pooling groups of patients with differing disorders is unclear. For example, numerous physiologic studies have found abnormalities in muscular coordination systems such as abnormal smooth-pursuit eye tracking patterns, abnormalities in muscle tissue, diminished arousal of the autonomic nervous system to stress, abnormal electroencephalogram (EEG) patterns, and "soft signs" of neurologic abnormality.

NEUROTRANSMITTER ABNORMALITIES

Much recent research has focused on the role of neurotransmitters in the etiology of schizophrenia. Since perception, cognition, memory, mood, and behavior all depend on the interaction of neurotransmitters and their receptors at the synapse, biochemical defects at this level could produce mental illness. Although a dopamine (DA) dysfunction is especially implicated in schizophrenia, evidence also points to a number of other neurotransmitters.

DOPAMINE

The "DA hypothesis of schizophrenia" is supported by indirect pharmacologic evidence. Drugs such as amphetamine and methylphenidate, which increase central DA function, can, in high and chronic doses, produce a paranoid schizophreniclike syndrome in normal subjects. These drugs also exacerbate positive symptoms (i.e., hallucinations, delusions) in schizophrenic patients. On the other hand, drugs that diminish (e.g., reserpine) or block (e.g., neuroleptics) central DA transmission produce a therapeutic effect. Furthermore, recent support of the DA hypothesis has derived from studies of the neuroleptic compounds which have shown that the drugs' clinical antipsychotic potencies are closely correlated with various measures of their anti-DA potency, such as their in vitro inhibition of DA receptor binding, their reversal of DA-related animal behaviors, and their elevation of human plasma prolactin (PRL). Thus if blocking DA receptors in the brain reduces schizophrenia symptoms, then schizophrenia may be caused by an excess of dopaminergic neurotransmission in some brain pathways.

Biological studies that test the "DA hypothesis" investigate: (1) presynaptic DA mechanisms (e.g., measurement of DA and its metabolites in cerebrospinal fluid [CSF], plasma, and postmortum brain tissue; enzymes of dopamine synthesis and degradation); (2) postsynaptic DA mechanisms (e.g., DA receptor binding; neuroendocrinology).

Dopamine and/or its primary metabolite, homovanillic acid (HVA) have been measured in the CSF, urine, and postmortem brains of schizophrenic patients. If schizophrenia is associated with a generalized increase in brain DA turnover, then HVA should be increased in unmedicated schizophrenic patients. Most recent CSF studies utilize the probenecid technique to inhibit egress of HVA from the CSF. Overall, the studies of lumbar CSF HVA in unmedicated schizophrenic patients find normal HVA levels. However, some differences are seen in patient subgroups. Bowers reports that schizophrenic patients with Schneiderian first-rank symptoms have lower HVA accumulations than patients without such symptoms, or than control subjects. In agreement with Bowers, Post and colleagues studied a population of generally good-prognosis schizophrenic patients and reported a similar decrease in HVA accumulations in the patients with more Schneiderian first-rank symptoms. In addition, they note that, following recovery from the acute psychosis, the accumulations of HVA are reduced compared to those measured in the acute stage. The findings of Bowers and Post of decreased DA turnover in remitted and chronic patients may be interpreted as a reflection of a trait-related increase in DA receptor sensitivity in schizophrenic patients. Dopamine receptor supersensitivity could produce via feedback inhibition the

lower DA turnover observed in chronic patients and during remission from psychosis. Increased DA turnover might occur
then only during the initial period of acute psychosis, through
an impairment of normal regulatory mechanisms. Both Bowers
and Curzon point out that if brain DA receptors are supersensitive in schizophrenic patients, then there could be increased
functional DA activity in the face of low or normal HVA levels.

Another test of the DA hypothesis, more direct than CSF
but with its own inherent complications, is examination of DA
and HVA levels in areas of postmortem schizophrenic brains.
Although investigations report increased levels in some areas
of schizophrenic brain, the effects are small and are not obtained in all studies. Bird and colleagues report that DA levels
are elevated in a group of psychotic patients only in the limbic
nucleus accumbens. After these investigators enlarged their
study they again note elevated DA concentrations in the nucleus
accumbens of the schizophrenic group and reports that this elevated DA concentration is especially marked in those patients
who had an early onset of psychosis and died at a young age.
Such patients also have elevated DA levels in the caudate. The
increases the authors noted in DA levels do not seem related to
treatment with neuroleptic medication. These results are not
widely replicated. Since the majority of patients investigated
received neuroleptics shortly before death, drug effects must
be considered in the interpretation of the results.

Monoamine oxidase (MAO) is the major means by which
many of the neurotransmitters, including DA, are broken down.
The observation of Murphy and Wyatt in 1972 that some schizophrenic patients (chronic, but not acute) had diminished platelet
MAO activity led to considerable research on this subject. In a
subsequent review of this research, Wyatt and associates noted
that while most studies had reported diminished MAO activity in
chronic schizophrenic patients, the data on its activity in acute
schizophrenic patients remained inconclusive, and an etiologic
relationship between low platelet MAO activity and schizophrenia
had not been demonstrated. In fact, low platelet MAO activity
has been observed to be significantly related to a variety of psychopathology and behavior pathology.

Dopamine-beta-hydroxylase (DBH), the enzyme that converts DA to norepinephrine (NE), is present in brain NE neurons but not in brain DA neurons. CSF DBH is in the normal
range in schizophrenic patients. However, when this measure
was examined within the schizophrenic group, it was significantly lower in those schizophrenic patients who became nonpsychotic during neuroleptic treatment than in those who remained
psychotic. Furthermore, the patients with better premorbid

socialization, better prognosis, and less psychopathology between psychotic episodes also tended to have lower levels of CSF DBH activity. Low CSF DBH activity thus appears to delineate a subgroup of schizophrenic patients with an acute "reactive" syndrome (characterized by episodic psychotic behavior in response to stress) which is very responsive to neuroleptic treatment. One may hypothesize that genetically determined low levels of DBH activity may lead, under stressful stimulation, to DBH becoming a rate-limiting enzyme in NE synthesis and thus to increased levels of DA in NE neurons. Low DBH may thus be characteristic of a schizophrenic subgroup who, as evidence by their responsiveness to neuroleptic treatment, may have a hyperdopaminergic disorder, as distinguished from patients who are not responsive to neuroleptic treatment and who may thus have different or additional pathophysiology.

Since most studies do not demonstrate increased DA turnover in schizophrenic patients, there is a recent trend in research to focus more on a postsynaptic DA pathophysiology in schizophrenia. Such investigations have included measurement of DA receptor binding in postmortem schizophrenic brain, as well as neuroendocrine strategies. With four out of five laboratories reporting postsynaptic DA receptor supersensitivity, the most reproducible finding in postmortem schizophrenic brain is an increase in the number of DA receptor binding sites of the D-2 type found in the caudate, nucleus accumbens, and olfactory tubercle. Because of the potential importance of these observations toward understanding etiology, it is essential to evaluate whether such differences reflect an intrinsic aspect of the disease process or are secondary to neuroleptic treatment which can itself augment the number of DA receptor binding sites.

Neuroendocrinologic methods are extensively used to test the DA hypothesis by examining DA activity in the hypothalamic-pituitary system. Investigations in schizophrenic patients of DA activity in this system have studied basal plasma PRL and growth hormone (GH) levels, as well as the effects of DA agonists and antagonists on PRL and GH levels. If schizophrenic patients are increased central DA activity, they might also have decreased levels of serum PRL. However, most studies of baseline PRL levels in unmedicated acute and chronic schizophrenics find no difference compared to control subjects. Severity of formal thought disorder does relate inversely to plasma PRL in unmedicated chronic patients. Kleinman recently reported that patients with normal cerebral ventricular size have reduced plasma PRL levels (compared to patients with enlarged ventricles) and that the PRL levels have a significant inverse correlation to the degree of psychotic symptomatology. These

studies suggest a relationship between DA activity and psychopathology, at least in some schizophrenic patients. No differences are documented in baseline GH levels between unmedicated schizophrenic patients and control subjects. Rotrosen,
studying the GH response to apomorphine in a group of floridly
psychotic schizophrenic patients, reports that although the
mean GH peak does not differ between the patients and controls,
the distribution of responses in the two groups differs significantly, with the schizophrenic patients tending toward a bimodal
distribution. Four separate investigations demonstrate, in comparison to control subjects, an exaggerated GH response to apomorphine in acute schizophrenics and a small number of chronic patients with little or no previous neuroleptic treatment. On
the other hand, most chronic schizophrenics show a blunting of
the GH response to apomorphine. One possible explanation for
these findings is that the exaggerated GH responses in the acute
patients may represent evidence of DA receptor supersensitivity that is characteristic of their disease process whereas the
blunted responses in the chronic patients are either secondary
to neuroleptic treatment or are evidence that the more chronically ill schizophrenics have subsensitive DA receptors. This
hypothesis is supported by the reports of different effects of DA
agonist drugs on the clinical state of acute compared to chronic
schizophrenic patients.

NOREPINEPHRINE

A number of studies have provided evidence of noradrenergic
hyperfunction in schizophrenia. Four groups of investigators
reported elevated levels of NE in areas of the limbic forebrain
of schizophrenic patients studied after death. Two groups found
concentrations of NE in CSF to be significantly higher in schizophrenic patients than in normal control subjects. Furthermore,
a recent study showed that chronic neuroleptic treatment of
schizophrenic patients produced a significant decrease in CSF
NE levels, that significantly correlated with the medication-
induced improvement of the psychotic state. Evidence that the
beta-adrenergic receptor blocker, propranolol, is an effective
antipsychotic drug for some schizophrenic patients also points
to the possible importance of noradrenergic hyperfunction in
schizophrenia. Norepinephrine release in the brain is regulated
by presynaptic alpha-1-receptors. Sternberg and colleagues
found that clonidine, an alpha-receptor stimulant, reduced plasma 3-methoxy, 4-hydroxy-phenylethyleneglycol—the primary
metabolite of NE—levels in normal persons but not in schizophrenic patients. This indicates a subsensitivity of presynaptic

receptors in these patients and therefore impaired regulation of NE release.

SEROTONIN

One of the earliest factors implicating serotonin in schizophrenia was the finding that the hallucinogenic compound lysergic acid diethylamide (LSD) binds to serotonergic receptors and appears to exert its hallucinogenic action there. However, schizophrenic patients given LSD reported that its effects, while interesting, were different from the hallucinations concomitant with their psychosis. Nevertheless, evidence that serotonergic neurotransmission is in some way abnormal in schizophrenia continues to crop up. Although antipsychotic drugs have been shown to bind serotonin receptors and to inhibit serotonin-stimulated production of cyclic AMP (cAMP), the hypothesis that overproduction of serotonin receptors is pathogenic in schizophrenia does not appear to fit with other evidence. For example, newly hospitalized schizophrenic patients were found to have lower plasma trytophan levels than control subjects before treatment, and their tryptophan levels increased with treatment. Treatment with L-5-hydroxytryptophan (another serotonin precursor) improved symptoms in six of seven chronic schizophrenic patients who had been resistant to phenothiazines and in one of four chronic paranoid schizophrenic patients. Choinard and co-workers treated 32 chronic schizophrenic patients with tryptophan and benserazide, an inhibitor of liver tryptophan pyrrolase, an enzyme that converts plasma tryptophan to niacin. These researchers found that although this combination was not as effective in symptom reduction as chlorpromazine, in general the tryptophan treatment did decrease psychotic symptoms and particularly decreased depressive mood and guilt feelings. Another suggestion that serotonin deficiency may be implicated in schizophrenic symptoms is that long-term amphetamine treatment decreases serotonin; it also produces a psychosis indistinguishable from paranoid schizophrenia as mentioned earlier.

GAMMA-AMINOBUTYRIC ACID

Although gamma-aminobutyric acid (GABA) has long been known to be a constituent of brain tissue by playing a role in normal brain functioning as part of carbohydrate metabolism through the Krebs cycle, this amino acid has more recently been found to act also as an inhibitory neurotransmitter in the mammalian central nervous system (CNS). While it is a widely distributed neurotransmitter, it appears to have a discrete distribution.

often in the areas of CNS with high DA concentration, and it seems to modulate the activity of dopaminergic neurons. This and other evidence suggests that the GABA system may have partial control over the DA system or vice versa. Roberts proposed that the basic biochemical fault in schizophrenia may arise from a defective GABA system. An underactive GABA system in schizophrenia would decrease the inhibitory influence of the GABA neurons on DA systems. Then, DA activities that should be suppressed are not, thus producing inappropriate behavior. Suggestive evidence for this hypothesis was provided by Stevens and colleagues, who found that injection of a GABA antagonist into a DA-rich area of a cat led to psychoticlike behavior. The report of Bird and coworkers of not only increased DA but also reduced glutamic acid decarboxylase in postmortem tissue samples from schizophrenic brains, created considerable interest in the possibility of a role for abnormal GABAergic transmission in schizophrenia. The reduction in glutamic acid decarboxylase was particularly striking in the nucleus accumbens, where DA concentrations were noted to be elevated. Perry and coworkers found significantly reduced levels of GABA itself, in comparisons with control subjects, in the nucleus accumbens in postmortem samples of brain tissue from both schizophrenic patients and patients with Huntington's chorea (a disorder also often accompanied by psychotic symptoms). However, Gold and associates found decreased levels of GABA in the CSF of depressed patients but not psychotic patients when compared with neurologic control subjects. Even though withdrawal from the GABA agonist drug baclofen has been rereported to result in hallucinations, trials of baclofen and other GABAergic agonists failed to produce evidence of significant antipsychotic effects in schizophrenic patients. Thus GABA joins the list of neurotransmitters apparently disordered in at least some schizophrenic patients, but this abnormality does not in itself appear sufficient to account for the disorder.

OPIATES AND ENDORPHINS

When it was discovered that a section of beta-lipotropin had many of the properties of opiate compounds, it was named beta-endorphin and the search was begun for its actions in the human nervous system. The fact that opiates affect many of the brain functions that are disordered in mental illness (such as mood, sleep, pain sensitivity, etc.) suggested the investigation of a possible role for the endorphins in mental illness.

Two main hypotheses have been researched: (1) that schizophrenia involves endorphin excess, which can be studied by assaying endorphin levels in patients compared with normal persons, by giving narcotic antagonists (opiate receptor-blocking agents) to schizophrenic patients; (2) that schizophrenia involves a deficit of endorphins, which can be investigated by administering opiate peptides to patients.

Endorphin Excess

Terenius developed several techniques for the analysis of opiate peptides from human serum and CSF. A number of reports of CSF sample analysis showed differences between patients and normal control subjects, with acute schizophrenic patients showing an excess of CSF opioids and chronic schizophrenic patients apparently deficient when compared with control subjects. However, not all studies found this; Naber and associates found that although schizophrenic men had higher levels of immunoreactive opioids (though not beta-endorphin) than normal men, they did not differ significantly from other patients. Another strategy for testing the hypothesis of excess endorphins in schizophrenic patients is to give opiate antagonists to patients and observe them for a potential reduction in symptoms. The two most commonly used of these are naloxone and naltrexone. An initial report of a therapeutic effect of naloxone in schizophrenia by Gunne and colleagues led to a number of attempts to replicate that finding, but the results were generally negative. Later studies using higher doses showed more significant reductions in symptoms, particularly hallucinations. Pickar and coworkers summarized these studies, and reported that in their own study, conducted with a large number of patients from World Health Organization centers, patients who were also receiving neuroleptic medication were more likely to show significant general symptom reduction with naloxone. Studies with naltrexone, a longer-lasting oral antagonist, have so far been negative.

Endorphin Deficiency

In the past, opiate drugs have generally not been used in the treatment of schizophrenia, primarily because of their high addiction potential, but also because they have not been reported to have significant therapeutic value. However, the synthesis of beta-endorphin in the laboratory was followed by research to determine whether it might have a therapeutic effect in schizophrenia. The initial study by Kline and colleagues produced mixed results in a single-blind design. Berger and associates found that schizophrenic patients injected intravenously with a bolus of beta-endorphin from an albumin-coated syringe showed an increase in serum prolactin (suggesting inhibition of dopamine neurotransmission); although in some of the patients there was a statistically significant reduction in symptoms of schizophrenia, the reduction was not clinically apparent. Pickar and colleagues did not observe beneficial effects of intravenous beta-endorphin in their schizophrenic or depressed patients. The most successful results of endorphin treatment of schizophrenic patients have been reported by researchers in the Netherlands. These researchers studied the activity of fragments of the beta-lipotropin chain in animals and found that the non-opiate-like peptide des-tyrosine-gamma-endorphin (DT-gamma-E), had neuroleptic-like activity. In the belief that this might constitute an "endogenous neuroleptic," they treated a group of otherwise neuroleptic-resistant schizophrenic patients with the compound. Positive results were also reported by Emrich and colleagues using the same compound. Further research with DT-gamma-E has indicated that although it provides a dramatic therapeutic effect it is essentially ineffective in schizo-affective patients with "residual" schizophrenic symptoms. These researchers noted that the effect of DT-gamma-E on various aspects of neural and endocrine function suggest that it has a major impact on the dopamine system in the brain and functions to some extent as a dopamine antagonist in some areas.

VIRAL AND IMMULOGIC ABNORMALITIES

It has been known for a long time that some kinds of viral infection, particularly meningeal or encephalitic infections, are frequently manifested with symptoms of psychosis. In addition, slow virus infections can result in diseases of the brain such as kuru or Creutzfeld-Jacob disease, in which psychosis is a major part of the symptomatology. This has led to speculation that the symptoms of schizophrenia may result from either viral infection, especially of a slow-acting type, or from destruction of brain tissue through an autoimmune process possibly triggered by a viral infection (such as is thought to be the etiologic factor in multiple sclerosis). One of the agents suspected has been herpes simplex virus, as a brain infection by this virus has been shown to be associated with significant alterations in neurotransmitters and their release. These researchers also investigated cytomegalovirus (CMV), varicella zoster virus, and measles virus, primarily by means of antibody levels in serum from patients and control subjects. Two studies demonstrated that levels of antibodies to CMV in schizophrenics were significantly higher than in control subjects or other mental patients.

The data indicate that the viral infection probably occurred years before the onset of schizophrenia. What we know about CMV makes it a likely candidate as a cause of schizophrenia. Cytomegalovirus, like the other herpes viruses, is neurotropic ¬i.e., it infects nervous tissue. More specifically, it infects the limbic system of the brain, an area thought to be affected in schizophrenia.

There is some evidence that schizophrenics were infected by viruses very early in life. Adult schizophrenics have a higher than expected incidence of dermatoglyphics, or abnormal fingerprints. Viruses attacking fetuses in the first few months of pregnancy are known to interfere with the formation of fingerprints. Thus, the high rate of dermatoglyphics in schizophrenics may indicate intrauterine viral infections. The viral hypothesis also fits in well with the seasonal effects in schizophrenia. Schizophrenics are more likely to have been born from January to March. Several viruses have seasonal peaks in the winter months. If viruses cause schizophrenia, it is logical to ask whether or not the disease can be transmitted between people. Evidence suggesting this possibility can be found in family and twin studies. Concordance rates for schizophrenics are higher in pairs of relatives when both members are of the same sex. This may be due to the fact that same-sex family members are in closer contact than opposite-sex pairs. Also, fraternal twins have a higher concordance rate for schizophrenia than siblings of different ages, even though they share genes to the same extent. Again, fraternal twins are more likely to be in closer contact with each other than with their older or younger siblings. And identical twins have a higher concordance rate for schizophrenia when they are living together at the time of onset. That is, when one identical twin becomes schizophrenic, the second twin is more likely to be affected if both live together than if they live apart.

Russian researchers have reported finding unusual immunoglobulins in the brains of schizophrenic patients. Heath and Krupp found a protein fraction in schizophrenic serum which they named "taraxein" which produced schizophreniform behavior in monkeys; however, this finding has not been duplicated. These reports have spurred further efforts to determine whether some cases of apparent schizophrenia could result from viral or autoimmune processes. These may result from unusual viruses, but it is also possible that they could result from common viruses that persist after primary infection in these patients and ultimately produce pathology by cell destruction or by autoimmune pathology after antigenic alteration of hos cells. Pulkkinen studied concentrations of immunoglobulin A (IgA), immunoglobulin G (IgG), and immunoglobulin M (IgM) in the serum of schizophrenic patients. He found the highest concentrations of IgM in the patients who were behaviorally withdrawn at the time of admission and the lowest in those with paranoid symptoms. Furthermore, elevations (relative to other patients) of IgA and IgM at admission predicted a shorter hospitalization. Low IgM in paranoid patients was hypothesized to be related to stress (presumably higher in these than other patients), which may result in hypofunction of their immune system. In a review of several studies on humoral and cellular immunity in schizophrenia done in their laboratory, Vartanian and associates reported several findings: the schizophrenic patients they studied had very high antibody titer against a brain alpha-glycoprotein found in glial cells—much higher than titers found in normal control subjects or in patients with other neurologic autoimmune disorders like multiple sclerosis or amyotrophic lateral sclerosis. The schizophrenic patients had more elevated levels of B lymphocytes and fewer than normal T lymphocytes. Stevens has reported that postmortem examination of tissue from schizophrenic brains has shown substantial fibrallary gliosis, which would be consistent with Vartanian and associates' report of antiglial antibodies. Stevens noted that glial cells are rarely examined in postmortem studies of schizophrenic brain tissue, yet alterations of the glia could have a tremendous impact on neural functioning. Pandey and colleagues replicated the finding of antibrain antibodies in nearly half of 54 schizophrenic patients. The antibodies were more likely to be found in patients with a positive family history of schizophrenia and in patients with several prior episodes of schizophrenia. These authors reasoned that their evidence is consistent with a process produced by a slow virus infection.

CAT SCAN AND PET SCAN

Before the advent of computer-assisted tomography (CAT) scans, the study of brain morphology in living patients required the performance of pneumoencephalography, a painful and risky procedure often very difficult to justify on grounds of the patient's diagnosis or treatment. In 1976, in one of the first studies to utilize the CAT scan, Johnstone and coworkers noted that those schizophrenic patients with the greatest evidence of cerebral atrophy also showed the greatest cognitive impairment. Weinberger and associates observed significant ventricular enlargement in chronic schizophrenic patients. Schizoaffective and nonschizophrenic patients did not show this abnormality. In further studies, these researchers also found that ventricular enlargement was associated with poor premorbid social adjustment and with poor response to treatment. They felt that this might identify a genetically separate group of patients. Also, those chronic schizophrenics with increased ventricular space appear to do poorly on various tests of intellectual ability. Andreason, studying a group of young, nonhospitalized patients meeting Diagnostic and Statistical Manual of Mental Disorders 3d ed. (DSM-III) criteria for schizophrenia, also found ventricular enlargement in this group. They also found that patients with ventricular enlargement showed a preponderance of the "negative" symptoms of schizophrenia (e.g., poverty of speech, affective flattening, anhedonia, and "avolition"). Patients with normal ventricles were characterized by the more "positive" symptoms of schizophrenia (hallucinations, delusions, bizarre behavior, formal thought disorder).

The recent development of positron-emission tomography (the PET scan) has permitted the study of cerebral glucose utilization similar to the use of the CAT scan to study brain tissue. As cerebral glucose utilization is believed to reflect the activity of various parts of the brain, this advance permits the observation of the actual functional activity of various brain regions. Ingvar and Franzen, using xenon radiography, had observed reduced blood flow to the frontal lobes of older chronic schizophrenic patients during mental activation. In a later review of this research, Ingvar postulated that this hypofrontal activity in deteriorated schizophrenic patients might be related to malfunction of dopaminergic projections to this region. This finding was dramatically verified with the development of the PET scan. Buchsbaum and colleagues measured glucose metabolism in the brains of schizophrenics and normal control subjects. They also found that the frontal cortex of schizophrenics was less active than in normal persons. This area of the brain is believed to be the center for goal-directed behavior. Thus, low activity in the frontal cortex may explain the lack of goal-directed behavior and deteriorated motor ability that are characteristic negative symptoms of schizophrenia. The researchers also found reduced activity in the left central gray matter in schizophrenic brains, an area thought to be involved in various schizophrenic symptoms, such as perceptual-cognitive disorders and motor-behavioral deterioration.

SUMMARY

We have reviewed the evidence of biological abnormalities associated with schizophrenia. Some of these biological abnormalities have generated various hypotheses and theories concerning the etiology of schizophrenia itself or at least of some of its symptoms. For various reasons, although some of these hypotheses are compelling in many ways, none has yet provided an adequate explanation for all or even most cases of schizophrenia.

For example, the theory of schizophrenia with the strongest evidence behind it is the theory that the symptoms of schizophrenia result from abnormal stimulation of DA receptors. The evidence favoring this theory is based on the fact that all drugs that have proved to reduce symptoms of schizophrenia act on the DA system, either directly or indirectly, to reduce stimulation of postsynaptic dopamine receptors. The problems with this theory are: (1) that the same drugs, apparently by the same mechanism, reduce psychotic symptoms in disorders other than schizophrenia, (2) that not all symptoms of schizophrenia can be demonstrated to result from abnormal dopaminergic neurotransmission, (3) that chronically schizophrenic patients show evidence of reduced, rather than excessive, DA turnover in the CNS, and (4) that schizophrenic patients whose overt psychosis is brought into remission by the use of DA receptor-blocking drugs continue to have other persistent symptoms of both a biological and a psychological-behavioral nature.

Modifications in the hypothesis that might lead to further understanding of the syndrome's pathogenesis include: (1) The DA abnormality may only occur in a very specific brain area (e.g., prefrontal cortex). (2) The primary disturbance in schizophrenia may occur in another neurotransmitter system that interacts with DA neurons. Neuroleptics may thus be operating on a "secondary" DA system. Similarly, although anticholinergic drugs are of clinical benefit in Parkinson's disease, the primary defect in parkinsonism lies in the nigrostriatal DA system rather than in a cholinergic system. Furthermore, although neuroleptics rapidly produce DA receptor blockade, as evidence by the rapid neuroleptic-induced rise in plasma PRL, the full clinical antipsychotic response requires a number of weeks. Thus, whereas DA receptor blockade does appear necessary for the antipsychotic effects of neuroleptic medication, that blockade may allow other slower processes to take place which are more directly responsible for the therapeutic change. (3) Several biochemical factors involved in central DA function (e.g., low MAO, low DBH, DA receptor supersensitivity) may each be a vulnerability factor toward the illness. That is, each abnormality may be a necessary but not sufficient element for the development of schizophrenia. (4) The heterogeneity of the clinical syndrome of schizophrenia itself may be responsible for the inconclusive results. Schizophrenia probably represents a variety of disease entities, each having a different biological dysfunction. Only some of these may entail a defect in DA systems. Thus, Crow has attempted to draw a neurobiological distinction between schizophrenic patients who have good antipsychotic responses to neuroleptic treatment and patients who remain psychotic during such treatment. He proposes that there are two syndromes with distinct disease processes: an acute episodic schizophrenic syndrome with positive symptoms reversed by neuroleptic treatment, the illness thus being associated with increased DA neurotransmission (type I syndrome); and a chronic deteriorating syndrome with negative symptoms not reversed by neuroleptic treatment, the illness thus being unrelated to DA transmission, but possibly related to structural brain changes (type II syndrome). Recent pharmacologic, neuroendocrinologic, and neuroradiologic reports provide preliminary support for this hypothesized distinction.

Clearly, much work remains to be done in the study of the causes of schizophrenia. Just as research on the DA system has been productive, especially for the development of new drugs, it is hoped that similar research on the many other neurotransmitter systems will be equally productive and may reveal selective abnormalities. The goal remains to prevent this devastating disorder.

BIBLIOGRAPHY

Burt, D. R., Creese, J., and Snyder, S. H.: Antischizophrenic drugs. Chronic treatment elevages dopamine receptor binding in brain. Science 196:326-328, 1977.

Bender, D. A.: Tryptophan and serotonin in schizophrenia: a clue to biochemical defects? In: Biological Basis of Schizophrenia (Edited by G. Hemmings and W. A. Hemmings). University Park Press, Baltimore, 1978, pp. 96-117.

Bird, E. D., Spokes, E. G., and Iversen, L. L.: Brain norepinephrine and dopamine in schizophrenia. Science 204:93-94, 1979.

Bowers, M. B.: Central dopamine turnover in schizophrenic syndromes. Arch Gen Psychiatry 31:50-54, 1974.

Buchsbaum, M. S., Ingvar, D. H., Kessler, R., et al.: Cerebral glucography with positron tomography. Arch Gen Psychiatry 39:251-259, 1982.

Creese, I., Burt, D. R., and Snyder, S. H.: Dopamine receptor binding predicts clinical and pharmacological potencies of antischizophrenic drugs. Science 192:481-483, 1976.

Crow, T. J.: Molecular pathology of schizophrenia: more than one disease process? Br Med J 280:66-68, 1980.

Davis, G. C., Buchsbaum, M. S., and Bunney, W. E., Jr.: Research in endorphins and schizophrenia. Schizophr Bull 5: 244-250, 1979.

Ingvar, D. H., and Franzen, G.: Abnormalities of cerebral blood flow distribution in patients with chronic schizophrenia. Acta Psychiatr Scand 50:425-462, 1974.

Janowsky, D. S., El-Yousef, M. K., David, I. M., and Sekerke, H. J.: Provocation of schizophrenia symptoms of intravenous administration of methylphenidate. Arch Gen Psychiatry 28:185-191, 1973.

Kleinman, J. E., Weinberger, D. R., Rogol, A. D., Bigelow, L. B., Klein, S. T., Gillin, J. C., and Wyatt, R. J.: Plasma prolactin concentrations and psychopathology in chronic schizophrenia. Arch Gen Psychiatry 39:655-657, 1982.

Lee, T., and Seeman, P.: Elevation of brain neuroleptic/dopamine receptors in schizophrenia. Am J Psychiatry 137:191-197, 1980.

Mackay, A. V. P., Iversen, L. L., Rossor, M., Spokes, F., Bird, E., Arregui, A., Creese, I., and Snyder, S. H.: Increased brain dopamine and dopamine receptors in schizophrenia. Arch Gen Psychiatry 39:991-997, 1982.

Mason, J. W., and Docherty, J. P.: Psychoendocrine research on schizophrenia: a need for reevaluation. In: Perspectives in Schizophrenia Research (Edited by C. Baxter and T. Melnechuk). Raven Press, New York, 1980, pp. 782-798.

Meltzer, H. Y.: Neuromuscular dysfunction in schizophrenia. Schizophr Bull 2:106-135, 1976.

Meltzer, H. Y., and Stahl, S. M.: The dopamine hypothesis of schizophrenia: a review. Schizophr Bull 2:19-76, 1976.

Pandey, R. S., Gupta, A. K., and Chaturvedi, U. C.: Auto-immune model of schizophrenia with special reference to anti-brain antibodies. Biol Psychiatry 16:1123-1136, 1981.

Pickar, D., Vartanian, F., Bunney, W. E., Jr., et al.: Short-term naloxone administration in schizophrenic and manic patients; a World Health Organization Collaborative Study. Arch Gen Psychiatry 39:313-319, 1982.

Post, R. M., Fink, F., Carpenter, W. T., and Goodwin, F. K.: Cerebrospinal fluid amine metabolites in acute schizophrenia. Arch Gen Psychiatry 32:1063-1069, 1975.

Rosenthal, D., and Kety, S. S. (Editors): The Transmission of Schizophrenia. Pergamon Press, London, 1968.

Rotrosen, J., Angrist, B., Gershon, S., Paquin, J., Branchey, L., Oleshansky, M., Halpern, F., and Sachar, E. J.: Neuro-endocrine effects of apomorphine: characterization of response patterns and application to schizophrenia research. Br J Psychiatry 135:444-456, 1979.

Sternberg, D. E., Charney, D. S., Heninger, G. R., et al.: Impaired presynaptic regulation of norepinephrine in schizo-phrenia: effects of clonidine in schizophrenic patients and normal controls. Arch Gen Psychiatry 39:285-289, 1982.

Sternberg, D. E., van Kammen, D. P., Lake, C. R., Ballenger, J. D., Post, R. M., and Bunney, W. E., Jr.: The effect of pimozide on cerebrospinal norepinephrine in schizo-phrenia. Am J Psychiatry 188:1045-1051, 1981.

Sternberg, D. E., van Kammen, D. P., Ballenger, J. C., Lerner, P., Marder, S. R., Post, R. M., and Bunney, W. E.: CSF dopamine-beta-hydroxylase in schizophrenia: low activity associated with good prognosis and good response to neuroleptic treatment. Arch Gen Psychiatry 40:743-747, 1983.

Torrey, E. F., Peterson, M. R., Brannon, W. L., et al.: Immunoglobulins and viral antibodies in psychiatric patients. Br J Psychiatry 132:342-348, 1978.

Van Kammen, D. P., Sternberg, D. E., Hare, T. A., Waters, R. N., and Bunney, W. E.: CSF levels of gamma-aminobuty-ric acid in schizophrenia. Arch Gen Psychiatry 39:91-97, 1982.

Verhoeven, W. M. A., van Praag, H. M., van Ree, I. M., et al.: Improvement of schizophrenic patients treated with (des-tyr[1])-gamma-endorphin (DT-E). Arch Gen Psychiatry 36:294-298, 1979.

Weinberger, D. R., Cannon-Spoor, E., Potkin, S. G., and Wyatt, R. J.: Poor premorbid adjustment and CT scan abnormalities in chronic schizophrenia. Am J Psychiatry 137:1410-1413, 1980.

Weinberger, D. R., Torrey, E. F., Neophytides, A. N., et al.: Lateral cerebral ventricular enlargement in chronic schizophrenia. Arch Gen Psychiatry 36:735-739, 1979.

Wyatt, R. J., Potkin, S. G., and Murphy, D. L.: Platelet monoamine oxidase activity in schizophrenia: a review of the data. Am J Psychiatry 136:377-385, 1979.

Chapter 16

HYPERACTIVITY AND LEARNING DISORDERS

Stephen M. Kalavsky, M.D.

Approximately 10-30% of children in school fail to learn ade-
quately. As a generalization, there are three reasons why children do not learn in an average classroom environment: organic central or peripheral nervous system lesions, psycho-social
problems, and learning disabilities.
    Organic lesions are causative in only a small proportion of
children with academic failures. Diffuse lesions of the cerebral
cortex (caused by infection, trauma, genetic conditions, etc.)
can cause mental retardation. Children with moderate to severe
mental retardation are usually diagnosed before school age, but
mild or borderline cases may be unrecognized. Either diffuse
or focal lesions of the cerebral cortex can cause seizures which
intermittently interrupt the learning process, and medications
used to control the seizures may also hamper learning. Generalized tonic-clonic seizures ("grand mal") are easily recognized, but other seizure types may be difficult to recognize.
These include partial complex seizures ("temporal lobe epilepsy" or "psychomotor seizures") which may cause recognizable
automatisms such as lip-smacking, chewing, or swallowing
movements but which may also cause alterations in consciousness which may be mistaken for daydreaming, drug abuse, or
psychiatric illness. They also include absence seizures ("petit
mal seizures") which cause sudden, brief episodes of uncon-
sciousness with little or no motor activity; these may occur
hundreds of times each day. Lesions that affect the visual or
auditory end organs or pathways and cause decreased visual
acuity or hearing can also interfere with the normal learning
process. Finally there are some conditions, such as Duchenne's
muscular dystrophy, which may mistakenly be considered to be
conditions that do not involve the central nervous system and
thus cannot affect learning but which are associated with a lower
mean intelligence.

Diagnostic evaluation should include:

Careful history (documenting any genetic predisposition, along with unusual incidents during gestation, delivery, or childhood, and including acquisition of developmental landmarks, and phenomena suggesting seizures)

General neurologic examination (including a careful examination of the skin for "birthmarks, " of the general habitus for recognizable patterns of genetic or congenital syndromes, and of behavior during the examination for any signs of seizures)

Vision and hearing screening

Electroencephalogram (EEG) (only in those patients in whom the history or physical examination suggest seizure activity)

Treatment must be individualized based on the specific underlying etiology. Children with mental retardation will need special classroom placement based on the results of psychological testing. Patients with seizures will require anticonvulsant medication. Children with vision or hearing problems may have a correctable condition but if not they will require special educational techniques.

Psychosocial problems are more common causes of school failure. These range from serious cases in which the child and/or parent has a primary psychiatric problem (e. g. , psychosis, substance abuse, character disorder, child abuse) to patients with inadequate parenting (absent or contradictory discipline, failure to recognize importance of formal education). Unfortunately, these conditions may be difficult to recognize because of a tendency to conceal or deny these problems and because of the common practice whereby only the mother and child present data to the physician, thus excluding input from the father and school.

Evaluation should include data from:

Both parents (including socioeconomic status, level of parental academic achievement, attitudes regarding discipline, and presence of stress factors)

Child (including attitude toward school and teachers, interaction with peers, and strengths and weaknesses in various academic areas)

Teacher (including perception of child's academic strengths and weaknesses, and his interaction with authority and peers)

Treatment will be determined by the underlying condition and may include counseling, medication, behavior modification, and/or special classroom placement.

Learning disabilities are also a common cause of academic failure. They usually occur in the absence of organic or primary psychosocial problems. They affect children with near-normal, normal, or above-normal intelligence. They occur more commonly in males than females and some may be at least partially inherited. They seem to result in subtle, partial dysfunction of higher cortical activities such as the processing and/or integration of visual and auditory stimuli, encoding or recalling memory of such data, and production of appropriate verbal or motor responses. However, these children have no abnormalities on "classic" neurologic examination which seems to exclude major organic pathology and for this reason these children are often said to have "minimal brain dysfunction."

Many investigators have looked for more subtle "organic" (either anatomic, developmental, or biochemical) lesions in the central nervous system that would be responsible for learning disabilities. Since the condition is not lethal and has only recently been recognized, very little postmortem data are available. Two patients with learning problems who died had abnormalities (in the parietal lobes in one patient, while the other had abnormalities in the left temporal speech area and dysplasia in limbic, primary, and association areas). However, both of these patients had seizures, which is not typical of the learning disabled child and therefore the autopsy findings may be related to the seizures and not the learning disability. Computerized tomographic scanning can then be used to detect gross anatomic detail in living subjects; reversed cerebral asymmetry has been reported in children with learning disabilities. However, this was present in less than half of the affected children and also in one-quarter of a group of normal children so the significant of this finding is uncertain. The EEG assesses a different aspect of the central nervous system: electrical activity. Early reports using traditional interpretation of the EEG suggested an increased incidence of abnormalities but these appear to be non-specific and may even be normal variations. More elaborate methods of reviewing the data generated by the EEG may be more helpful. Power spectrum analysis has shown abnormalities in parietal theta activity, less attenuation of alpha rhythm in the parietooccipital area during learning tasks, and greater energy in theta and beta rates in the left parietooccipital region. Visual evoked response testing assesses only that part of the EEG that is time-linked to visual stimuli, and initial reports suggest this may be abnormal in children with learning disabilities. An even more elaborate method is brain electrical activity mapping (BEAM); reports suggest abnormalities in the posterior regions may better predict underlying pathology in children with learning disabilities. Much more work with better-defined populations and control populations will have to be done before the pathophysiology of learning disabled children can be understood.

Children with learning disabilities are not a homogeneous group; different children appear to have defects in different parts of the learning process. Unfortunately, a universally acceptable classification system does not exist and may await a better understanding of learning. At present an attempt should be made to categorize as precisely as possible the specific deficit. Some of the deficits appear to improve with time while others present a life-long problem. The most serious complication is the development of psychological problems (the most important of which is loss of self-esteem) which may result from the experience of repeated failures.

An adequate evaluation should include:

History (including specific areas of failure and other family members with similar problems)

Neurologic examination (including the presence or absence of "soft neurologic signs" such as synkinesis ("mirror movements"), mixed dominance (e.g., left-eyed, right-handed, and left-footed), or fine motor incoordination and/or gross motor clumsiness; these signs are a normal part of early development but should disappear as the child matures: e.g., the speed of finger tapping reaches a plateau at about 8 years of age, mirror movements disappear in 86% of normal 9-10-year-olds, and backward tandem gait is mastered by 90% of 7-year-olds. These signs are of no "localizing" value; no one has been able to correlate these signs with an organic lesion in a specific part of the brain. They are seen in higher frequency in children with learning disabilities, but are not seen in all affected children)

Formal psychological testing, including at least a WISC-R, which can help predict school performance. Other tests that may be helpful include the Peabody Individual Achievement Test, which can be used in spite of motor or speech

problems, the Wide Range Achievement Test, and others—
unfortunately, none of these tests is universally recognized
as a test that can definitively establish the diagnosis of a
learning disability, however, these tests can be helpful in
formulating a plan of treatment.

Visual and auditory evoked potentials have been reported
to differ from those in normal children; use of these tests
is investigational.

Treatment includes education of child and family about the
problem, and modification of curriculum to allow additional
help in areas of deficiency which frequently requires a low
teacher/student ratio.

Although the majority of patients will have only one cause
of learning failure—either organic, psychosocial, or learning
disability—some children may have combinations of causes. The
child with primary psychosocial problems may also have a
learning disability. A problem that frequently causes difficulty
involves the intellectually gifted child who also has a learning
disability. The child may function far below his potential, but
his potential may be so high that even with defective learning
skills "average" scholastic performance is achieved. This child
will receive "average" grades and the school may be unwilling
to commit resources to deal with his deficits. In this and other
cases of learning problems the patient is legally aided by Public
Law 94-142, passed by the federal government in 1975, which
provides for free and appropriate education for all handicapped
children and establishes the Individual Education Program to
monitor the services to children.

HYPERACTIVITY

Excessive motor activity, inability to attend to a task long
enough for successful completion, or "overactivity" is a frequent complaint about some children and has been estimated to
affect 3-15% of school age children. The problem may occur
only at home, only at school, or as a constant problem and may
be associated with decreased total sleep. The symptom has
been a difficult one to objectively assess quantitatively. Several
questionnaires have been developed but pragmatically the problem will have to be dealt with if it causes failure in school work
or play.
   Hyperactivity can be seen in children with very different

underlying illness (organic central or peripheral nervous system lesions, psychosocial problems, or learning disabilities) or in children with no other apparent problem. For example, children who are vision or hearing impaired may appear to excessively explore the environment with a sense that is not impaired (touch) or fail to modulate activity based on stimuli sensed by the impaired organ (e.g., a hearing impaired child's failure to modulate activity based on auditory stimuli). A retarded child may have excessive motor activity (hand wringing, rocking, jumping) or an inability to attend to any task for a significant length of time. Some children with seizures who are treated with barbiturates may have the "paradoxical" symptom of hyperactivity. Children with primary psychiatric problems (such as autism) may be unable to perform successfully and exhibit excessive motor activity. Children whose parents or siblings have primary psychiatric problems may develop anxiety which interferes with their ability to complete tasks. Patients with manic illness will also show signs of overactivity. Children with learning disabilities may have difficulty in focusing their attention long enough to complete a task or may be unable to "filter out" extraneous sensory stimuli. The intellectually "gifted" child may be bored with normal classwork and disrupt the class once he has completed his assigned tasks. Finally, some children with no underlying problem appear to be unable to control their activity. The type of behavior identified as "hyperactivity" may not be characteristic of any underlying disorder and it is therefore necessary to first establish the presence (or absence) of any of the above associated conditions. This is necessary not only for diagnostic clarity but because the different types of hyperactivity require different types of therapy.

Special interest has been focused on the hyperactivity of children with learning disabilities. These individuals seem to have abnormal processes necessary for attention. In order to "pay attention" to something, the individual must first sense the stimulus; the stimulus must then pass through lower levels of the brain (brain stem) without distortion, and arrive at the cortex where it can be interpreted and a decision made if it is important; other stimuli must be then "filtered out" by the individuals. The person must then be able to sustain attention as long as necessary. There are several anatomic sites at which dysfunction could disrupt attention. Numerous attempts have been made to better define the level of dysfunction and the possible pathophysiology. Behavioral studies indicate that these children are less task oriented and more distractible and that they are less able to selectively attend to relevant stimuli in a learning task. The term "attention deficit disorder" has been used for these children. It has been reported that these children have EEG abnormalities with some of them having hypoaroused physiologic patterns including higher-amplitude evoked potentials and reduced galvanic skin conductance.

There has been much discussion about the role of biogenic amines in attention deficit disorders. Since these chemicals are neurotransmitters it seems to be a reasonable hypothesis that abnormalities in their concentrations might be causal or at least reflect underlying causes. Each neuron appears to produce a single type of chemical neurotransmitter. A large number of norepinephrine neurons are found in the locus ceruleus and a large number of dopamine neurons are found in the substantia nigra. Both types of neurons utilize tyrosine to form their neurotransmitter but the degradation products of each type of neuron are unique. The major degradation product of norepinephrine is 3-methoxy-4-hydroxy-phenylglycol (MHPG) and the major degradation product of dopamine is homovanillic acid (HVA). Measurement of these products in urine, serum, and cerebrospinal fluid (CSF), using various techniques, has been performed in hope of finding consistent abnormalities in hyperactive children. Urinary MHPG was found to be higher than controls in some children with hyperactivity but lower in other children, also with hyperactivity. These may represent two different types of hyperactivity or the presence of a fluctuation imbalance. Other workers have demonstrated low levels of HVA in the CSF of hyperactive children and suggested that dopamine deficiency may play a role. It is of interest that treatment of hyperactive children with D-amphetamine (which increases the release of norepinephrine and also blocks its reuptake inactivation) has been an effective treatment and has been shown to lower levels of urinary MHPG and HVA and also CSF HVA. Furthermore, at low dosage this drug appears to inhibit the firing of dopamine and norepinephrine neurons. These data seem to contradict the basal monamine abnormalities. One theory suggests that the amphetamine exerts its effect via an acute increase of monamine followed by a longer reactive decrease in the neurotransmitters. It is difficult to determine how levels of metabolites in urine or CSF relate to levels of activity in specific subdivisions of the central nervous system, and these results must be interpreted with caution. It is equally difficult to interpret the results of studies reporting a correlation with minor congenital anomalies. Much work remains to be done before an understanding of the pathophysiology of this condition is understood.

The treatment of a child who is overactive will depend upon an accurate diagnosis of any underlying condition. If a child has mental retardation, the family will have to be informed of the diagnosis and prognosis. Feelings of denial and/or anger are common and must be resolved before any effective treatment can be undertaken. Special education classes must be arranged based on the child's level of function; behavior modification techniques are frequently helpful. If medication is necessary minor or major tranquilizers may be necessary for these children.

Children whose hyperactivity is a side effect of a medication will preferably be switched to an alternative medication or if this is impossible, have the dose lowered. Adding another medication to try to counteract the initial medication is to be avoided.

Children with primary psychosocial problems will have to have their basic problem treated by appropriate methods. Attempts to simply sedate the child without addressing the underlying problem are inappropriate.

The intellectually "gifted" child will have to have his curriculum modified to provide a more challenging and satisfying experience. Behavior modification techniques may also be helpful.

Although the pathophysiology of the attention deficit disorder is not understood, several therapeutic alternatives are available. The most important is to be sure that everyone involved—the patient, parents, and teacher—understand as much as possible about the condition. Behavior modification techniques may be helpful; it is necessary to be firm and, more importantly, consistent. Modifying the classroom environment may be most important; the child may require a smaller classroom, at least in those subjects in which he is having difficulty. This may be all that is necessary and, if possible, should be instituted before any medication is started. If medication is necessary, 75% of these patients have been found to have an increase in their attention span and decrease in their impulsivity with the use of stimulant medication. Methylphenidate (Ritalin) at low dosage (0.3 mg/kg/day) has been reported to improve social behavior, learning, and impulsive behavior but at higher dosage (1 mg/kg/day) social behavior may continue to improve but learning and impulsive behavior may worsen. Dextroamphetamine has also been used (5-40 mg/day). Pemoline (Cylert) has also been shown to be effective (starting at 37.5 mg/day and increasing as needed by 18.75-mg increments each week to a maximum of 112.5 mg). It has the advantage of being effective with a "once in the morning" dosage. The development of "tics" has been reported following the administration of stimulant medication and is a reason for discontinuing the medication.

There are conflicting reports of growth suppression in children receiving this class of medication and growth should be monitored.

As an alternative to medication the use of a diet avoiding artificial additives ("Feingold diet") has been recommended. Support for theory includes in vitro studies which demonstrated acetylcholine release from synapses and inhibition of uptake of dopamine and norepinephrine by synaptosomes; this is consistent with baseline neurotransmitter abnormalities seen in children with hyperactivity. Another theoretical reason for dietary control invokes the concept of foods causing "allergic-tension-fatigue" syndrome. A meeting was held at the National Institutes of Health in 1982 to develop a consensus about the use of dietary management of hyperactivity. No well-controlled studies have been presented to provide a scientific basis for the numerous personal reports of success with the diet. The panel recommended that a trial of the diet did not appear to be harmful.

Megavitamin therapy invokes the hypothesis that hyperactive children have a genetic defect which can be corrected by very large doses of vitamins. There has been no substantiation of the presence of such a defect and no reliable studies confirming the efficacy of the treatment. Furthermore, giving large doses of vitamins involves running the risk of toxicity.

Another theory postulates the deficiency of minerals. A study of children treated with the Feingold diet demonstrated low serum copper levels and normal serum zinc levels. Other studies are based on the analysis of mineral concentrations in hair. Uncertain normative values and the risk of contamination make hair analysis of uncertain significance. No correlation of serum mineral levels and central nervous system concentrations have been demonstrated.

Dietary sugar has also been suggested as a cause of hyperactivity. Interestingly both reactive hypoglycemia and hyperglycemia have been postulated. There are no supporting data for either theory.

Both "patterning" and optometric training have been reviewed by the American Academy of Pediatrics, however, neither method has been proven to have any effect by itself.

BIBLIOGRAPHY

Colon, E. F., Notermans, S. L. H., deWeerd, J. P. C., and Kap, J.: The discriminating role of EEG power spectra in dyslexic children. J Neurol 221:257-262, 1979.

Duffy, F. H., Denckla, M. B., Bartels, P. H., and Sandini, G.: Dyslexia: regional differences in brain electrical activity by topographic mapping. Ann Neurol 7:421-428, 1980.

Feagans, L.: A current view of learning disabilities. J Pediatr 102:487-493, 1983.

Fuller, P. W.: Computer estimated alpha attenuation during problem solving in children with learning disabilities. Electroencephalogr Clin Neurophysiol 42:149-156, 1977.

Golden, G. S.: Neurobiological correlation of learning disabilities. Ann Neurol 12:409-418, 1982.

Golden, G. S.: Controversial therapies. Pediatr Clin N Am 31(2):459-469, 1984.

Hastings, J. E., and Barkley, R. A.: A review of psychopharmacological research with hyperkinetic children. J Abnorm Child Psychol 6:413-447, 1978.

Kandt, R. S.: Neurologic examination of children with learning disorders. Pediatr Clin N Am 31(2):297-316, 1984.

Kolata, G.: Consensus on diets and hyperactivity. Science 215: 958, 1982.

Leisman, G., and Ashkenazi, M.: Aetiological factors in dyslexia. IV. Cerebral hemispheres are functionally equivalent. Neuroscience 11:157-164, 1980.

Mattes, J. A., and Gittelman, R.: Growth of hyperactive children on maintenance regimen of methylphenidate. Gen Psychol 40:317-321, 1983.

McMahon, R. C.: Biological factors in childhood hyperkinesis: a review of genetic and biochemical hypothesis. J Clin Psychol 37:12-21, 1981.

Quinn, P. O., and Rapoport, J. L.: Minor physical anomalies and neurologic status in hyperactive boys. Pediatrics 53:742-747, 1974.

Raskin, L., Shaywitz, S. E., Shaywitz, B. A., Anderson, G., and Cohen, D. J.: Neurochemical correlates of attention deficit disorder. Pediatr Clin N Am 31(2):387-396, 1984.

Rebert, C. S., Wexler, B. N., and Sproul, A.: EEG asymmetry in educationally handicapped children. Electroencephalogr Clin Neurophysiol 45:436-442, 1978.

Rosenberger, P. B., and Hier, D. B.: Cerebral asymmetry and verbal intellectual deficits. Ann Neurol 8:300-304, 1980.

Taylor, R., and Warren, S. A.: Educational and psychological assessment of children with learning disorders. Pediatr Clin N Am 31(2):281-296, 1984.

Waldrop, M. F., Bell, R. Q., McLaughlin, B., and Halverson, C. F.: Newborn minor physical anomalies predict short attention span, peer aggression and impulsivity at age 3. Science 199:563-565, 1978.

Wright, F. S., Schain, R. J., Weinberg, W. A., and Rapin, I.: Learning disabilities and associated conditions. In: The Practice of Pediatric Neurology, 2d ed. (Edited by K. F. Swaiman and F. S. Wright). C. V. Mosby, St. Louis, 1982, pp. 1083-1138.

Chapter 17

ALZHEIMER'S DISEASE

Robert L. Gilliland, M.D.

Alzheimer's disease is one of the senile dementias occurring in the older population with a prevalence rate of about 1% at age 65, increasing to 15% by age 85. The appearance of the symptoms of this disorder may be as early as 50 years of age. This disease has been characterized as the epidemic of the 20th century.

Although more than 50 diseases have been identified as causing dementia, Alzheimer's is the leading cause. In published postmortem studies, 60% of patients dying with dementia have this disease.

ETIOLOGY

The etiology is unknown. Genetic factors have been implicated. Studies with a small number of families would suggest that a pattern of autosomal dominant transmission may be present in the early-onset group of Alzheimer patients. This does not hold true for the late-onset group. A definite pattern of association is seen in the chromosomal abnormality of trisomy 21 which produces Down's syndrome. These patients will have the pathologic findings characteristic of Alzheimer's disease if they live past the age of 40. No chromosomal abnormality has been identified in the general population of patients with Alzheimer's disease. Infective agents have been implicated in the etiology without success.

The observation that high aluminum concentrations are found in the cortex of degenerating brains of Alzheimer's disease patients has produced a suspicion that ingestion of this metal in the water supply may be a cause of the biochemical abnormalities. Other sources of aluminum used in everyday life have been suggested as causative factors.

176

It should be noted that Alzheimer's disease is different than the normal attritional type of aging because of the genetic factors involved.

DIAGNOSIS

The diagnosis of Alzheimer's disease is still a clinical one supported with some laboratory findings. Dementia is the cardinal manifestation. The early detection of dementia becomes the challenge. Differentiating this dementia from affective disorders and from other organic brain syndromes is difficult. Further separating out the group of patients with pseudodementing functional illnesses from those with psychological depression makes the diagnosis more difficult.

A careful history and a thorough mental status examination is necessary. Survey of the patient for possible drug toxicity, metabolic or nutritional disorders particularly related to thyroid disturbances, and vitamin B_{12}, folic acid, and thiamine deficiencies is necessary. Often forgotten is the laboratory examination for neurosyphilis, a condition producing dementia. It is essential for the diagnosing physician to look for reversible conditions producing dementia.

The availability of the computerized axial tomography (CAT) scan makes it easier to eliminate those patients with hydrocephalus or mass lesions who may initially present as having dementia. This test will also identify the patient with multiple cerebral infarcts.

A careful neurological examination along with the history will identify other disease states presenting as dementia, e.g., progressive supranuclear palsy, Parkinson's disease, Huntington's disease, and spinocerebellar degeneration.

The dementia presenting in Alzheimer's disease is not specific for this condition but may be seen in many of the previously mentioned conditions. The neuropathologic findings are the final determinants of this diagnosis. These are not available to the clinician at the beginning of the illness.

PROGRESSION

The stages of Alzheimer's disease follow a usual course from an asymptomatic to a terminal illness. The early stage of disease is characterized by changes in mood, along with loss of judgment, spatial orientation, and memory. There is usually a collapse of social relationships, accompanied by depression.

This gives way to a more childlike state requiring specialized care. The patient's command over speech and gait suffers and continued deterioration is noted in these areas. Bouts of irritability characterize the intermediate stage. Communication is lost and the patient becomes uncooperative; disruption of sleep and restlessness are also often noted at this stage.

The late stage is characterized by marked apathy, with loss of response to most stimuli. This is followed by the terminal stage of the illness.

When a patient presents with these signs and other possible causes have been eliminated, the most likely diagnosis is Alzheimer's disease. A period of careful follow-up lasting 1 or 2 years is required before the diagnosis can be certain. Frequent attempts should be made to identify and eliminate the treatable dementias.

NEUROLOGIC EXAMINATION

Focal findings are absent. The usual findings are of diffuse cortical function loss with mental status changes being the most prominent. Mental status changes may be grouped into abnormalities of: (1) arousal, attention, concentration, and motivation; (2) perception; (3) mood and affect; (4) language and memory; and (5) personality.

Motor signs will be late and limited to progressive clumsiness in walking; loss of motor power; increased hyperreflexia; the appearance of a snout reflex, and the presence of the palmomomental reflex.

PATHOLOGY

Pathologic and biochemical abnormalities that contribute to the diagnosis are well studied. There is widespread, diffuse symmetrical loss of neurons in the frontal, parietal, and temporal lobes of the brain. This neuronal degeneration will also be seen in the limbic system. In addition, neurofibrillary tangles and neuritic plaques are observed in the same region. The precise identity of the neuritic plaques has not been established in spite of many biochemical studies. Increase in fibrous astrocytes has been observed in the same regions. Recent observations have shown a consistent loss of neurons in the nucleus basalis of Meynert. These neurons are cholinergic and have an influence on the production of choline acetyltransferase of the neocortex. The loss of this enzyme decreases the amount of acetylcholine, a neurotransmitter that is important in the function of this part of the cortex. In Alzheimer's disease, there is a 60-90% drop in the amount of choline acetyltransferase produced.

Electron microscopic and biochemical studies have focused on the neurofibrillary tangle that is so prominent in the brains of Alzheimer's disease patients. Identification of the filamentous protein does not differ from that found in aging brains.

Noted on electron microscopic studies is the marked loss of dendritic connections. This is of significant functional importance.

The widespread degenerative changes of the brain result in a decrease in its mass which may be noted on the CAT scan performed at the time of the intermediate stage.

LABORATORY STUDIES

The most practical laboratory finding for clinical application in Alzheimer's disease is the consistent slowing of the rhythm of the electroencephalogram. The resting alpha rhythm decreases and the appearance of more theta rhythm is observed. Progression of the disease produces a mixture of theta and delta rhythms.

Findings of decreased cerebral blood flow and decreased glucose metabolism in such patients may relate to the loss of cholinergic influences over the cerebral blood flow regulation and may also contribute to the progression of the disease by decreasing the oxygen and glucose supply to the cortical neurons.

The CAT scan will show changes of diffuse loss of the neurons. Increase in ventricular size and widening of the sulci reflect the loss of brain mass. Direct correlation with the CAT scan findings and the accompanying neuropsychological changes may not be possible until late in the course of the disease. The functional loss will usually be much greater than the anatomic loss observed on the CAT scan.

TREATMENT

There is no specific treatment for Alzheimer's disease. Family education and reassurance is important. Drugs for the treatment of symptomatic problems such as anxiety, sleeplessness, depression, agitation, and paranoia are useful. Depression does occur frequently in the early stages of Alzheimer's disease and may be relieved by tricyclic antidepressants.

Reducing agitation is frequently the most difficult part of patient management. Neuroleptic drugs can help reduce the degree of agitation. This may postpone the need for institutional care.

The physician faces a challenging task in the diagnosis and management of this disease; much clinical skill is required and little laboratory help may be available. Growing interest in the causative factors of Alzheimer's disease has sparked widespread research; it is hoped that the end result for the future will be a better preventive program and a better treatment plan.

BIBLIOGRAPHY

Albert, M. L.: Changes in language with aging. Semin Neurol 1(1):43-46, 1981.

Alzheimer's Disease and Related Disorders Association Newsletter. Winter 1982.

Bennett, D. R.: Electroencephalographic and evoked potential changes with aging. Semin Neurol 1(1):47-52, 1981.

Buell, S. J., and McNeill, T. H.: New thoughts on old neurons. Semin Neurol 1(1):31-35, 1981.

Caine, E. D.: Mental status changes with aging. Semin Neurol 1(1):36-42, 1981.

Cohen, D., Eisdorfer, C., and Walford, R.: HLA antigens and patterns of cognitive loss in dementia of the Alzheimer's type. Neurol Aging 2:27, 1981.

Goldstein, S.: The biology of aging. N Engl J Med 285(20):1120-1129, 1971.

Greenhouse, A. H.: Neurologic disability in normal aging. Semin Neurol 1(1):13-19, 1981.

Honch, G. W., and Spitzer, R. M.: Radiographic aids to the diagnosis of dementia in the elderly. Semin Neurol 1(1):53-59, 1981.

Jenkyn, L. R., and Reeves, A. G.: Neurologic finds in uncomplicated aging (senescence). Semin Neurol 1(1):21-30, 1981.

Joynt, R. J.: Senility – a look at your future? Semin Neurol 1(1):1-4, 1981.

Schoenberg, B. S.: Neurologic disease in the elderly; epidemiologic considerations. Semin Neurol 1(1):5-12, 1981.

Part III

BIOLOGICAL TESTING

Chapter 18

DEXAMETHASONE SUPPRESSION TEST

Mark S. Gold, M. D. and Cary L. Hamlin, M. D.

A major goal of research in biological psychiatry has been to
identify measurable biological abnormalities that would reliably
confirm a psychiatric diagnosis, identify the major psychiatric
disorders, and aid in differential diagnosis and choice of treatment. One strategy for augmenting clinical diagnosis is to
measure neuroendocrine and other biological correlates that,
in addition to helping to elucidate the biological mechanisms of
psychiatric disorders, may define more homogenous groups of
psychiatric patients and guide the choice of pharmacotherapy.
Despite the advances of clinical nosology that The Diagnostic
and Statistical Manual of Mental Disorders, 3rd ed. (DSM III)
offers, the use of biological markers may define more clearly
homogenous groups of psychiatric patients and guide choice of
treatment.
      For example, the term "depression" can be applied to a
spectrum of clinical presentations that may appear similar but
which may respond differently to antidepressant medications. In
particular, it is important to identify patients with the full-
blown medical syndrome of depression, called "endogenous depression" in the older literature and called "major depressive
disorder" in DSM III. In this subgroup of depressives with major depression the clinician would think in terms of genetic and
other biological predispositions as of etiological significance.
Most importantly, in this subgroup, somatic treatment, usually
antidepressant medications, would usually be the initial focus of
treatment.

THE NEUROENDOCRINE STRATEGY

The neuroendocrine strategy involves measuring changes in

185

peripheral hormone concentrations, sometimes after provocation, as markers of major psychiatric disorders. Because the monoamine neurotransmitters norepinephrine (NE), serotonin (5HT), and dopamine (DA) regulate the hypothalamic factors that control the pituitary and hence other glands, changes in neuroendocrine systems reflect changes in the monoamine systems thought to be involved in mood disorders. For this reason, the neuroendocrine strategy has been called the "window into the brain."

The vegetative symptoms of depression, including disturbances in sleep, appetite, weight, and libido—the hypothalamic symptoms of depression—have long suggested neuroendocrine abnormalities in depression. Patients with major depression have a decreased growth hormone (GH) response to a number of provocative stimuli, including insulin-induced hypoglycemia, L-dopa, clonidine, and amphetamine and an augmented GH response to thyrotropin-releasing hormone (TRH). Other neuroendocrine abnormalities reported in major depression included increased prolactin (PRL) secretion, decreased luteinizing hormone (LH), decreased LH response to gonadotropin releasing hormone (LHRH), increased cortisol secretion, failure to suppress cortisol production on the dexamethasone suppression test (DST), decreased cortisol secretion in response to dextroamphetamine, and decreased thyroid-stimulating hormone (TSH) and PRL response to TRH. Neuroendocrine tests may have multiple uses in the diagnosis and treatment of the depressed patient (Table 18-1).

The focus of this and the next chapters will be on two neuroendocrine challenge tests—the DST and the TRH test—which have been shown to be useful markers for major depression and with which our group has considerable experience.

HYPERCORTISOL SECRETION AND THE DST

It has been well documented that a significant proportion of patients with major depressions secrete abnormally high amounts of cortisol from the adrenal gland. This has been reported by measurement of the serum cortisol at multiple time points throughout the 24-hour period, as well as by more integrated measures such as 24-hour urinary-free cortisol secretion.

Secretion of cortisol by the adrenal is stimulated by the pituitary hormone adrenocorticotrophic hormone (ACTH). ACTH production is in turn controlled by corticotropin-releasing hormone (CRH). This hypothalamic-pituitary-adrenal (HPA) axis shows inhibitory feedback control, which is utilized in the DST, a test of HPA regulation.

Table 18-1   Clinical Uses of Neuroendocrine Tests
                       in Depression

Diagnosis
Prediction of treatment response
Documentation of biological state change with treatment
Prediction of relapse

In the DST 1 mg (or 2 mg) of the synthetic corticosteroid
dexamethasone is administered orally at about 11 P.M. The
normal response is that this excess corticosteroid is "read" by
the pituitary and hypothalamus like an excess of cortisol, and
cortisol production is suppressed for at least 24 hours. Failure
to suppress on this DST was first used as a diagnostic test for
Cushing's syndrome. The finding of importance to psychiatry is
that approximately 45% of major depressives fail to suppress
cortisol production on the standard DST. Failure to suppress is
defined as any cortisol value $\geq 5.0\,\mu g\%$ at any time in the 24
hours after dexamethasone administration.

Carroll and colleagues, who have pioneered the use of the
DST as a laboratory test in psychiatry, have reported a rate of
nonsuppression as high as 67% in a melancholic subgroup of
major depressives and have proposed the DST as a diagnostic
test for this disorder. The DST does not seem to differentiate
between unipolar and bipolar depression. However, DST nonsuppression seems clearly to differentiate major depression
from nonmajor depressions, and primary from secondary depressions. Failure to suppress on the DST has been reported
to be rare in psychiatric disorders other than major depression,
with a false-positive rate of less than 5% in appropriately pre-
screened populations. However, some recent studies suggest
higher levels of nonsuppression in certain subgroups of patients
with psychiatric disorders other than major depression.

Carroll and associates and others have utilized two postdexamethasone time points for determination of cortisol: 4 P.M.
and 11 P.M. We have reported that by increasing the number of
time points in the 24-hours postdexamethasone to 6, the sensitivity of the test for major depression is increased by about 40%,
with only a small loss of specificity. Specificity has been reported increased and sensitivity decreased with increase in dosage
of dexamethasone from 1 to 2 mg. It has been suggested that a
cutoff of $4\,\mu g\%$ or lower for nonsuppression may be optimal, depending on the assay. The optimal parameters for the DST in
psychiatry need to be studied further.

Which testing protocol if any is suited for the patient you
are currently evaluating remains to be defined. I have always

been biased toward the power of markers to confirm in my
mind that I am treating what I think I am treating and to help
me control for the placebo or avoid diagnosing according to the
"famous depression expert" response. The DST is extremely
useful in both regards. The test is extremely well-suited for
inpatient neuropsychiatric evaluation units where the patient is
taken off all medications and given a thorough medical, neurologic, endocrinologic, social, employment, family, neuropsychological, psychological, and psychopharmacologic evaluation.
The physician who is attempting to maximize the possibility of
a positive test result will order a 1 mg DST with samples taken
before the dose at 11:59 and after the dose at 8AM, 12 midnight,
4PM, 6PM, 8PM, 10PM and/or 12. In an outpatient setting it is
frequently difficult to get the patient to the laboratory for all of
these appointments. However, the physician who does not order
enough time points may quickly lose interest in the DST as a
confirmatory test since as few as one in three patients with a
one-time point test who meet clinical criteria for a major depressive disorder will have an abnormal DST. Like all tests in
medicine the DST has false-positive and false-negative results
and is only as good as the protocol, laboratory, drug-free
washout, and physician at interpreting the significance of the
test vis-a-vis the clinical evaluation.

Certain factors that can affect the validity of the DST must
be taken into account in screening psychiatric patients appropriate for the DST. While usual therapeutic doses of benzodiazepines, neuroleptics, tricyclics, and lithium do not affect the
DST, other medications can. Barbiturates, phenytoin, carbamazepine, and other medications that induce hepatic enzymes
and hence speed the metabolism of dexamethasone can cause
false-positive results. It is noteworthy, however, that a recent
study showed that the DST can be useful in alcoholics 3-4 weeks
after detoxification in identifying patients with major depression.

Failure to suppress on the DST and hypercortisol secretion
are dissociated in some patients. In other words, some major
depressives have elevated diurnal cortisols while showing normal suppression on the DST, and some felt to suppress on the
DST despite normal diurnal cortisols. The DST has also been
suggested as a test that can help differentiate patients with so-
called "depressive pseudomentia" who may respond to antidepressant treatment from patients with true dementia.

The DST has been suggested by some researchers as identifying patients with good-prognosis schizophrenia, and a whole
list of psychiatric illnesses and syndromes which might be better
treated with antidepressants. DST false-positive results in so-
called normal subjects may really point to covert affectively ill

persons or persons with genetic loading for depressive disorders. We all know that depressions are complex and multifac-
torily determined so it is naive to expect the DST to solve all of
the problems we have had with the syndrome. From my point of
view a patient who has a positive DST is in a common, biologically relevant subgroup with other patients and nonpatients who
have a positive DST. In addition, the presence of a positive DST
suggests likely response to antidepressant pharmacotherapy. A
negative DST in a patient with the clinical diagnosis of major
depressive disorder may suggest the need to perform other
tests to establish that the patient has an active neurobiological
disease. A negative DST may mean that the disease is in the
self-correction phase and that supportive measures may be
enough to enable the patient to spontaneously remit.

Failure to suppress on the DST and blunted TSH responses
on the TRH test in major depressions tend to normalize with
clinical and neurobiological improvement during the course of
treatment. By repeating the DST and TRH test during the course
of treatment the clinician can obtain initial prognostic information about when the neurobiological abnormalities of depression
are in remission. This information may help determine when
antidepressant medications or electroconvulsive therapy (ECT)
is no longer needed, and when continued or different treatment
is needed. This use for the DST and TRH test in confirming successful treatment is particularly important in psychiatry, where
efficacy has been questioned.

The DST is a useful test in tertiary and neurodiagnostic
centers which are populated by patients who have had persistent
symptoms in the face of standard treatment. The DST has as its
main virtues, simplicity and reliability. A positive test once
repeated will enable the clinician to have some external validation of how well he is succeeding and will enable the physician
to decide on additional therapies if any. The test does not replace psychiatrists; on the contrary, the DST is difficult to integrate into the care of the patient without a thorough understanding of the test and affective illnesses. The DST is the most widely studied of the currently available interim measures that psychiatrists and other physicians are using to confirm the presence
of an active major depression and establish response to treatment.

BIBLIOGRAPHY

Carroll, B. J., Feinberg, M., Greden, J. F., Tarika, J., Albala, A. A., Haskett, R. F., James, N. M., Kronfol, Z., Lohr, N., Stiner, M., DeVigne, J. P., and Young, E.: A specific laboratory test for the diagnosis of melancholia. Arch Gen Psychiatry 38:15, 1981.

Dackis, C. A., Bailey, J., Gold, M. S., Extein, I., Pottash, A. L. C., and Stuckey, R.: Neuroendocrine tests in alcoholics with and without major depression. In: Problems of Drug Dependence (Edited by L. S. Harris). Proceedings of the 43rd annual scientific meeting, The Committee on Problems of Drug Dependence. NIDA Research Monograph Series. National Institute on Drug Abuse, Rockville, MD (in press).

Gold, M. S., Pottash, A. L. C., Extein, I., and Sweeney, D. R.: Dexamethasone suppression tests in depression and response to treatment. Lancet 1:1190, 1980.

Extein, I., Pottash, A. L. C., Gold, M. S., and Silver, J. M.: Thyroid-stimulating hormone in unipolar depression before and after clinical improvement. Psychiatry Res 6:161, 1982.

Greden, J. F., Albala, A. A., Haskett, R. F., James, N. M., Goodman, L., Steiner, M., and Carroll, B. J.: Normalization of dexamethasone suppression test: a laboratory index of recovery from endogenous depression. Biol Psychiatry 15:449, 1980.

Martin, J. P., Reichlin, S., and Brown, G. M.: Clinical Neuroendocrinology. F. A. Davis, Philadelphia, 1977, p. 201.

Sternbach, H., Extein, I., and Gold, M. S.: Diurnal cortisol: DST and TRH tests in depression. In: Continuing Medical Education Syllabus and Scientific Proceedings in Summary Form, The One Hundred and Thirty-Fifth Annual Meeting of the American Psychiatric Association, Toronto, Canada, 1982, p. 223.

Chapter 19

PROTIRELIN TESTING IN PSYCHIATRY

Mark S. Gold, M.D., Cary L. Hamlin, M.D., and Charles A. Dackis, M.D.

TRH TESTING

Thyrotropin-releasing hormone (TRH) is a naturally occurring tripeptide which has an extensive extrahypothalamic distribution and has been identified as binding to thyrotrophs on the anterior pituitary to produce the release of thyroid-stimulating hormone (TSH). The TRH test has been widely used in both endocrinology and psychiatry to identify grades of thyroid failure and to confirm a diagnosis of active major depressive disorder or confirm a neurobiological response to treatment of a major depressive disorder. We will briefly review the use of the TRH test in psychiatry, and then present data suggesting that the endocrinologist's use of the test to evaluate thyroid function is also of considerable psychiatric value.

Many independent investigators have confirmed the finding that patients with major depression have blunted response of the pituitary hormone TSH to an infusion of the hypothalamic tripeptide TRH. There is some controversy as to whether unipolar and bipolar depressives differ on the TRH test. The TRH test is a standard endocrinologic procedure which was first used in the diagnosis of thyroid disease. We have suggested that the TRH test has utility as a psychiatric diagnostic test in euthyroid patients with affective disorders.

The TRH test consists of measurement of TSH response to infusion of TRH. An indwelling venous catheter is placed in patients who are at bedrest at 8 A.M. after an overnight fast. At 9 A.M. 500 μg of synthetic TRH is administered over 30 seconds through the catheter. The patient experiences only mild, transient autonomic symptoms such as the urge to urinate. Before and 15, 30, 60 and 90 minutes after TRH administration small samples of blood are obtained via the catheter for measurement of serum TSH in duplicate by radioimmunassay (RIA). The maximum TSH response (ΔTSH) is determined for each patient by subtracting the baseline TSH from the peak TSH level after TRH infusion.

Several factors can decrease the TSH response to TRH and they must be taken into account in interpreting TRH test results in depression. Many commonly used psychotropics, including benzodiazepines, neuroleptics, and tricyclic antidepressants do not significantly interfere with the TRH test.

TRH TEST AND DEPRESSION

We have found the definition of $\Delta TSH \leqslant 7.0 \, \mu IU/ml$ as a blunted TSH response to TRH useful in discriminating subgroups of depression. In one study we administered the TRH test to 145 consecutive patients who met research diagnostic criteria (RDC) for major depression, primary unipolar subtype, or nonmajor depressions (minor or intermittent depression). The mean ΔTSH 7.3 $\pm$ 0.5 $\mu IU/ml$ in the 105 unipolar patients was significantly lower (p $\geqslant$ 0.01 by t test) than that of 10.9 $\pm$ 0.7 $\mu IU/ml$ in the 40 patients with nonmajor depressions. Sixty-five of the unipolar depressed patients, but only four of the nonmajor depressed patients and none of the control subjects showed a $\Delta TSH < 7.0 \, \mu IU/ml$.

If a $\Delta TSH \, \mu 7.0 \quad IU/ml$ is used as a diagnostic test to identify patients with a clinical diagnosis of major unipolar depression in this group of patients and control subjects, the sensitivity is 56%, the specificity is 93%, and the diagnostic confidence level is 91%. In many respects the TRH test is the ideal confirmatory test for major depression. A blunted response to TRH confirms the presence of active major depression and allows the physician to follow the state marker throughout the course of treatment. A blunted response should return to normal after successful treatment, and failure of a blunted test to return to normal is a poor prognostic sign which in many patients will outweigh clinical judgement and demand a change of therapy regardless of the patient's state. The TRH test is relatively easy to perform and interpret. Finally, as we will discuss below, the test also rules out the presence of subclinical, mild, or overt hypothyroidism which are frequently causes of misdiagnosis in tertiary or evaluation centers. We studied 124 consecutive euthyroid, nonalcoholic, or drug-abusing inpatients with major depressive disorder, primary unipolar subtype who had a 1-mg DST following a TRH test. Of these, 51% failed to suppress on the dexamethasone suppression test (DST) and 50% had a blunted TSH response to TRH. There was no relationship between these abnormalities by chi-square test. Twenty-three percent had an abnormality on the TRH test only, 24% on the DST only, 27% on both, and 26% on neither. Thus, each of the two tests seem necessary and complementary in the neuroendocrine evaluation of the depressed patient. Using both tests, 74% of the unipolar patients could be identified on having a neuroendocrine abnormality.

TRH TEST IN MANIA AND COCAINE INTOXICATION

We have also found that manic patients tend to have blunted TSH response to TRH, whereas patients with schizophrenic psychosis tend to have a normal response. It is important to differentiate these two groups of patients, who can appear similar in the acute phase of illness due to the better prognosis and response to lithium of the manic patient. Clinical manifestations of cocaine intoxication, such as increased energy, weight loss, hyperactivity, diaphoresis, hyperthermia, and cardiovascular arousal are remarkably similar to symptoms of hyperthyroidism. Conversely, the abrupt cessation of cocaine abuse often results in symptoms resembling hypothyroidism, such as fatigue, depression, psychomotor retardation, weight gain, and hypersomnia. Since cocaine has profound noradrenergic effects, and norepinephrine (NE) is involved in TRH regulation, it is plausible that thyroid axis disruptions contribute to the neurovegetative changes found in cocaine abuse patients. Recent data demonstrating inadequate TSH responses to infused TRH in cocaine abusers support this hypothesis.

We studied 17 consecutive patients admitted with cocaine abuse by Diagnostic and Statistical Manual of Mental Disorders, 3d ed. (DSM-III) criteria, along with confirmatory plasma or urinary cocaine titers demonstrated at the time of admission to a local hospital ward. Patients were excluded if they met DSM-III criteria for other substance abuse or for major affective disorders. Twenty normal control subjects, similar in age and sex and without substance abuse or major affective illness were also studied. Each subject received a TRH test as previously described with baseline T_3 and T_4 levels by RIA. Cocaine patients received TRH testing during their first week of hospitalization. The TSH response to TRH ($500 \mu g$ intravenously) was calculated as peak minus baseline TSH (ΔTSH).

There were not significant differences in baseline T_3, T_4, and TSH between the two groups. However, the TSH scores of

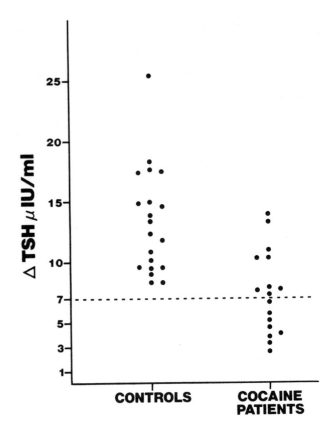

Figure 19-1   TSH responses to TRH (ΔTSH) in 20 normals and 17 cocaine patients.

cocaine patients (7. 4 + 3. 3 μIU/ml) were significantly lower (p <0. 001, degrees of freedom (df) = 35, t = 4. 59 when compared to the control subjects (13. 4 + 4. 2 μIU/ml). In addition, 8 of 17 cocaine patients (47%) had a blunted ΔTSH (<7 μIU/ml), compared to none of the control subjects (chi-square = 9. 27, p > 0. 01) (Fig. 19-1).

Our data demonstrate inadequate TSH responses to TRH in patients with cocaine abuse. This finding is consistent with our present knowledge regarding TRH regulation by biogenic amines. Direct hypothalamic administration of norepinephrine results in TRH release. Chronic cocaine abuse could lead to chronically elevated TRH, down-regulation of the receptors for TRH in the anterior pituitary, and subsequent blunting of the TSH response to TRH. This response is exquisitely sensitive to thyroid axis changes and involved in the maintenance of homeostasis. Cocaine intoxication could produce a state of compensated hyperthyroidism which is only evident on TRH testing.

While cocaine intoxication could produce thyroid axis activation by releasing TRH, sudden cessation of cocaine use might result in thyroid axis inhibition due to the presence of desensitized thyrotroph TRH receptors. Thyroid axis inhibition at the level of the pituitary thyrotroph was found in our cocaine patients, and could make a major contribution to the neurovegetative symptoms associated with the cessation of cocaine abuse. Reversal of cocaine abstinence symptoms may depend upon normalization of the thyroid axis and NE neuronal systems. Why mania, unipolar depression, hyperthyroidism, and cocaine intoxication share TSH blunting will be a very important discovery for the future of chemical theories of affective illness.

THYROID FAILURE: IMPROVING TREATMENT RESPONSE IN DEPRESSION BY IDENTIFYING HYPOTHYROIDISM

In the absence of a neuropsychiatric evaluation unit program the physician must rule out known and likely illnesses that may manifest symptoms similar to or indistinguishable from major depressive disorders, anxiety disorders, thought disorders, and others. One of the most common illnesses imitating naturally occurring psychiatric illness is thyroid dysfunction. Excess thyroid activity (e.g., over the person's own normal) can produce anxiety, panic, and even delusions and hallucinations. Reductions in thyroid function can induce dementia, depression, and problems in living and thinking. In this chapter we will focus on the failing thyroid gland and its relevance to psychiatric diagnosis and maximizing treatment response. The importance of this syndrome becomes clearer when we recognize that patients with even the mildest forms of subclinical hypothyroidism present with major depressive symptomatology.

Early thyroid failure with its predilection for behavioral symptoms is much more likely to present as depression, anergia, or as problems in concentrating and the patient may present with these difficulties to a generalist or psychiatrist. Even when overt or classical hypothyroidism is present it is usually diagnosed well before the patient is referred to a psychiatrist. With advances in thyroid testing, and given that our clinical data suggesting early thyroid failure may preferentially appear as a behavioral syndrome, testing depressed patients for evidence of covert, mild, or overt hypothyroidism has become more routine. This notion is supported by evidence that small decreases in thyroid hormone production may change adrenergic receptor sensitivities in the brain and thus modify behavior. Studies have demonstrated that DSM-III or RDC psychiatric diagnosis did not rule out thyroid failure as the primary diagnosis. In other words, without instituting comprehensive thyroid testing, clinicians cannot differentiate primary thyroid from primary affective disorder. In addition, TRH testing has identified two new patient group that were previously included in the descriptive diagnosis of major depression – thyroid hormone responders and thyroid plus antidepressant responders. In our studies, the incidence of hypothyroidism in patients with a chief complaint of depression or anergia who meet the criteria for major depressive disorder, unipolar subtype, appeared to be greater than previously believed, and this finding has been recently supported by additional studies in both inpatient and outpatient populations.

Over the past decade it has been increasingly recognized that there is a spectrum of thyroid dysfunction. Recognition of this continuum has led to development of systems for grading degrees of hypothyroidism. Development of this system has been aided by the more widespread availability of TRH testing which allows laboratory detection of hypothyroidism at a much earlier stage (Table 19-1). The diagnosis of overt hypothyroidism (grade 1) designates patients with classic clinical signs and symptoms of hypothyroidism along with the typical pattern of laboratory abnormalities $\downarrow T_4$, $\uparrow TSH$, $\uparrow \Delta TSH$. Mild hypothyroidism (grade 2) includes patients with only a few minor or early clinical symptoms, perhaps accompanied by additional nonspecific complaints and signs, plus normal T_4 or T_3 and borderline basal TSH and $\uparrow \Delta TSH$ on TRH testing. Patients with subclinical hypothyroidism (grade 3) have few if any clinical signs and normal T_4, T_3, and TSH, however, the ΔTSH is increased on TRH testing. In a study of 250 consecutive inpatients admitted for evaluation of depression or anergia, we found that 20 patients (8%) showed some degree of hypothyroidism on comprehensive clinical evaluation and thyroid testing including the TRH test. Of these 20 patients, only 2 (<1%) had grade 1, overt hypothyroidism with positive clinical findings and the typical laboratory

Table 19-1   Grades of Hypothyroidism

Grade 1	Overt	Classic clinical symptoms: anergia, weight gain, cold intolerance, constipation, hoarseness, etc.	$\downarrow$ T$_4$, TSH, $\uparrow$ TSH
Grade 2	Mild	Mild or few symptoms (fatigue, dry skin, constipation)	T$_4$ normal, borderline or $\uparrow$ TSH, $\uparrow\Delta$ TSH
Grade 3	Subclinical	No specific thyroid symptoms, some symptoms of anergia or depression	T$_4$, TSH normal, $\uparrow\Delta$ TSH

pattern. Eight patients (3%) had evidence of mild hypothyroidism with only a few clinical symptoms, such as dry skin, weight gain, and fatigue, normal thyroid hormone levels, mildly elevated TSH, and increased Δ TSH. Ten patients (4%) had no clinical symptoms of hypothyroidism other than complaints of anergia or depressed mood with normal T$_4$ and TSH but Δ TSH values of greater than 30 mIu. These findings suggested hypothyroidism can be detected at a much higher rate among depressed patients than had previously been appreciated. In our experience with 400 depressed patients, hypothyroidism was a significant and important cause of misdiagnosis (Table 19-2).

While there are numerous potential etiologies for hypothyroidism; autoimmune mechanisms are frequently implicated and can be screened for with relative ease. Additional testing for the presence of antibodies to either thyroglobulin or thyroid microsomes showed that 9 of 15 hypothyroid patients (60%) had positive titers of antimicrosomal antibodies. The presence of antibodies suggests an autoimmune etiology for 60% of the patients with thyroid dysfunction.

In patients without other evidence of thyroid disease, the name symptomless autoimmune thyroiditis (SAT) has been proposed for patients with augmented TSH response to TRH and circulating thyroid antibodies. We have found that SAT is an illness characterized by normal thyroid indices (T$_4$, T$_3$) elevated TSH, clinical symptoms of anergia or depression, and the presence of antithyroid antibodies.

Evaluation of the thyroid gland of the depressed or anergic patient in clinical practice requires that the psychiatrist be

Table 19-2   Summary of Inpatient and Outpatient Data
             on Hypothyroidism

N	Grade 1	Grade 2	Grade 3
Total 400	3 (1%)	16 (4%)	24 (6%)

aware of and focus attention on, three aspects of evaluation —
clinical history, physical examination, and laboratory testing.
All of these components are mandatory. Overreliance on or ne-
glect of any major area increases the risk of neglecting the presence of hypothyroidism in patients.

The most useful laboratory tests for hypothyroidism are
total T_4, T_3, T_3 RIA, T_3 RU, TSH, and TRH stimulation test.
More recently the T_3 RU has been replaced by the T_4 TBG
ratio. The T_3 uptake test has long been used as an indirect esti-
mate of TBG concentrations and when included in the calculation
of a "free thyroxine index" has proven to be useful in correcting
T_4 concentrations for mild or moderate changes in TBG levels.
The T_3 uptake test is, however, an indirect and imperfect esti-
mate of TBG concentrations and the "free thyroxine index" fails
to correct serum T_4 levels for extremes in TBG concentrations.
By replacing the T_3 uptake test with the TBG RIA, actual TBG
concentrations are measured and a new index, the T_4/TBG ratio
can replace the older "free thyroxine index." In patients with
evidence of overt, grade 1 hypothyroidism, T_4 and TSH will both
be abnormal thus confirming the clinical diagnosis. Patients
with possible grade 2 or 3 hypothyroidism should have the TRH
stimulation test to establish the diagnosis. All patients with a
TSH of $\geq$ 20 mIu should be tested for thyroid antibodies. Our data
suggest that roughly half of the identified hypothyroid patients
have positive thyroid antibodies and that the primary etiology
for our findings is autoimmune in nature. The etiology of the
other 50% who are nonautoimmune needs to be clarified.

SUMMARY

The protirelin or TRH test is one of the most useful testing procedures in psychiatry. The test is essential in the differential
diagnosis of affective states. With psychiatry relying on an entirely descriptive nosology, the burden is on the physician to
rule out from active consideration all competing diagnoses.
Meeting DSM-III criteria does not rule in a diagnosis of major
depressive disorder but only allows the physician to make a diagnosis after all viable competing medical, neurologic,

endocrinologic, vitaminologic, and other diagnoses are eliminated from active consideration by formal evaluation and testing. The TRH test eliminates from consideration the most important cause of secondary affective disorder presenting as anergia, depression, or failure to respond to standard pharmacotherapy. In addition, a blunted test can serve as a state marker enabling the physician to form an impartial "third party" opinion as to whether the patient is phenomenologically and neurobiologically improved or not.

When a patient is identified as having a grade of thyroid failure the treatment of that patient will change. Generally those patients with SAT will be given a formal trial on thyroid hormone. Those patients without antithyroid antibodies but in whom the TRH test has identified grade 1 (overt) or grade 2 (mild) hypothyroidism will be given a formal thyroid hormone trial for their behavioral complaints. Finally, patients with grade 3 (subclinical) hypothyroidism may also be given a trial of thyroid hormone to which an antidepressant can be added if the response to thyroid is not adequate or complete. The TRH test is a powerful diagnostic tool which complements the clinical interview and examination skills of the modern biopsychiatrist. The TRH test results can dramatically alter the course of an inpatient hospitalization or outpatient treatment trial. Thus, the TRH test is recommended when the physician's differential diagnosis includes hypothyroidism and when the clinical evaluation and examination suggest the possibility of hypothyroidism, when the patient has not responded to an adequate antidepressant trial, or when the patient is seen in a tertiary or evaluation center.

BIBLIOGRAPHY

Berens, S. C., Bernstein, R. S., Robbins, J., and Wolff, J.: Antithyroid effects of lithium. J Clin Invest 49:1357, 1970.

Evered, D. E., Ormston, B. J., Smith, P. A., Hall, R., and Bird, T.: Grades of hypothyroidism. Br J Med 1:657, 1973.

Extein, I., Pottash, A. L. C., and Gold, M. S.: Relationship of thyrotropin releasing hormone test and dexamethasone suppression test abnormalities in unipolar depression. Psychiatry Res 4:49, 1981.

Extein, I., Pottash, A. L. C., Gold, M. S., and Cowdry, R. W.: Using the protirelin test to distinguish mania from schizophrenia. Arch Gen Psychiatry 39:77-81, 1982.

Extein, I., Pottash, A. L. C., Gold, M. S., Cadet, J., Sweeney, D. R., Davies, R. K., and Martin, D.: The thyroid stimulating hormone response to thyrotropin releasing hormone in mania and bipolar depression. Psychiatry Res 2:199, 1980.

Gold, M. S., and Byck, R.: Endorphins, lithium, and naloxone: their relationship to pathological and drug-induced manic-euphoric states. In: National Institute on Drug Abuse Research Monograph 19: The International Challenge of Drug Abuse (Edited by R. C. Petersen). National Institute on Drug Abuse, U.S. Government Printing Office, Rockville, MD, 1978, pp. 192-209.

Gold, M. S., Pottash, A. L. C., and Extein, I.: Hypothyroidism and depression. JAMA 245(19):1919, 1981.

Gold, M. S., Pottash, A. L. C., and Extein, I.: "Symptomless: autoimmune thyroiditis in depression. Psychiatry Res 6: 261, 1982.

Gold, P. W., Goodwin, F. K., Wehr, T., and Rebar, R.: Pituitary thyrotropin response to thyrotropin releasing hormone in affective illness: relationship to spiral fluid amine metabolites. Am J Psychiatry 139:1028-1029, 1977.

Gold, M. S., Pottash, A. L. C., Davies, R. K., Ryan, N., Sweeney, D. R., and Martin, D. M.: Distinguishing unipolar and bipolar depression by thyrotropin release test. Lancet 2: 411-413, 1979.

Gordin, A., and Lamberg, B. A.: Natural course of symptomless autoimmune thyroiditis. Lancet 2:1234, 1975.

Grimm, Y., and Reichlin, S.: Thyrotropin releasing hormone (TRH): neurotransmitter regulation of secretion by mouse hypothalamic tissue in vitro. Endocrinology 93:626-631, 1973.

Kim, H. J., and Cereo, E.: Interferences by NaCl with the emit method of analyses for drugs of abuse. Clin Chem 22:1935-1936, 1976.

Reichlin, S.: Regulation of the hypophysiotropic secretions of the brain. Arch Intern Med 135:1350-1361, 1975.

Saberi, M., and Utiger, R. D.: Augmentation of thyrotropin response to thyrotropin-releasing hormone following small decreases in serum thyroid hormone concentrations. J Clin Endocrinol Metab 40:435, 1975.

Van Dyke, C., Jatlow, P., Ungerer, J., Barash, P. G., and Byck, R.: Oral cocaine: plasma concentrations and central effects. Science 200:211-213, 1978.

Whybrow, P. C., and Prange, A. J.: A hypothesis of thyroid-catecholamine receptor interaction. Arch Gen Psychiatry 38: 106, 1981.

Chapter 20

ADVANCED TECHNOLOGY AND PSYCHIATRIC DIAGNOSIS

Steven M. Kalavsky, M.D.

Recent technological advances have led to new methods of assessing the brain. They include computerized tomography (CT
scanning of the brain), nuclear magnetic resonance (NMR scanning), positron emission tomography (PET scanning), and brain
electrical activity mapping (BEAM). The availability of the
equipment needed for such testing is variable; many hospitals
have CT scanners but very few have the equipment necessary
for the other techniques.
    Computerized tomography employs the projection of narrow
beams of x-rays through the head onto detectors which "feed"
information to a computer which mathematically constructs a
cross-sectional picture of the head and its contents as "slices"
of varying thickness. Conventional neuroradiography (skull
radiographs, pneumoencephalography, cerebral angiography)
could distinguish only three densities ("bone," "tissue," and
"air") but CT can distinguish a greater number of and much
smaller variations in density allowing the identification of cerebrospinal fluid, white matter, grey matter, clotted blood and,
with contrast injection, blood vessels. Newer scanners can construct cross-sections in coronal, saggital, and even oblique
planes allowing the formation of three-dimensional representa-
tions. The patient must remain motionless during the scan or
"movement" artifact will be introduced; scanning during periods
of acute agitation is impossible unless the patient is sedated.
This is not a major limitation because the test demonstrates
structure (not function) of the brain and the state of the patient's
functioning will not alter the results. A more important problem
is the limit of resolution. The test can only demonstrate gross
anatomic abnormalities similar to those seen at gross inspection
at an autopsy and years of experience with autopsies have failed
to demonstrate consistent gross anatomic abnormalities in

patients with schizophrenia. The advantages are that the CT scan can view the brain in a more "physiologic" state and can follow changes over time.

Patients with cerebral atrophy have reduced brain volume which is seen by CT scanning as enlarged ventricles and enlarged sulci over the cortical surface (as opposed to hydrocephalus which also shows enlarged ventricles but sulci are not seen because the pressure forces the surface of the cortex against the inner table of the skull). Early studies of patients with schizophrenia demonstrated enlarged lateral ventricles, enlarged cortical sulci, and an increased frequency of reversed cerebral asymmetry. Atrophy of the cerebellar vermis which may have links to the limbic forebrain has also been demonstrated by CT scan and postmortem examination in patients with schizophrenia. Up to 60% of certain populations of patients with schizophrenia were reported to have abnormal CT scans. More recent reports have failed to confirm these findings. These differences may be explained by differences in measurement techniques, differences in CT equipment and scanning technique, or differences in patient populations. Patients who did not respond to conventional therapy and were in locked inpatient wards as well as those with deficits on the Luria-Nebraska Neuropsychological Battery and those with low cerebrospinal fluid concentrations of 5-hyproxyindoleacetic acid may have been more likely to show such changes than those who appear to be more mildly affected. Further studies will require careful control of such factors.

Some patients with anorexia nervosa have also been reported to have abnormal CT scans with enlarged cerebral sulci which return toward normal as the patients gained weight.

Nuclear magnetic resonance scanning involves placing the patient in a strong magnetic field (which aligns hydrogen nuclei — primarily in tissue water molecules) and then displacing the alignment with an energizing radio signal that excites the nuclei. As the signal is stopped, the nuclei fall back into alignment emitting energy which can be detected and processed by a computer to construct visual "slices" of the head. The images produced resemble CT scans but NMR differentiates white matter and grey matter more clearly and does not demonstrate bone which contains much less water. The test does not employ any ionizing radiation. However, the patient must also remain motionless during the examination and only gross anatomic detail can be demonstrated. Once again, this test does not measure function of the central nervous system.

It has been reported that manic-depressive patients' hydrogen protons react differently to nuclear magnetic resonance (NMR) scanning before and after treatment with lithium carbonate.

Positron emission tomography uses positron-emitting isotopes which are injected into the patient's vasculature. Various isotopes have been used and their distribution in the brain are affected by cerebral blood flow and the local metabolism of the isotope. The positrons that are emitted can be detected and an image of the brain based on varying concentrations of isotopes in different parts of the brain can be constructed. The test is unlikely to be widely available because a cyclotron must be available to generate the isotopes. This test has the advantage over those discussed previously of measuring some aspect of central nervous system function as opposed to gross anatomic detail. For example, the test can give some indication of glucose utilization which is an indirect measure of metabolism. However, the test involves a rather long "scan time" and rapid fluctuations of function will not be detected. Possible harmful effects of the isotopes will limit the number of times a patient can be scanned.

It has been reported that patients with acute schizophrenia with positive symptoms have asymmetries of glucose uptake in subcortical structures such as the basal ganglia with a left sided predominance. Patients with schizophrenia of long duration and with negative symptoms have a lowered blood flow and lowered glucose metabolism in the frontal lobes.

Brain electrical activity mapping is a refinement of electroencephalographic (EEG) and evoked potential recording. It involves topographically mapping EEG and evoked potential data derived from multiple scalp electrodes producing colored images on a computer-driven video screen representing ranges of voltage. This test also gives some estimation of one of the functions of the central nervous system — generation of electrical potentials. However, it assays only the superficial layer of about one-third of the cortex. Electrical abnormalities on the undersurface of the brain are not assayed and abnormalities in deeper, subcortical structures may be missed unless they affect the function of the cortex.

It has been reported that a small number of schizophrenics have large bilateral, frontally maximal increases in EEG 1- to 3- Hz (delta) activity in both medicated and drug-free patients which extends to involve the entire cortex during eye-opening. A large bifrontal abnormality was also seen late in the visual evoked potential for medicated schizophrenics. There was also increased fast (beta) activity in the left parietal region with greater amplitude of the late visual evoked potential in the left posterior quadrant of medicated and drug-free schizophrenic patients.

None of the tests above allow an assessment of microscopic anatomy or biochemical status of an intact, living brain. It is too early to determine if these tests will be of value in diagnosing schizophrenia patients, monitoring their treatment or even in classifying these patients.

BIBLIOGRAPHY

Awad, A. G.: Schizophrenia and multiple sclerosis. J Nerv Ment Dis 171:323-324, 1983.

Gunby, P.: Scanning the field of neuroradiology. JAMA 249: 857-867, 1983.

Jernigan, J. L., Zatz, L. M., Moses, J. A., and Berger, P. A.: Computed tomography in schizophrenics and normal volunteers II. cranial asymmetry. Arch Gen Psychiatry 39:771-773, 1982.

Jernigan, J. L., Zatz, L. M., Moses, J. A., and Cardellino, J. P.: Computed tomography in schizophrenics and normal volunteers. I. Fluid volume. Arch Gen Psychiatry 39:765-770, 1982.

Luchins, D. J.: Computed tomography in schizophrenia. Disparities in the prevalence of abnormalities. Arch Gen Psychiatry 39:859-860, 1982.

Morihisa, J. M., Duffy, F. H., and Wyatt, R. J.: Brain electrical activity mapping (BEAM) in schizophrenic patients. Arch Gen Psychiatry 40:719-728, 1983.

Nasrallah, H. A., Jacoby, C. G.: McCalley-Whitters, M., and Kuperman, S.: Cerebral ventricular enlargement in subtypes of chronic schizophrenia. Arch Gen Psychiatry 39:774-777, 1982.

Potkin, S. G., Weinberger, D. R., Linnoila, M., and Wyatt, R. J.: Low CSF 5-hydroxyindoleacetic acid in schizophrenic patients with enlarged cerebral ventricles. Am J Psychiatry 140:21-25, 1983.

Part IV

PSYCHOPHARMACOLOGY

Chapter 21

TRICYCLIC AND TETRACYCLIC ANTIDEPRESSANTS

Mark S. Gold, M.D. and Cary L. Hamlin, M.D.

Since the discovery of the antidepressant (AD) properties of imipramine (IMI) by Kuhn there have been considerable advances
of the pharmacotherapy of depression. The efficacy of tricyclic
antidepressants (TCA) in treating depressive illness has been
established beyond doubt. The spectrum of conditions to which
the term "depression" is applied ranges from a dysphoric response to adverse environmental events, to a medical syndrome
that occurs spontaneously and is characterized by fixed, depressed mood and physiologic symptoms such as disturbed sleep
and appetite patterns. The former set of conditions is often referred to as "reactive" or "neurotic" depression; while the latter set of conditions, often termed "endogenous" depression, is
approximately equivalent to the category of major depressive
disorder with melancholia. While there is some controversy as
to whether all types of depressive illness respond to pharmacologic treatment, it is generally accepted that patients who meet
descriptive criteria for endogenous depression or who have neurobiological evidence for an active major depression, are most
likely to respond to somatic treatments.

However, within the descriptively homogeneous endogenous
subgroup of depressives, 35-50% of patients fail to respond to
treatment with standard dosages of TCA. Among many of the
"responders" the quality of response is quite variable. Furthermore, many "responders" in a research study relapse within 6
months and some are even included in another study. Others are
treated and studied by other physicians. Undoubtedly, some patients are treatment-resistant because they have been misdiag-
nosed and suffer from medical illness but other factors may be
equally important.

Given the probable biochemical heterogeneity of endogenous
depression, it is no more reasonable to expect that every

individual will respond to a given AD than it is to assume that all patients who have sore throats and fever will respond to the same pharmacologic treatment. Another reason why many patients fail to respond to treatment is that they have not received an adequate therapeutic trial of AD drug therapy. Most physicians do not even know what constitutes an AD trial. Other, less-obvious factors may contribute to inadequate drug treatment and include interpatient pharmacokinetic variability resulting in nontherapeutic blood levels, drug-drug interactions, generic substitution, noncompliance, and inadequate duration of drug treatment. Since the majority of depressed patients do not seek treatment and those who do seek treatment feel a stigma upon filling a prescription, medical factors are less important than patient attitudes.

The pharmacologic treatment of the depressed patient can be one of the most rewarding aspects of psychiatric practice. When used properly in the depressed patient likely to respond — even the severely depressed patient — improvement can be striking and patients can be returned to their previous level of functioning within a matter of weeks with a minimum of side effects. However, it has been well documented that many depressed patients, including those with major depressive disorders, receive far from optimal treatment with AD medications. Treatment can be enhanced by attention to appropriate target symptoms and knowledge of the spectrum of side effects. The physician can be guided in efforts to insure adequate trials of AD medication by monitoring of blood levels, and can potentiate unsuccessful AD trials by several new and safe pharmacologic methods. Neuroendocrine markers can help in proving response or lack of response and in assessing prognosis after a course of treatment.

Given the clinical and biological heterogeneity of Diagnostic and Statistical Manual of Mental Disorders, 3d ed (DSM-III)-diagnosed patients along the depressive spectrum, it is not surprising that there is much variation in response rates of different subgroups of depressives to AD. There is a high rate of spontaneous remission as well as placebo response in depressive illness. Up to 50% of a mixed group of depressives will improve over several months without specific treatment. One clinically useful approach to the problem of variability in response is to apply, when practical, a drug-free "washout" or evaluation period when initially assessing the depressed patient. Not only does this allow for a careful psychiatric and medical assessment and relief from the ill effects of medication, but it also insures that patients with spontaneous remissions or response to psychosocial support will be spared unnecessary labeling and medication.

Table 21-1   Comparison of Antidepressants for Clinical Use

	Therapeutic Plasma Level (mg/ml)	Average Daily Maintenance Dose (mg)
Imipramine (Tofranil, Janimine, SK-Pramine)	With desipramine 180	75-200
Amitriptyline (Elavil, Endep)	With nortriptyline 120	75-200
Desipramine (Norpramine, Pertofrane)	>125	75-100
Nortriptyline (Pamelor)	50-140	50-100
Doxepin (Adapin, Sinequan)	With desmethyldoxepin 110	150-250
Protriptyline (Vivactil)	90-170	20-40
Maprotiline (Ludiomil)	180-300	75-125
Amoxapine (Asendin)	30-120 (150-450)[a]	200-300
Trazodone (Desyrel)	750	100-500

[a]8-Hydroxyamoxapine.

ANTIDEPRESSANT THERAPY

The physician may begin treatment with any AD, since no clinical differences in response to various ADs have been demonstrated conclusively. In general, in the absence of a positive personal
or family history of clear response we prefer to begin therapy
with nortriptyline (NT) or imipramine (IMI) and to monitor the
plasma level closely to insure trial at a therapeutic level for 21
days or longer. It is usually advisable to begin therapy with a
NT or IMI dose prediction test. If this is not possible, therapy
begins at a fairly low dosage and the dosage is increased

gradually over a number of days to a therapeutically effective level as defined in Table 21-1. Plasma level of AD should also be used as a check of compliance, since most patients do not take the medication as prescribed. Medications given in an amount sufficient to maintain therapeutic plasma levels should, if effective, produce within 10 days some improvement in sleep, appetite, and even mood. However, the full effect does not appear until the end of the third week or occasionally even later. If response to 21 days at a consistent therapeutic plasma AD level is negligible or minimal, a change to another AD is recommended. Therapeutic plasma level monitoring has been useful in helping to define an adequate AD trial. In light of the high proportion of treated depressives who have inadequate pharmacologic treatment, criteria for adequacy are important. We define and consider an adequate AD trial to consist of maintaining the patient at dosage adequate to achieve therapeutic plasma levels for a minimum of 21 days with documented compliance (Table 21-2).

There are many ADs on the market currently. The commercially available TCAs consist of IMI, desipramine, amitriptyline, NT, doxepin, protriptyline, and trimipramine. The new generation of ADs includes maprotiline, trazodone, buproprion, and amoxapine. Tranylcypromine, phenelzine, and isocardoxazid are the commercially available monoamine oxidase inhibitors (MAOI). Lithium is available in regular and slow-release forms. Carbamazepine and alprazolam are also reported to have AD effects. All the ADs are reported to have about equal AD effects, but wide variation in side effects. Important side effects include sedation, anticholinergic effects, and postural hypotension. These side effects should be considered when making the initial choice for treatment, and can often be tailored to suit a particular patient's requirements. Orthostatic hypotension is probably the most frequently encountered adverse effect resulting from alpha-adrenergic receptor blockade. For patients who are sensitive to this effect, agents such as desipramine or NT may be indicated, while highly anti-alpha-adrenergic agents such as doxepin, trimipramine, or amitriptyline should be avoided.

Amoxapine is a new antidepressant designated chemically as 2-chloro-11-(1-piperazinyl) dibenz (b, f) (1, 4) oxazepine. The antidepressant activity of amoxapine is related to the blockade of norepinephrine and serotonin uptake. Amoxapine has two major metabolites, 7-OH-amoxapine and 8-OH-amoxapine, and it appears that these metabolites are responsible, more so than the parent compound, for pharmacologic effects. 8-OH-Amoxapine is comparable to the parent compound's norepinephrine reuptake blocking properties, however, it is extremely potent in serotonin

Table 21-2   Adequacy of an Antidepressant Trial

Documenting with plasma levels a minimum trial of 21 consecutive days at therapeutic plasma levels controls for:

1. Dosage
2. Duration
3. Compliance

reuptake blockade. It has been demonstrated that 7-OH-amoxapine has significant dopamine receptor blockade in laboratory animals and as such its dopamine (DA) blocking and neuroleptic activity in humans should be studied. However, amoxapine is a very useful novel AD as is the DA agonist buproprion.

OTHER ANTIDEPRESSANTS

While the relationship between blood levels of NT or IMI and response are very clear, doxepin (plus desmethyldoxepin) levels and clinical response have been reported by only a few investigators. Friedel and Raskind reported that a minimum concentration of doxepin plus desmethyldoxepin of 125 ng/ml. Ward and associates replicated this finding and suggested an upper limit of 250 ng/ml. Two studies have reported the relationship between protriptyline and clinical response. Biggs and Ziegler reported that plasma levels of greater than 70 ng/ml are necessary for a clinical response. In this small group of patients, it was not possible to ascertain a therapeutic ceiling level. Whyte and coworkers reported a curvilinear relationship for protriptyline (165-240 ng/ml). For the newer ADs, trazodone, maprotiline, bupropion, and amoxapine, there are insufficient data on the relationship between blood levels and clinical response to guide therapeutic drug level monitoring. At the present time, blood levels of these newer AD can be useful in determining whether patients are complying with treatment or whether extremely low or excessively high blood levels are resulting from the regimen being prescribed.

CLINICAL USE

Antidepressants are the mainstay of the pharmacologic treatment of uncomplicated, nonpsychotic major unipolar depression. The TCAs are all effective ADs, with their main differences being side effects. Some researchers have tried to provide guidelines for choice of TCA based on potentiation of brain noradrenergic versus serotonergic neurotransmission, or based on neurobiological markers. More research needs to be done in these areas. In view of the limiting anticholinergic and sedative effects of the tertiary tricyclics and the major advantages of a medication with a defined window, our first choice generally is the tricyclic NT. In our experience, NT is generally well tolerated and therapeutic levels can be achieved and the trial established and maintained without side effects. Low doses of benzodiazepines and neuroleptics can be added in unusual circumstances if needed for anxiety, agitation, or sleeplessness. I would reserve the "second-generation" ADs for patients who have real and severe low plasma levels side effects. We will reconsider this judgment when there is better documentation that these newer ADs have efficacy equal to the TCAs and efficacy equal to NT with typically prescribed NT levels in the blood.

Much attention has been focused on the old and new ADs. However, a psychopharmacologist is not a physician who uses medication no one has ever heard of but rather an expert who uses medications everyone has heard of in the optimal clinical syndrome in a manner that maximizes efficacy and reduces risks. For the psychopharmacologist, learning how to use two or at the most three ADs is important but it is more important that he learn how to identify potential responders. Only through a meticulous, rigorous psychiatric and medical assessment can a diagnosis be made that results in a viable pharmacologic treatment plan.

To avoid the pitfalls of prescribing via the Physicians' Desk Reference ("PDR prescribing"), medications should be used that have well-understood plasma levels and response relationship. There are no alternatives to starting most patients on NT or at least IMI or desmethylimipramine (DMI). In order to prescribe ADs properly, it is important to define target symptoms to be treated. In many clear-cut cases of major depressive episodes with good premorbid functioning one can aim for virtually an absolute and complete remission of the depressive syndrome. In cases that are less clear-cut, especially where there are characterologic and other long-standing problems that may be difficult to sort out from the depression in question, one may aim for improvement and symptom reduction without expecting remission from all the depressive symptomatology. As a general rule, the physician can expect ADs at best to return the patient to his baseline level of functioning as it existed before the depression, but administering ADs seldom affects baseline character structure or functioning. Well-designed studies of female outpatients with major depression have shown that AD medications and psychotherapy have additive benefits, but on different target symptoms. The ADs were necessary to alleviate depression symptoms, whereas psychotherapy was necessary to improve the patients' social functioning.

BIBLIOGRAPHY

Amsterdam, J., Brunswick, D., and Mendels, J.: The clinical application of tricyclic antidepressant, pharmacokinetics and plasma levels. Am J Psychiatry 137:653, 1980.

DeMontigney, C., Grunberg, F., and Mayer, A.: Lithium induces rapid relief of depression in tricyclic antidepressant drug nonresponders. Br J Psychiatry 138:252, 1981.

Diagnostic and Statistical Manual of Mental Disorders--Third Edition. American Psychiatric Assoc., Washington, D.C., 1980, pp. 205-224.

Goodwin, F. K., Prange, A. J., Post, R. M., Muscettola, G., and Lipton, M. A.: Potentiation of antidepressant effects of L-triiodothyronine in tricyclic nonresponders. Am J Psychiatry 139:34, 1982.

Heninger, G. R., and Charney, D. S.: Lithium potentiation of antidepressant treatment. New Research Abstracts, 135th Annual Meeting of the American Psychiatric Association, Toronto, N.R. 66, 1982.

Klein, D. F., Gittelman, R., Quitkin, F., and Rifkin, A.: Diagnosis and Drug Treatment of Psychiatric Disorders. Williams & Wilkins, Baltimore and London, 1980, pp. 461-470.

Kuhn, R.: The treatment of depressive states with imipramine. Am J Psychiatry 115:459, 1958.

Lipton, M. A., and DiMascio, A. A.: Psychopharmacology, Raven Press, NY, 1977, p. 371.

Maas, J. W.: Biogenic amines and depression. Arch Gen Psychiatry 32:1357, 1975.

Prange, A. J., Wilson, I. C., Rabon, A. M., and Lipton, M. A.: Enhancement of imipramine antidepressant activity by thyroid hormone. Am J Psychiatry 126:457, 1969.

Risch, S. C., Huey, L. Y., and Janowsky, D. S.: Plasma levels of tricyclic antidepressants and clinical efficacy: a review of the literature, Parts I and II. J Clin Psychiatry 40:6, 58, 1979.

Chapter 22

MONOAMINE OXIDASE INHIBITORS

Ana E. Dvoredsky, M.D. and Conrad Swartz, M.D., Ph.D.

In 1951, isoniazid and iproniazid were developed as agents to treat tuberculosis. Although these compounds were significantly successful in achieving this end, it was soon evident that patients treated with them developed bacterial resistance. However, it did not go unnoticed that the treatment also caused an improvement in the patient's mood. Zeller (1952) described the inhibiting effect of these drugs on monoamine oxidase (MAO). Less toxic monoamine oxidase inhibitors (MAOIs) were soon developed.

ACTION

Monoamine oxidases are ubiquitous enzymes found almost exclusively in the outer layer of the mitochondrial membrane. Their main known action is in the metabolic degradation of non-methylated amines by oxidative deamination (Cohen et al., 1980). Monoamine oxidase heterogeneity has been long recognized. In the past, brain MAO was known to be different from liver MAO. At present, the enzymes are classified according to substrate and specific inhibitor. Type-A monoamine oxidase (MAO-A) deaminates norepinephrine and serotonin; it is inhibited by clorgyline. Type B monoamine oxidase (MAO-B) deaminates phenylethylamine and benzylamine; it is inhibited by pargyline and deprenyl [see work by Davidson and associates (1978) in Bibliography]. Clinically used MAOIs are drugs that block MAO irreversibly, leading to increased levels of norepinephrine, dopamine, and serotonin in brain and other tissues.

Table 22-1   Monoamine Oxidase Inhibitors Available for
              Clinical Use

Generic Name	Brand Name	Usual Therapeutic Dosage
Hydrazines		
Phenelzine	Nardil	0. 75-1. 0 mg/kg/day
Nonhydrazines		
Tranylcypromine	Parnate	10-60 mg/day
Selective inhibitor	Eutonyl	25-200 mg/day

AVAILABLE COMPOUNDS

The first MAOI was derived from hydrazine, a highly hepatotoxic substance. Newer products are more effective and present fewer toxic side effects. Table 22-1 shows the MAOIs available in the United States. Their chemical structure is shown in Figure 22-1.

CLINICAL STUDIES

As with many medications in the human pharmacopoaeia, MAOIs have been tried in the treatment of many known behavioral conditions: research on the effects of MAOIs has been complicated by high variability of diagnosis, diversity of dosage, and variability of age groups. It is difficult to compare studies. Available data are summarized in the discussion of pharmacokinetics below.

PHARMACOKINETICS

Robinson and coworkers (1972) suggest that MAO levels in plasma, platelets, and particularly in brain increase with age. No standardized dose-response relationships for MAOIs among patients in different age groups have been developed. Metabolic rates of removal vary among patients. Patients who are slower acetylators have been found to respond better to phenelzine; however, in Davidson and colleagues' group (1978) the metabolic acetylation rate was found to be independent of the MAOI's clinical effect. Since the inhibiting effect of phenelzine upon the MAO system persists after the drug is eliminated, metabolic removal only partially describes the effects of phenelzine over the course of time. In sum, the mechanisms of action of MAOIs remain unclear.

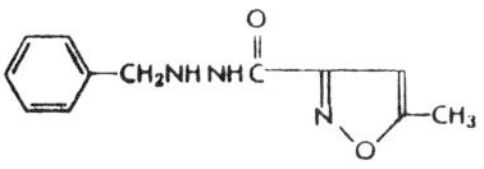

Isocarboxazid

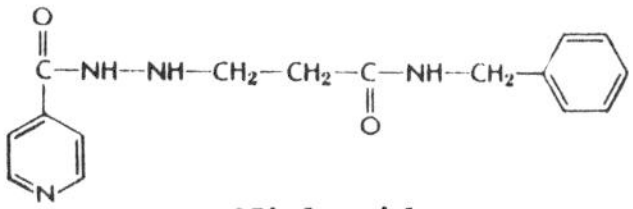

Nialamide

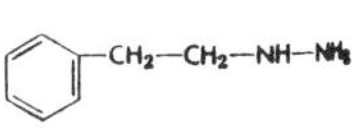

Phenelzine

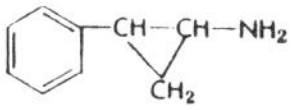

Tranylcypromine

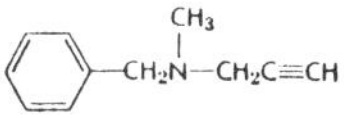

Pargyline

Figure 22-1.

CLINICAL TRIALS

In the treatment of endogenous depression with MAOIs, underdosage may be the most common cause of response failure. Considering the dictum that therapeutic effects and side effects occur at about the same dose, if no side effects are apparent the dose may be too low.

If underdosage indeed is common, then responses should tend to be seen mostly in mildly ill patients (who require less drug) and in patients who metabolize the drug slowly. Robinson (1973) found that MAOIs were specifically effective in patients with nonendogenous depressions; his 60 patients were treated with 60 mg/day phenelzine. Raskin (1974) and also Ravaris and colleagues (1976) also found phenelzine to be equal to placebo in dosages of 45 mg/day or less. Though not mentioning the dose, Himmelhoch and associates (1982) observed rapid and intense efficacy of tranylcypromine relative to placebo in a group of 40 patients with clearly endogenous depressive illness with motor retardation. Though effective for most of their patients, drug response was claimed to be somewhat better among those patients without character disorders. In a later study, Robinson (1978) found that patients did not show clear symptomatic relief until at least 80% of their platelet MAO was inhibited; this effect was seen between 2 and 4 weeks of treatment in dosage of

1 mg/kg/day. This dependency on the intensity of MAO inhibition may account for the lack of efficacy for severely ill patients reported in studies using lower doses.

Monoamine oxidase activity is generally measured in terms of the effect on platelets. The relationship between this activity and that of brain MAO is not established, but some correlation has been reported.

DIAGNOSTIC CRITERIA

The question of diagnostic specificity of MAOIs remains unanswered. Although several reports claim specific MAOI effectiveness for nonendogenous depression, the definition of this MAOI subtype is not clear as no criteria such as research diagnostic criteria [RDC] or Diagnostic and Statistical Manual of Mental Disorders, 3d ed. DSM-III were applied. Some attempts to define the nonendogenous syndrome involve symptom clusters of hypochondriasis, somatic anxiety, social phobia, and anergia or irritability, hypochondriasis, and psychomotor retardation. Still other patients with clinical pictures not defined as depression have been shown to be responsive to MAOIs. Among these patients, those with the following clinical pictures have been found most constant in their response to MAOIs: agoraphobia, phobic depersonalization, phobic anxiety, somatic delusional syndromes, and depressive anxiety states.

CLINICAL USE

Suboptimal dosages and early reports of catastrophic paroxysmal hypertension have given MAOIs an undeserved bad reputation; we believe that MAOIs are no less safe than other antidepressants so long as precautions on their use are followed. We suggest the following guidelines:

CASE SELECTION

As noted above, MAOIs are more effective in patients who suffer from severe anxiety, somatic symptoms, weight gain, hypersomnia, and little guilt. Failure to respond to tricyclics, lithium, and even electroconvulsive therapy (ECT) does not preclude successful treatment with MAOIs. Patients must be reliable in following dietary and medical restrictions (see Table 22-2). Old age is not a contraindication; although cognitive skills of demented patients might not improve, both demented and intact patients show mood improvement.

Table 22-2
_____
Dietary precautions for MAOI use

Cheese, aged	Blue cheese, brie, camembert, cheddar, emmenthaler, stilton, and so forth
Meats, fermented	Herring, dried or pickled Sausages Caviar Liver
Vegetables	Fava beans Avocados, ripe
Fruits	Figs
Other	Caffeine[a] Chocolate[a] Yeast Wine, especially aged

Pharmacologic precautions for MAOI

Sympathomimetic amine (cold prescriptions, appetite
  suppressors)
L-DOPA
Meperidine
Tricyclic antidepressants[a]
_____
[a]Often cited in the literature, although data are not conclusive.

ADEQUATE DOSAGE

Table 22-1 summarizes recommended dosages for each MAOI
according to recent studies. Because of the multiplicity and un-
predictability of side effects it is preferable to approach full
therapeutic dosages slowly.

INSTRUCTION

Patients should be well instructed in the correct use of the medication, given a list of foods and medications to avoid, and re-
assured about their safety if the precautions are followed. Table
22-2 lists the substances patients should avoid.

CLINICAL PROGRESSION

Clinical progression should be monitored. About half the total therapeutic effect of phenelzine is reached within 1 week of dose initiation and three-fourths within 2 weeks; maximal effect occurs after about 4 weeks of treatment. Higher doses may shorten this period of latency but are seldom well tolerated by patients.

It is important to remember that patients receiving MAOIs are typically suffering from severe anxiety and somatic depressive symptoms. They will require more than usual reassurance to comply with therapy during periods of slow clinical improvement, while the medication effects are accumulating.

SIDE EFFECTS

Two toxic effects of MAOIs are dangerous. The best known one is acute hypertension, which can cause a stroke. These episodes, which are not necessarily silent, can include severe occipital headache and the symptoms of raised intracranial pressure and meningeal irritation (such as nausea, vomiting, photophobia, and stiff neck). Such hypertension can follow ingestion of sympathomimetic agents or the consumption of foods high in tyramine or dopamine.

Acute management of this complication is achieved with gradual intravenous administration of an alpha-adrenergic antagonist (as 5 mg phentolamine) titrated against blood pressure (precautions for must be taken for emergency resuscitation). Another risk for MAOI use involves the simultaneous administration of meperidine (Demerol); this mixture can precipitate a hyperpyrexic episode and death.

The side effect most likely to limit the prescribed dose of phenelzine and tranylcypromine is orthostatic hypotension. Support stockings and instructions to make postural changes gradually can help in the management of mild cases.

Other side effects can occur with these drugs. Symptoms of hypomania have been seen, including one or more of: hyperactivity, irritability, insomnia, confusion, and paranoia. Rapid-cycling bipolar illness has been reported. The arousing nature of these drugs can lead to early insomnia if they are given near bedtime. Neither phenelzine nor tranylcypromine has been shown to lead to liver damage, but the hydrazine, phenelzine, can cause a lupuslike reaction. Sexual dysfunctions have been described including ejaculatory problems in men and anorgasmia in women. Withdrawal symptoms following abrupt discontinuation of the drug have been reported.

Another area of concern involves drug interaction. Monoamine oxidase inhibitors have an effect on the metabolism of other compounds, either by blocking enzymes other than MAO (such as those involved in N-dealkylation or hydroxylation), or through other chemical reactions unrelated to hepatic enzymes. As a consequence, they will retard clearance of drugs such as phenothiazines, barbiturates, narcotics, ethanol, antihistamines, and antiparkinsonian (anticholinergic) agents.

DRUG HOLIDAY

Since patients treated with MAOIs experience marked symptomatic relief, these individuals often are reluctant to discontinue the medication. There are no sufficient data regarding chronic treatment; it seems reasonable to attempt a drug holiday at least once a year.

SUMMARY

MAOIs are very effective drugs which have not been used properly because of underdosage and dietary transgressions. The clinical results following MAOI administration can be strikingly positive, as long as the appropriate dietary precautions are observed.

BIBLIOGRAPHY

Ashford, J. W., and Ford, C. V.: Use of MAOI in elderly patients. Am J Psychiatry 136:1466-1467, 1979.

Cohen, R. M., Pickar, D., and Murphy, D. L.: Myoclonus-associated hypomania during MAO-inhibitor treatment. Am J Psychiatry 137:105-106, 1980.

Davidson, J., McLeod, M. N., and Blum, M.: Acetylation phenotype, platelet monoamine oxidase inhibition and the effectiveness of phenelzine in depression. Am J Psychiatry 135:467-469, 1978.

Diagnostic and Statistical Manual of Mental Disorders--Third Edition. American Psychiatric Assoc., Washington, D.C., 1980, pp. 218-222.

Feinberg, M., DeVigne, J. P., Kronfol, Z., and Young, E.:
Duration of action of phenelzine in two patients. Am J Psychiatry 138:379-380, 1981.

Goodman, L. S., and Gillman, E.: The Pharmacological Basis
of Therapeutics, 5th ed. Macmillan, New York, 1972.

Gualtieri, C. T., and Powell, S. F.: Psychoactive drug interactions. J Clin Psychiatry 39:62-71, 1978.

Himmelhoch, J. M., Fuchs, C. Z., and Symons, B. J.: A
double blind study of tranylcypromine treatment of major anergic depression. J Nerv Ment Dis 170:628-634, 1982.

Johnstone, E. C., and Marsh, W.: Acetylator status and response to phenelzine in depressed patients. Lancet 1:567-570,
1973.

Lesko, L. M.: Three cases of female anorgasmia associated
with MAOIs. Am J Psychiatry 139:1353-1355, 1982.

Liebowitz, M. R., Neutzel, E. J., Bowser, A. E., and Klein,
D. F.: Phenelzine and delusions of parasitosis: a case report.
Am J Psychiatry 135:1565-1566, 1978.

Matteson, A., and Seltzer, R. L.: MAOI-induced rapid cycling
bipolar affective disorder in an adolescent. Am J Psychiatry
138:677-679, 1981.

Mountjoy, C. Q., Roth, M., Gurside, R. F., et al.: A clinical
trial of phenelzine in anxiety depressive and phobic neurosis.
Br J Psychiatry 131:486-492, 1977.

Murphy, D. L.: The behavioral toxicity of monoamine oxidase –
inhibiting antidepressants. Adv Pharmacol Chemother 14:72-
105, 1977.

Palladino, A.: Adverse reactions to abrupt discontinuation of
phenelzine. J Clin Psychopharmacol 3:206-207, 1983.

Paykel, E. S., West, P. S., Rowan, P. R., and Parker, R.
R.: Influence of acetylator phenotype on antidepressant effect of
phenelzine. Br J Psychol 141:243-248, 1982.

Physicians' Desk Reference, 37th ed. Medical Economics Co.,
Oradell, NJ, 1983.

Rapp, M.: Two cases of ejaculatory impairment related to phenelzine. Am J Psychiatry 136:1200-1201, 1979.

Raskin, A., Schulterbrandt, J. G., Reatig, N., et al.: Depression subtypes and response to phenelzine, diazepam and a placebo. Arch Gen Psychiatry 30:66-75, 1974.

Ravaris, C. L., Nies, A., Robinson, D. S., et al.: A multiple dose, controlled study of phenelzine in depression-anxiety states. Arch Gen Psychiatry 33:347-350, 1976.

Robinson, D. S., Davis, J. M., Nies, A., et al.: Aging, monoamines, and monoamine-oxidase levels. Lancet 1:290-291, 1972.

Robinson, D. S., Nies, A., Ravaris, L., et al.: Clinical pharmacology of phenelzine. Arch Gen Psychiatry 35:629-635, 1978.

Robinson, D. S., Nies, A., Ravaris, C. L., and Lamborn, K. R.: The monoamine oxidase inhibitor, phenelzine, in the treatment of depressive-anxiety states. Arch Gen Psychiatry 29: 407-413, 1973.

Swartz, C.: Depression with non-auditory hallucinations: success with phenelzine. Psychosomatics 20:286-287, 1979.

Swartz, C.: Lupus-like reaction to phenelzine. JAMA 239:2693, 1978.

Teychenne, P. F., Calne, D. B., Lewis, P. J., and Findley, F. J.: Interactions of levodopa with inhibitors of monoamine oxidase and L-aromatic amine acid decarboxylase. Clin Pharmacol Ther 18:273-277, 1975.

Tyrer, P.: Towards rational therapy with monoamine oxidase inhibitors. Br J Psychiatry 128:354-370, 1976.

Tyrer, P., and Steinberg, D.: Symptomatic treatment of agoraphobia and social phobias: a follow-up study. Br J Psychiatry 127:163-168, 1975.

Youdim, M.: Multiple forms of monoamine oxidase and their properties. In Pharmacology (Edited by E. Costa and M. Sandler). Raven Press, New York, 1972, pp. 67-77.

Zeller, E. A., Barsky, J., Fouts, J. R., Dvorak, A.: Influence of isonicotinic acid hydrazide (INH) and I-isonicotinyl-2-isopropyl hydrazide (IIH) on bacterial and mammalian enzymes. Experientia 8:349-350, 1952.

Chapter 23

ISSUES IN LITHIUM THERAPY

A. L. C. Pottash, M.D. and Mark S. Gold, M.D.

MODE OF ACTION

While researchers have learned a great deal about various effects of lithium and have formulated various theories to explain these effects and in particular lithium's mode or modes of action, we still cannot describe with certainty lithium's actual mechanism of action.

Lithium interacts with the common cations sodium and potassium, as well as calcium and magnesium. The primary mechanism controlling distribution of lithium is a lithium-sodium flow-transport system in which lithium is transported against its electrochemical potential gradient, while sodium is transported in an opposite electrochemical potential gradient. In this sodium-lithium countertransport system lithium is removed from the cell in exchange for extracellular sodium, which is then transported inward.

There are other processes involved in the transportation of lithium across the cell membrane, including movement via a sodium-potassium pump, a "voltage-dependent" channel available during a nerve impulse, and passive diffusion.

Lithium inhibits the sodium-lithium countertransport system, although this effect does not appear in vitro in erythrocytes for 4-7 days, regardless of whether the erythrocytes are exposed to therapeutic levels of lithium from the outset. This may explain the delay in clinical response when lithium is used to treat manic symptomatology.

Lithium may compete with other ions for binding sites and influence ion-sensitive reactions. For example, by occupying calcium sites, lithium could affect calcium-dependent cyclic AMP production or neurotransmitter release. Lithium inhibits hormonal stimulated adenylate cyclases. For example, lithium inhibits vasopressin-stimulated adenylate cyclase, which can lead to polyuria or nephrogenic diabetes insipidus. Lithium blocks prostaglandin-E1-stimulated adenylate cyclase and prostaglandin-E1-synthesis. Lithium may exert antimanic effects through any number or combination of these effects.

LITHIUM AND NEUROTRANSMITTERS

There have been numerous reports, some of them conflicting, concerning lithium's effects on neurotransmitters. It elevates red blood cell (RBC) intracellular levels of choline, the metabolic precursor of acetylcholine, and also inhibits choline transport across the RBC membrane. Increased rate of synthesis of acetylcholine is seen after lithium treatment. The dopamine system seems to be affected by lithium in varying ways depending on the area of the brain being studied. Lithium's effect on the norepinephrine system shows a similar regional pattern. Norepinephrine uptake may be affected differently at various times during treatment with lithium. Similarly, lithium's effects on serotonin change with duration of treatment. Serotonin turnover appears to increase during the first days of treatment. Lithium treatment leads to a decrease in plasma levels of some amino acids which complete with tryptophan at the blood-brain barrier, suggesting that enhancement of brain serotonin may be one effect. Intracellular levels of glycine, which may be a central nervous system (CNS) neurotransmitter, are increased by lithium.

In the area of effects on receptor sensitivity, lithium prevents dopamine receptor supersensitivity, perhaps by reducing the number of brain dopamine receptors. This effect may be dependent on lithium level. Lithium prevents the development of tolerance to the effects of haloperidol on cerebrospinal fluid (CSF) homovanillic acid (HVA) in schizophrenic patients and prevents neuroleptic-induced functional supersensitivity of dopamine receptors.

Clinically, this may mean that lithium combined with neuroleptics may lead to a synergistic reaction through lithium's enhancement and prolongation of neuroleptic blockade of dopamine receptors by preventing functional supersensitivity of dopamine receptor systems. Also, if tardive dyskinesia is related to neuroleptic-induced dopamine supersensitivity, then perhaps this may mean that lithium treatment combined with neuroleptics will help prevent some or all cases of tardive dyskinesia.

Lithium decreases the number of 5-hydroxytryptamine binding sites and gamma-aminobutyric acid (GABA) receptors and has mixed effects on alpha- and beta-adrenergic receptors.

LITHIUM-INDUCED HYPOTHYROIDISM

Lithium is known to have a direct antithyroid effect, although the reasons why only some patients develop goiter during treatment with lithium remain unclear. Thyroid hormone release is inhibited by lithium through stabilization of the microtubules in the gland. In addition, lithium may affect iodide concentrating capacity and biosynthesis of iodotyrosines and iodothyronines. It is unclear whether peripheral degradation of thyroid hormones is increased or decreased. It is also possible that lithium has a direct pituitary effect or that it interferes with the actions of thyroid stimulating hormone (TSH) that are mediated by cyclic AMP.

It has been common practice to follow peripheral thyroid hormones or TSH as indicators of failing thyroid function in patients receiving lithium as if hypothyroidism was either present or absent. However, more recently it has become clear that hypothyroidism is a progressive illness which develops in a stepwise fashion, slowly over time. The thyrotropin-releasing hormone (TRH) test appears to be a more sensitive and earlier indicator of impaired thyroid function in these patients.

In a recent study by our group (Gold, Pottash, Lydiard in press) at Fair Oaks Hospital, 12 euthyroid patients were studied before, and then again 4 to 8 weeks after starting lithium. While none had abnormal TRH tests prior to lithium treatment, 3 of the 12 patients developed abnormally augmented TSH responses to TRH after being on lithium.

Other studies have followed patients for longer periods, finding abnormal TRH tests in nearly 50% of patients maintained on lithium an average of 3 years. Only 20% of the patients on lithium had abnormal baseline TRH tests. These and other data indicate that TRH abnormalities precede elevation in basal TSH and decrease in peripheral thyroid hormone. Lithium's ability to slow functional thyroid status in all patients may be a major part of its mechanism of action.

Early diagnosis of this group of hypothyroid patients on lithium is necessary in order to reduce patient suffering and the tendency to treat the symptoms of undiagnosed lithium-induced hypothyroidism with antidepressants. Symptoms may include atypical depression, anergy, and psychomotor changes. It may be more advisable to treat such complaints with thyroid supplements.

LITHIUM AND THE KIDNEY

Lithium, which is not metabolized, is almost completely eliminated by the kidneys. Investigators have especially been trying to definitively answer the question of whether lithium causes renal damage since 1977, when the first major report of apparently irreversible structural changes in the biopsied kidneys of patients on lithium was published by Danish researchers (Hestbech, et al., 1977). Since then, numerous studies have been done which examined the question further. Interestingly, one group found tubular and other renal pathology, including many of the changes supposedly caused by lithium, in a group of patients with affective disorders prior to their even starting on lithium.

A review of previous reports shows clear decrease in renal concentrating capacity which may correlate with length of lithium usage and may persist for months after lithium is discontinued. However, once again, patients with affective disorders who had never been on lithium also had a decreased concentrating capacity as compared to normal subjects. Polyuria appeared in 2-35% of lithium-treated patients. In patients without previous renal disease, glomerular filtration rate was affected much less often. Occasionally irreversible nephrogenic diabetes insipidus (NDI) has been reported. While the mechanism of lithium-induced NDI is unclear, it may be related to inhibition of the adenyl cyclate system. The vasopressin unresponsiveness seen in NDI could be caused by decreased cyclic AMP, acting as the mediator.

Histopathologic studies show renal changes in essentially all patients with decreased renal function and in approximately 15% of other patients, including interstitial fibrosis as well as tubular atrophy, epithelial degeneration, and sclerotic glomeruli. The structural changes appear primarily in the distal tubules and collecting ducts. The degree of tubular damage appeared to be correlated with the decrease in renal concentrating capacity.

In summary, decrease in renal tubular function is the most common renal change seen in lithium treatment, and may be irreversible in perhaps 5-10% of the patients, although measurement of maximum concentrating ability may be abnormal in up to half the patients while on lithium. There is a possibility that the impairment may be less in patients on sustained release lithium preparations, and damage does not appear to be increased by concomitant neuroleptic use. A history of higher average serum lithium levels led to greater changes in renal concentrating ability.

Two points limit definitive conclusions about the matter:

first, since there is considerable renal reserve and since therefore renal function tests may not be changed even in the face of significant histopathologic changes, we cannot say with certainty how great the danger is, since most studies rely on testing of renal functions. Second, we cannot answer the question definitively until we have observed large numbers of patients after long periods on lithium, since in many patients lithium is intended to be prescribed for decades. Lithium has only been used in psychiatry since 1949, and large numbers of patients have only been on the medication for a limited period. No one can say what the future holds, even though current information supports continued, though carefully monitored, use of lithium.

Clinically, a careful screening with a thorough medical history and physical examination prior to starting lithium is required with special attention paid to history of renal disease or exposure to nephrotoxins. For the renal part of this workup, laboratory testing should be performed, including a urinalysis, blood urea nitrogen (BUN) and serum creatinine tests, serum electrolytes test, 24-hr urinary volume and creatinine clearance tests, and perhaps a test of urinary ability. The evaluation should be repeated at regular intervals.

LITHIUM AND PREGNANCY

Since lithium freely crosses the placenta, maternal and fetal serum lithium concentrations are essentially equal. The question of whether lithium is a teratogen is controversial and no certain answer emerges. There appears to be a significant increase in the incidence of congenital heart disease among children born to mothers who took lithium during the pregnancy. An international Register of Lithium Babies has been developed for mothers who were on lithium during the first trimester or longer. As of 1980, there were 225 reports on births. It should be emphasized that abnormal births may be reported more often than normal ones. In addition, there is no control group, and some mothers took other medications in addition to lithium during pregnancy. The data can only suggest a trend rather than yield a true incidence of pathology. The most common cardiovascular complication was Ebstein's anomaly. This unusual disorder can be identified prenatally by echocardiography.

In the neonate, hypotonia, hypothyroidism, and goiter have been reported. A study of children exposed to lithium during the first trimester of pregnancy who were apparently normal at birth has shown no obvious developmental problems in their early years, based on subjective reports.

Although it is probable that lithium is a teratogen, in many cases it is still necessary for lithium to be used in pregnant women, even in the first trimester. In such cases the patient needs to be made aware of the risks, and lithium levels should be monitored frequently in order to maintain lower levels.

An alternative plan would be to take the risk of discontinuing lithium temporarily during the first trimester while closely observing the carefully informed patient.

LITHIUM LEVELS

While measurement of serum lithium is by far the most frequently used laboratory test to monitor lithium concentration, lithium has been measured in various other bodily fluids and blood components. For example, due to the need for frequent venipuncture in order to obtain serum for analysis in patients on maintenance doses of lithium, researchers have attempted to use saliva lithium levels as an alternative.

The results of attempts to correlate serum and saliva levels of lithium have been mixed. While some studies showed a constant ratio of saliva to serum lithium levels, others found poor correlation and widely fluctuating ratios of saliva to serum concentrations both between different patients and in the same patients over multiple sampling times. Theoretical explanations for this variability have included adrenocortical influences and changes in salivary secretion caused by individual variations, psychotropic medications, or psychosomatic influences. At this time, saliva lithium levels are not a substitute for serum levels.

As an alternative, one study suggested measurement of lithium concentrations in human tears and reported strong correlation with serum levels.

Since it has been reported that brain lithium levels in rats correlated better with erythrocyte lithium concentrations than with serum lithium concentration, other investigators have attempted to determine whether patients with higher erythrocyte to serum lithium ratios (the "lithium ratio" or "index") would have better clinical outcomes during lithium treatment. While study designs were limited, in general it appeared that lithium ratio did not predict response to lithium maintenance.

An alternative use for the lithium ratio would be to use it to gauge compliance. Since the erythrocyte level is slower to increase than the serum level of lithium, patients who take lithium irregularly and, especially, immediately prior to the blood sampling, may show a normal lithium level, while the erythrocyte level will be decreased, changing the lithium index. In some centers this is now a routine measurement, although other researchers have criticized the cost and the reliability of erythrocyte lithium measurements in inexperienced laboratories. Nonetheless, the test may turn out to be of value in clinical practice in selected patients, and further experience with the lithium ratio in the clinical setting is indicated.

BIBLIOGRAPHY

Amdisen, A., and Andersen, C. J.: Lithium treatment and thyroid function: a survey of 237 patients in long-term lithium treatment. Pharmacopsychiatry 15:149-155, 1982.

Bendz, H.: Kidney function in lithium-treatment patients. Acta Psychiatr Scand 68:303-324, 1983.

Brenner, R., Cooper, T. B., Yablonski, M. E., and Siefert, M. L.: Measurement of lithium concentrations in human tears. Am J Psychiatry 139(5):678-679, 1982.

Bunney, W. D., and Garland, B. L.: Lithium and its possible modes of action. In Neurobiology of Mood Disorders (Edited by R. Post and J. Ballenger). Williams & Wilkins, Baltimore, 1984, pp. 731-743.

Deutsche, S. I., Stanley, M., Peselow, E. D., et al.: Glycine: a possible role in lithium's action and affective illness. Neuropsychobiology 9:215-218, 1983.

Gold, M. S., Pottash, A. L. C., Lydiard, R. B., et al.: Lithium-induced hypothyroidism. In: American Psychiatric Association New Research (in press).

Hestbech, J., Munsen, H. E., Amidsen, A., and Olson, S.: Chronic lesions following long-term treatment with lithium. Kidney Int 12:205-207, 1977.

Jefferson, J. W., Greist, J. H., and Ackerman, D. L.: Lithium: Encyclopedia for Clinical Practice. American Psychiatric Press, Washington, D.C., 1983.

Kocsis, J. H., Kantor, J. S., Lieberman, K. W., et al.: Lithium ratio and maintenance treatment response. J Affect Dis 4:213-218, 1982.

Lazarus, J. H., John, R., Bennie, E. H., and Pritchard, T. F.: Lithium therapy and thyroid function: a long-term study. Psychol Med 11:85-92, 1981.

Linden, S., and Rich, C. J.: The use of lithium during pregnancy and lactation. J Clin Psychiatry 44(10):358-360, 1983.

Lydiard, R. B., and Pearsall, R.: Lithium: predicting response/maximizing efficacy. In: Advances in Psychopharmacology (Edited by M. S. Gold and R. B. Lydiard). CRC Press, Boca Raton, FL (in press).

Pottash, A. L. C.: Clinical use of lithium. In: Psychiatric, Psychogenic, and Somatopsychic Disorders Handbook (Edited by A. J. Giannini, H. R. Black, and R. L. Goettsche). Medical Examination Publishing, New York, 1978, pp. 277-280.

Pottash, A. L. C., Gold, M. S., and Extein, I.: The use of the clinical laboratory. In: Inpatient Psychiatry: Diagnosis and Treatment (Edited by L. I. Sederer). Williams & Wilkins, Baltimore, 1983, pp. 205-221.

Ramsey, T. A., and Cox, M.: Lithium and the kidney: a review. Am J Psychiatry 139(4):443-449, 1982.

Sternberg, D. E., Bowers, M. B., Jr., Heninger, G. R., and Bunney, B.: Lithium prevents adaptation of brain dopamine systems to haloperidol in schizophrenic patients. Psychiatry Res 10:79-86, 1983.

Vlaar, H., Bleeker, J. A. C., and Schalken, H. F. A.: Comparison between saliva and serum lithium concentrations in patients treated with lithium carbonate. Acta Psychiatr Scand 60: 423-426, 1979.

Wallin, L., Alling, C., and Aurell, M.: Impairment of renal function in patients on long-term lithium treatment. Clin Nephrol 18:23-28, 1982.

Chapter 24

BENZODIAZEPINES, NEUROTRANSMITTERS, AND THE
NEUROBIOLOGY OF ANXIETY

Daniel W. Hommer, M.D. and Steven M. Paul, M.D.

The benzodiazepines (BZ's) are among the most widely prescribed medications in the world today (Tallman, et al. , 1980).
Their superiority to older anxiolytics such as the barbiturates
or propanediol carbamates and their value in the treatment of
generalized anxiety and insomnia is without question (Greenblatt,
et al. , 1983). These qualities alone would make an understanding
of the BZ's mode of action of considerable interest, but in addition to their clinical utility it is now also apparent that the BZ's
represent valuable molecular probes for studying the biochemical and neurophysiologic basis of anxiety.
    In order to be able to use the BZ's as tools exploring the
brain mechnnisms underlying anxiety, it is first necessary to
have a clear idea of what we mean by anxiety as a disorder or
syndrome, and second to demonstrate that the BZs decrease the
specific symptoms that characterize this syndrome. Despite the
ubiquitous nature of anxiety, it has been a difficult term to define. Most authors have considered anxiety as being similar to
fear; the difference being that in the latter the precipitating
stimulus is clearly apparent, while in the former it is not
(Klein, et al. , 1980). Since anxiety and fear differ solely in the
ability to define their precipitating object or stimuli it seems
reasonable to assume that their underlying biology may be quite
similar. This is a critical assumption since all of the animal
models of anxiety are really techniques that produce or classically "condition" fear.
    What then are the characteristics of fear and how do BZs
affect them? Darwin (1965) describes fear as being "preceded
by astonishment, and is so far akin to it, that both lead to the
senses of sight and hearing being instantly aroused. In both
cases the eyes and mouth are widely opened, and the eyebrows

235

raised. The frightened man at first stands like a statue motionless and breathless or crouches down as if instinctively to es-
cape observation. " Darwin's description contains most of the
features that Gray has suggested constitute the behavioral essence of anxiety (Gray, 1982). These are: the inhibition of ongoing behavior, an increase in attention, and an increase in
arousal. Considered in this way it is easy to see the adaptive
value of fear. It seems likely that natural selection would favor
an animal that when confronted with an indication of danger
stops, looks, listens, and prepares to react rapidly. It also
seems apparent that excessive arousal, attention, and behavioral inhibition, particularly when the stimuli leading to these responses is not identified, could lead to the motor tension, autonomic hyperactivity, apprehension, hyperattentiveness, and the
sense of helpless paralysis that we recognize as clinically apparent anxiety.

In the clinical setting anxiety may occur in association with
various psychiatric and medical disorders and thus the accurate
diagnosis and treatment of such conditions is critical for the
management of associated symptoms of anxiety. In recently devised nosologic schemes (Diagnostic and Statistical Manual of
Mental Disorders, 3d ed. [DSM-III]) for the various anxiety
disorders, fear seems to provide a reasonable diagnostic cor-
nerstone for separating these disorders from many other psychiatric conditions. Phobias, for example, clearly involve fear
while generalized anxiety disorder also is characterized by apprehension or fear with no definite precipitating environmental
stimulus. Similarly, spontaneous panic attacks resemble sudden
episodes of terror but again, without an objective precipitating
stimulus. Whether or not fear is a specific enough symptom for
diagnosing anxiety in a clinical sense remains to be determined.
The fact that the preferred treatment for panic attacks are the
tricyclic antidepressants or monoamine oxidase inhibitors
(Klein, 1964) while BZs are more effective in the treatment of
generalized anxiety disorders (Greenblatt and Shader, 1974)
does not necessarily invalidate the role of fear for making a diagnosis of anxiety. The brain mechanisms that mediate fear
may represent a sort of final common pathway in all of the anxiety disorders. The recent observations that alprazolam
(Chouinard, et al., 1982, Sheehan, 1982) and diazepam (Noyes,
et al., 1983) have some efficacy in the treatment of panic attacks supports this notion. However, just because a group of
disorders share a final common pathway, does not necessarily
mean that they share the same etiology or that this final common
pathway represents the best site for medical intervention. Phobias seem to respond best to behavior techniques that act

psychologically at the level of the feared stimuli (O'Brien, 1981). Similarly, antidepressants may be more effective than BZs in treating panic disorder because they act neurochemically on brain events that precede and possibly trigger the panic attack.

THE EFFECTS OF BENZODIAZEPINES ON FEAR

Among the components of "fear" as conceptualized by Gray (1982), the effects of the BZs on behavioral inhibition have been the most widely studied. In fact, the ability of BZs to attenuate the suppression of behavior by punishment is the most widely used screening test for uncovering the anxiolytic properties of new drugs (Lippa, et al., 1979).

In one variation of this procedure animals are deprived of either food and/or water and then given access to a sucrose solution delivered through an electrified drinking spout. When hungry or thirsty rats are placed in this so-called "conflict" situation they generally respond to the punishment by not eating or drinking. Thus, the fear induced by punishment inhibits the animals' ongoing behavior (i. e., drinking). Animals given BZs, on the other hand, are more resistant to the effects of punishment in suppressing behavior.

The relative potencies of a large series of BZs in preventing the behavioral inhibition induced by punishment is highly correlated with their potencies as anxiolytics in man (Lippa, et al., 1979). This effect is not simply a reflection of sedation since sedation will decrease both punished and nonpunished behavior in the "conflict test" and therefore will antagonize the observed actions of BZs. Furthermore, the tolerance that has been shown to develop to the sedative actions of BZs during chronic administration does not develop to their anxiolytic actions in man (Greenblatt and Shader, 1974) or to their "anticonflict" preparation in animals. A variety of psychotropic drugs including stimulants, antidepressants, antipsychotics, and opiates have been tested for their ability to prevent the behavioral inhibition induced by punishment and have been found to be devoid of "anticonflict" activity at pharmacologically relevant doses. In addition, drugs that specifically block or enhance noradrenergic, dopaminergic, cholinergic, or glycinergic neurotransmission fail to produce or alter "anticonflict" activity in animals. Other drugs, however, that show cross-dependence with the BZs, including the barbiturates, propanediol carbamates, and ethanol reduce the behavioral inhibition by punishment in a variety of species, albeit at relatively high doses.

Benzodiazepines also decrease the increased arousal component of fear. This is demonstrated by their ability to block the stress-induced rises in cortisol, adrenocorticotropic hormone (ACTH), and plasma catecholamines in both humans and animals (Butler, et al., 1968; Rees, 1970; LeFur, et al., 1979). Similarly, BZs decrease vigilance in man (Linnoila, et al., 1983; Hommer, et al., 1984). As with the reduction of behavioral inhibition, these effects also occur at doses that are lower than those needed to produce sedation. Thus, BZs possess the ability to decrease the major behavioral and physiologic components of fear.

THE DISCOVERY OF BENZODIAZEPINE RECEPTORS

Although it has been known for years that BZs decrease the various behavioral aspects of fear as described above, it was not until 1977 that definite data on the mechanisms of action of these drugs began to accumulate. In that year, two groups of investigators (Mohler and Okada, 1977; Squires and Braestrup, 1977) discovered the presence of high-affinity, saturable, and stereospecific binding sites for BZs in membranes derived from the central nervous system (CNS) of a variety of species, including man. This observation sparked a flurry of activity since it indicated for the first time that a highly specific locus of action for these drugs existed in the brain. Furthermore, the excellent correlations between the potencies of a large series of BZs in displacing [^{3}H]diazepam binding from these sites in vitro and their potencies as anticonflict agents in animals and anxiolytics in man, strongly suggested that these binding sites were indeed pharmacologic receptors. Subsequent studies by many laboratories have confirmed and extended the initial findings on the importance of BZ receptors in mediating the pharmacologic actions of BZs. Several groups (Williamson, et al., 1978) have also demonstrated the presence of BZ receptors using in vivo labeling techniques and have shown that the potencies of various BZs for displacing the specific binding of [^{3}H]diazepam and of [^{3}H]flunitrazepam in vivo is also highly correlated with their behavioral and clinical potencies (Chang and Snyder, 1978). Similarly there is a high correlation between BZ receptor occupancy and facilitation of behavior inhibited by punishment in the paradigm already described (Lippa, et al., 1978).

Using a variety of lesioning techniques, BZ receptors have been shown to be localized almost exclusively to neurons, and predominantly to areas of synaptic contact (Chung and Snyder, 1978).

THE BENZODIAZEPINE/GABA RECEPTOR COMPLEX

Even prior to the discovery of the BZ receptor it was known the BZ's potentiate the inhibitory action of gamma-aminobutyric acid (GABA) as measured by electrophysiologic techniques (Haefely, et al., 1975). GABA is one of the most common inhibitory neurotransmitters. It has been estimated to be present in as many as 30% of the synapses in the brain (Roberts, et al., 1976). The definite link between BZ receptors and GABA came when Tallman and colleagues (1978) found that GABA increased the affinity of BZ for its receptor. One year later Costa and associates (1979) reported that small permeable anions such as chloride and bromide also enhanced the affinity of BZ receptors.

It is now generally accepted that BZ receptors are functionally and structurally coupled to the GABA receptor and along with an associated chloride channel form a "supramolecular receptor complex, " whose ultimate function is to regulate the transport or permeability of chloride ions across neuronal membranes (Skolnick and Paul, 1982). In the unstimulated state neuronal membranes are relatively impermeable to chloride ions. However, when GABA activates its receptor, the chloride channel "opens" and allows chloride ions to move more readily from the extracellular space to the inside of the neuron. The net effect of enhanced chloride permeability is to increase the negative potential across the neuronal membrane making the neuron less likely to generate an action potential (hyperpolarization). Benzodiazepines when applied to neurons alone produced very little effect on chloride permeability (Study and Barker, 1982). However, in the presence of GABA, BZs markedly potentiate the GABA-stimulated increases in chloride permeability. This effect appears to be due to an increase in the frequency of GABA-mediated chloride channel opening and not to an enhanced conductance of chloride by each channel. Thus, BZs increase GABA-mediated neuronal inhibition.

Other drugs may also produce their anxiolytic effects through an action on the "benzodiazepine/GABA receptor complex" although not by directly interacting with the recognition site for BZs (Olsen, 1981; Skolnick, et al., 1981). Barbiturates, for example, appear to interact directly with a chloride channel (coupled to BZ receptors), resulting in an increase in the time (rather than frequency) of channel opening. In this way barbiturates (like BZs) enhance GABA-mediated chloride permeability; but their direct (rather than allosteric) effects on chloride channels probably explain their far greater toxicity when compared to the BZs. Moreover, the common actions of BZs and barbiturates in enhancing GABA-mediated chloride permeability is believed to explain the development of cross-dependence and cross-tolerance between these two classes of drugs.

Ethanol, another drug that decreases the behavioral inhibition produced by punishment, also has been reported to increase BZ binding and thereby increase GABA's inhibitory action (Skolnick and Paul, 1982).

THE ANATOMY OF BRAIN BENZODIAZEPINE RECEPTORS

Following the demonstration of the BZ receptor in brain homogeneates, an autoradiographic technique to actually visualize and map the distribution of BZ receptors in brain was developed (Young and Kuhar, 1979). This technique permits us to tentatively identify brain regions that are targets for the BZs and may mediate their pharmacologic effects. For example, the frontal cortical and the hippocampal regions which have high densities of BZ receptors may mediate the anxiolytic effects or amnestic properties of BZs (Ghoneim, et al., 1984). Similarly, BZ receptors in the amygdala may also mediate BZ neuroendocrine effects and cerebellar BZ receptors are probably the site at which BZs produce ataxia in high doses. The function of BZ receptors in other brain regions such as the substantia nigra zona reticulata and superior colliculus is not so readily apparent. However, the substantia nigra zona reticulata is one of the two major outputs of the basal ganglia and as such it is possible that BZ receptors here could be involved in fear-induced motor inhibition. Also the neurons of the zona reticulata markedly increase their activity with increasing arousal (Miller, et al., 1983) and these neurons are inhibited by BZs (Ross, et al., 1982). Thus, the substantia nigra zona reticulata may also be one site at which BZs act to decrease certain kinds of arousal. The superior colliculus is involved in the control of visual and auditory attention (Wurtz and Goldberg, 1980). It is possible that the ability of BZs to reduce the increased vigilance induced by fear may be mediated through receptors in the superior colliculus. These anatomic speculations notwithstanding, the actual differences in BZ receptor density among various brain regions is relatively small and does not vary by more than an order of magnitude. The rather diffuse distribution of BZ receptors in brain suggests, therefore, that such receptors may, in fact, regulate a number of neuronal systems in addition to those described above.

Several investigators have attempted to localize the anticonflict actions (namely, anxiolytic) of BZs to a specific brain region. Preliminary results suggest that the local injection of BZs

into the amygdala (Scheel-Kruger and Petersen, 1982) hippocampus, or midbrain raphe (Tallman, et al., 1980) all can
mimic the effects of parenterally administered BZs on punished
behavior in rats. This approach will undoubtedly prove useful
in delineating the neuroanatomic pathways that mediate the anxiolytic actions of BZs in animals and perhaps help to define an-
alogous systems in man.

BENZODIAZEPINE AGONISTS AND ANTAGONISTS

The presence of specific receptors for BZs in brain prompted a
search for an endogenous or naturally occurring ligand for the
receptor (i.e., the brain's own anxiolytic or anxiogenic substance). Braestrup and colleagues (1980) isolated a novel high-
affinity BZ receptor ligand from human urine that was subsequently identified as beta-carboline-3-carboxylic acid ethyl
ester (beta-CCE). Although first thought to be a naturally occurring compound, beta-CCE has since been shown to be produced
artifactually by a Pictet-Spengler condensation of tryptophan
during the extraction process. Although beta-CCE cannot be
considered an endogenous ligand, its extremely high affinity for
the BZ receptor, combined with its unique pharmacologic properties, have made it (and chemically related beta-carboline derivatives) an extremely valuable tool for studying the BZ receptor.
    Unlike BZs, beta-CCE has no anticonvulsant or anticonflict
activity in animals but instead blocks the anticonvulsant, anticonflict, and sedative-hypnotic actions of BZs (Tenen and
Hirsch, 1980; Cowen, et al., 1981). These observations were
the first indication that compounds such as beta-CCE could be
developed that antagonize the pharmacologic properties of BZs.
Since the initial discovery of beta-CCE, several other beta-
carboline derivatives, as well as novel BZs (e.g., Ro-15-1788)
and chemically unrelated compounds (e.g., CGS-8216), have
been discovered that antagonize all of the pharmacologic (including anxiolytic) actions of the BZs (Hunkeler, et al., 1981;
Czernik, et al., 1982). In addition to blocking the effects of the
BZs, beta-CCE and several other beta-carboline derivatives
possess potent intrinsic pharmacologic properties of their own
which seem to be the opposite of those of the BZs. These intrinsic properties are not possessed by other BZ receptor ligands,
such as Ro-15-1788, which appears to be a relatively selective
antagonist. In a modified version of the behavioral inhibition
test previously described, beta-CCE was reported to increase
the behavior inhibition produced by mild punishment (Costa and

Biggio, 1983). Furthermore, when beta-CCE is administered
to rhesus monkeys it produces dramatic behavioral effects
which include piloerection, generalized arousal, and "vigilance."
Higher doses of beta-CCE result in behavioral "agitation"
(struggling in the restraint chair) which is accompanied by
marked autonomic and endocrine changes. These include an immediate rise in heart rate and blood pressure. Activation of the
hypothalamic-pituitary-adrenal axis also occurs following beta-
CCE administration. Plasma concentrations of ACTH, cortisol,
and the catecholamines, epinephrine and norepinephrine, are
all significantly increased following administration of beta-CCE
at doses as low as 100 μg/kg. That the effects of beta-CCE are
mediated via the BZ receptor complex is supported by their
complete blockade following pretreatment with BZs such as diazepam as well as the specific BZ receptor antagonist Ro-15-1788
(Ninan, et al. , 1982).

The behavioral, physiologic, and endocrine effects of beta-
CCE in subhuman primates are reminiscent of those seen in extremely anxious patients and in animals or humans exposed to
fear-provoking situations (Rose and Sachar, 1981). The reversal of beta-CCE's effects by BZs supports the hypothesis that
this syndrome may represent a reliable pharmacologic model
of human anxiety or fear. Nevertheless, it is impossible to conclusively demonstrate the presence or absence of anxiety in any
animal other than man. Therefore, a key question is whether
the beta-CCE-induced syndrome is a valid model of anxiety,
and, if so, what kind of anxiety.

Several lines of evidence support the validity of the "BZ/
GABA receptor model" of anxiety. For one, the symptoms of
generalized anxiety disorders that were obtained from epidemiologic studies of anxious patients (American Psychiatric Association, 1980) are selectively ameliorated by BZs (Table 24-1). It
may not be a coincidence that the major pharmacologic properties of BZ (which is a muscle relaxant, anxiolytic, and hypnotic)
are essentially mirror images of the major symptoms reported
by patients with generalized anxiety disorders. Furthermore, in
recent studies by Dorow and associates (1983) a beta-carboline
derivative chemically similar to beta-CCE (FG 7142) was administered to human volunteers. Administration of this compound
resulted in symptoms of motor tension, autonomic hyperactivity,
and extreme apprehension. These effects were interpreted sub-
jectively as being identical to severe anxiety with "inner tension, excitation, and sensations of physical disturbance," and as
in the monkey studies with beta-CCE, were accompanied by increases in blood pressure, heart rate, and plasma cortisol. In
one subject these symptoms were so severe that intravenous

Table 24-1   Effects of Benzodiazepines and Beta-CCE on the
              Symptoms of Fear and Anxiety

DSM-III Criteria for Generalized Anxiety Disorder	Benzodiazepine Effects[a]	Beta-CCE Effects[b]
Motor tension		
Shakiness, jitteriness, trembling		
Muscle aches, tension		
Fatigability	−	−
Fidgeting, restlessness		
Autonomic hyperactivity		
Heart pounding, racing		
Dizziness	−	−
Light headedness		−
High respiratory rate	?	−
Paresthesias	?	−
Upset stomach	?	
Frequent urination	?	
Sweaty, cold, clammy hands	−	−
Flushing	−	
Apprehensive expectation		
Anxiety		
Fear, worry		
Anticipation of misfortune		
Vigilance and scanning		
Insomnia		

[a]Adapted from Greenblatt and Shader (1974).
[b]Adapted from Hendelson and colleagues (1982), Dorow and co-workers (1983), and Insel and associates (1984).

lormetazepam was administered and all symptoms were reported to subside within a few minutes. Beta-CCE, in addition to producing the opposite behavioral effects from the BZs, also seems to produce opposite biochemical effects. For example, while BZs potentiate the inhibitory action of GABA (Study and Barker, 1982), in contrast, beta-CCE antagonizes GABAergic neuronal inhibition (Polc, et al., 1981).

The ability of the BZs to potentiate GABAergic neurotransmission and of beta-CCE to attentuate GABAergic events suggests that other drugs that affect GABAergic neurotransmission might also possess anxiolytic or anxiogenic properties. This appears to be the case. Pentylenetetrazole (PTZ), a convulsant which antagonizes GABA-mediated postsynaptic inhibition

(MacDonald and Barker, 1979), also potentiates punishment-induced behavioral inhibition (Corda, et al. , 1983) and produces
anxiety in humans (Rodin, 1958). Muscimol, a GABA receptor
agonist, has been reported to mimic the ability of the BZs to
prevent punishment-induced behavioral inhibition (Canarzi, et
al., 1980). Since neither PTZ or muscimol act through BZ receptors, it is apparent that both anxiolytic and anxiogenic effects
can be produced through an action at various sites on the
benzodiazepines/GABA receptor complex. Thus, PTZ and beta-
CCE both may provide models of fear and anxiety although they
act through somewhat different recognition sites on the GABA/
BZ receptor complex.

RELATIONSHIP OF THE BENZODIAZEPINE/GABA RECEPTOR MODEL OF ANXIETY TO OTHER PHARMACOLOGIC MODELS OF ANXIETY

Redmond (1977) showed in nonhuman primates that stimulation
of the locus coeruleus either electrophysiologically or pharmacologically by administration of alpha-2-adrenoreceptor antagonists such as piperoxane or yohimbine results in "anxiety" or
"alarmlike" behaviors accompanied by elevations in plasma 3-
methoxy-4-hydroxyphenylglycol (MHPG). These effects were
blocked by clonidine. Charney and associates (1983) also showed
that yohimbine produced "anxiety" and an elevation in plasma
MHPG in healthy human volunteers. Curiously, although the
anxiogenic effect of yohimbine in man are blocked by both clonidine and diazepam, only clonidine blocked the rise in plasma
MHPG. The observation that diazepam did not block the rise in
MHPG indicates that diazepam may have anxiolytic effects without significantly altering norepinephrine turnover.
    Other evidence against the involvement of the locus coerul-
eus in anxiety has been recently reviewed by Insel and coworkers (1984), who also found that clonidine only partially blocked
the behavioral activation caused by beta-CCE in nonhuman primates. Destruction of the locus coeruleus does not affect social
models of anxiety in rodents (File, et al. , 1979). Also the novel
anxiolytic buspirone actually increases locus coeruleus activity (Sanghera, et al. , 1983). Furthermore, clonidine does not
consistently prevent punishment-induced behavioral inhibition as
do BZs (Patel and Malick, 1983). Clinically, distinctions are
also seen between clonidine and diazepam. Clonidine is effective
in treating panic attacks (Hoehn-Saric, et al., 1981) whereas
BZs like diazepam are generally ineffective, though recently
this specificity has been questioned (Noyes, 1983). Also, unlike

diazepam, rapid tolerance (2-3 weeks) develops to clonidine's anxiolytic actions in at least a subpopulation of patients and this may parallel the development of tolerance to clonidine's actions in inhibiting the firing rate of locus coeruleus neurons (Uhde, et al., 1984)

It is likely that the locus coeruleus and the BZ/GABA receptor "models" of anxiety describe somewhat different phenomena: the former more alarm and arousal, the latter more fear and conflict. Of course, in many conditions these systems probably overlap and symptoms might merge. For example, in panic disorder the locus coeruleus may provide the triggering stimulus that sets off the panic attack, but the associated anticipatory and residual anxiety as well as some aspects of the panic itself may in part be mediated through BZ/GABA receptor containing neural systems.

A different model of anxiety involves adenosine, a powerful CNS depressant (Phillis, et al., 1979). Caffeine, an adenosine receptor antagonist, at the usual doses consumed by human beings (Mattila, et al., 1982) can be anxiogenic. "Caffeinism" or the consumption of greater than 500-1000 mg caffeine (roughly 5-10 cups of coffee) daily may present with a clinical picture nearly indistinguishable from generalized anxiety disorder or panic (Greden, 1974; American Psychiatric Association, 1980). Symptoms may include restlessness, nervousness, insomnia, psychomotor agitation, flushed face, diuresis, gastrointestinal complaints, and cardiac arrhythmias. At toxic doses seizures may result. Levels of caffeine achieved in the brain and blood after a few cups of coffee are in the micromolar range and are sufficient to block 50% of brain adenosine receptors (Snyder and Sklar, in press). In contrast, much higher concentrations (in the millimolar range) are required to antagonize BZ receptors (Snyder and Sklar, in press). Furthermore, caffeine at doses up to 32 mg/kg has been reported to show no in vivo inhibition of [3H] flunitrazepam binding (Weir and Hruska, 1983). Concentrations achieved by considerably higher (namely, toxic or convulsant) doses may however, judging from in vitro competitive binding studies, interact with the BZ receptor (Weir and Hruska, 1983).

Despite the apparent lack of a conspecific locus of action of BZ and caffeine at usual doses, a pharmacologic antagonism between these two classes of drugs is clearly seen. Caffeine has been reported to counteract the anxiolytic as well as the cognitive, psychomotor, and muscle relaxant effects of the BZs (File, et al., 1982; Mattilla, et al., 1982). It seems likely that the CNS has redundant inhibitory systems, two of which involve GABA and adenosine, and that either system may be anxiolytic.

Potentiation of one inhibitory system may effectively antagonize disinhibition in the other (e.g. , diazepam versus caffeine).

FUTURE RESEARCH

Certainly one of the most exciting research pursuits now is the search for the presumed endogenous ligand(s) for the BZ receptor. If present, these ligands might help explain various psycho-pathologic states and offer new therapeutic methods. The purines inosine and hypoxanthine as well as nicotinamide have been proposed as endogenous ligands (Skolnick and Paul, 1982). More recently, "tribulin" (Sandler, et al. , 1984) and "diazepam binding inhibitor" (DBI) (Guidotti, et al. , 1983) have been identified, but their physiologic roles are still uncertain. Interestingly, both of these latter compounds have been shown to be "anxiogenic" in animal behavioral paradigms.

Other areas of future research interest include the effects of stress on the BZ/GABA receptor system. Stress-induced changes have been reported for both BZ (Medine, et al. , 1983) and GABA (Costa and Biggio, 1983) receptors. The relationship between stress, anxiety, and depression can also be investigated using BZ receptor ligands. Recently, Drugan and colleagues (submitted), reported that a beta-carboline derivative produced the same learning deficit as seen in "learned helplessness" induced by inescapable shock. "Learned helplessness" has been proposed as an animal model of human depression (Seligman, 1975).

We have recently begun to study in vivo BZ receptor sensitivity in healthy volunteers and patients (Hommer, et al. , 1984). These studies may determine if anxiety and affective disorders are characterized by alterations in BZ receptor sensitivity.

The explosion of research on the BZs and their receptors has provided us with new and far more sophisticated tools to understand the biochemical and physiologic basis of one of humankind's most common maladies, anxiety.

BIBLIOGRAPHY

APA Task Force on Diagnosis and Nomenclature: Diagnostic and Statistical Manual of Mental Disorders, 3d ed. American Psychiatric Association, Washington, D.C. , 1980.

Braestrup, C., Nielsen, M., and Olsen, C. F.: Urinary and brain β-carboline-3-carboxylates as potent inhibitors of brain benzodiazepine receptors. Proc Natl Acad Sci (USA) 77:2288-2292, 1980.

Butler, P. W., Besser, G. M., and Steinberg, H.: Changes in plasma cortisol-induced by dexamphetamine and chlordiazepoxide given alone and in combination in man. J Endocrinol 40:391-392, 1968.

Canarzi, A., Costa, E., and Guidotti, A.: Potentiation by intraventricular muscimol of the anticonflict effect of benzodiazepines. Brain Res 196:447-453, 1980.

Chang, R. S. L., and Snyder, S. H.: Benzodiazepine receptors: labeling in intact animals with ^{3}H-flunitrazepam. Eur J Pharmacol 48:213-218, 1978.

Charney, D. S., Heninger, G. R., and Redmond, D. E.: Yohimbine induced anxiety and increased noradrenergic function in humans: effects of diazepam and clonidine. Life Sci 33:19-24, 1983.

Chouinand, G., Annable, L., and Fontaine, R.: Alprazolam in the treatment of generalized anxiety and panic disorder: a double-blind placebo controlled study. Psychopharmacology 77:229-233, 1982.

Cowen, P. J., Green, A. R., Nutt, D. J., and Martin, I. L.: Ethyl β-carboline carboxylate lowers seizure threshold and antagonizes flurazepam-induced sedation in rats. Nature 290:54-55, 1981.

Costa, E., Biggio, G.: The action of stress β-carbolines, diazepam and Ro-15-1788 on GABA receptors in the rat brain. In: Advances in Biochemical Psychopharmacology, Vol. 38 (Edited by G. Biggio and E. Costa). Raven Press, New York, 1983, pp. 87-122.

Czernik, A. J., Petrack, B., Kalinsky, H. J., Psychoyos, S., Cash, W. D., Tsai, C., Rinehart, R. K., Granat, F. R., Loell, R. A., Brundish, D. E., and Wade, R.: CGS 8216: Receptor binding characteristics of a potent benzodiazepine antagonist. Life Sci 30:363-372, 1982.

Darwin, C.: The Expression of the Emotions in Man and Animals. University of Chicago Press, Chicago, 1965.

Dorow, R., Horowski, R., Pashelke, G., Amin, M., and Braestrup, C.: Severe anxiety induced by FG-7142, a β-carboline ligand for benzodiazepine receptors. Lancet 2:98-99, 1983.

Drugan, R. C., Maier, S. F., Skolnick, P., Paul, S. M., and Crawley, J. N.: An anxiogenic benzodiazepine receptor ligand induces learned helplessness. (Submitted for publication.)

File, S. E., Deakin, J. F. W., Longden, A., and Crow, T. J.: Investigation of the role of the locus coeruleus in anxiety and antagonistic behavior. Brain Res 169:411, 1979.

Ghoneim, M. M., Hinrichs, J. V., and Menaldt, S. P.: Dose-response analysis of the behavioral effects of diazepam: I. Learning and memory. Psychopharmacology 82:291-295, 1984.

Gray, J. A.: The Neuropsychology of Anxiety: An Enquiry into the Functions of the Septo-hippocampal System. Oxford University Press, New York, 1982.

Greden, J. F.: Anxiety or caffeinism: a diagnostic dilemma. Am J Psychiatry 131:1089-1092, 1974.

Greenblatt, D. J., and Shader, R. I.: Benzodiazepines in Clinical Practice. Raven Press, New York, 1974.

Greenblatt, D. J., Shader, R. I., and Abernathy, D. R.: Current status of benzodiazepines. N Engl J Med 309:354-358, 1983a.

Greenblatt, D. J., Shader, R. I., and Abernathy, D. R.: Current status of benzodiazepines. N Engl Med 309:410-416, 1983b.

Guidotti, A., Forchetti, C. M., Corda, M. G., Konkel, D., Bennett, C. D., and Costa, E.: Isolation, characterization, and purification to homogeneity of an endogenous polypeptide with agonistic action on benzodiazepine receptors. Proc Natl Acad Sci USA 80:3531-3535, 1983.

Haefely, W., Kulcsar, R., Mohler, H., Pieri, L., Polc, P., and Schaffner, R.: Possible involvement of GABA in the central actions of benzodiazepines. Adv Biochem Psychopharmacol 14: 131-151, 1975.

Hoehn-Saric, R., Merchant, A. F., Keyser, M. L., and Smith, V. K.: Effects of clonidine on anxiety disorders. Arch Gen Psychiatry 38:1278-1282, 1981.

Hommer, D. W., Wolkowitz, O. M., Chrousos, G. A., Matsuo, V., Goldstein, D., and Weingartner, H.: Benzodiazepine receptor sensitivity in humans. Presented at the New Research Session of the 137th Annual Meeting of the American Psychiatric Association, Los Angeles, May 5-11, 1984.

Hunkeler, W., Mohler, H., Pieri, L., Polc, P., Bonetti, E. P., Cumin, R., Schaffner, R., and Haefely, W.: Selective antagonists of benzodiazepines. Nature 290:514-516, 1981.

Insel, T. R., Ninan, P. T., Aloi, J., Jimerson, D. C., Skolnick, P., and Paul, S. M.: A benzodiazepine receptor-mediated model of anxiety: studies in non-human primates and clinical implications. Arch Gen Psychiatry 41:741-750, 1984.

Klein, D. F.: Delineation of two drug-responsive anxiety syndromes. Psychopharmacologia 5:397-408, 1964.

Klein, D. F., Gittelman, R., Quitkin, F., and Rifkin, A.: Diagnosis and Drug Treatment of Psychiatric Disorders: Adults and Children, 2d ed. Williams & Wilkins, Baltimore, 1980.

LeFur, G., Guilloux, F., Mitrani, N., Mizoule, J., and Uzan, A.: Relationships between plasma corticosteroids and benzodiazepines in stress. J Pharmacol Exp Ther 211:305-308, 1979.

Linnoila, M., Erwin, C. W., Brendle, A., and Simpson, D.: Psychomotor effects of diazepam in anxious patients and healthy volunteers. J Clin Psychopharmacol 3:88-96, 1983.

Lippa, A., Greenblatt, E., and Pelham, R.: The use of animal models for delineating the mechanisms of action of anxiolytic agents. In: Animal Models in Psychiatry and Neurology (Edited by I. Hanin and E. Usdin). Pergamon Press, Oxford, 1978.

Lippa, A. S., Nash, P. A., and Greenblatt, E. N.: Pre-clinical neuro-psychopharmacological testing procedures for anxiolytic drugs. In: Anxiolytics (Edited by S. Fielding and H. Lal). Futura, New York, 1979, pp. 41-81.

250 / The Biological Foundations of Clinical Psychiatry

MacDonald, J. F., and Barker, J. L. : Enhancement of GABA-mediated postsynaptic inhibition in cultured mammalian spinal cord neurons: a common mode of anti-convulsant action. Brain Res 167:323, 1979.

Mattila, M. J., Palva, E., and Savolainen, K. : Caffeine antagonizes diazepam effects in man. Med Biol 60:121-123, 1982.

Medina, J., Novas, M., and deRobertis, E. : Changes in benzodiazepine receptors by acute stress: different effect of chronic diazepam or Ro 15-1788 treatment. Eur J Pharmacol 96:181-185, 1983.

Miller, J., Farber, J., Gatz, P., Roffwarg, H., and German, D. : Activity of mesencephalic dopamine and non-dopamine neurons across stages of sleep and waking in the rat. Brain Res 273:133-141, 1983.

Mohler, H., and Okada, T. : Benzodiazepine receptor: demonstration in the central nervous system. Science 198:849-851, 1977.

Ninan, P. T., Insel, T. M., Cohen, R. M., Cook, J. M., Skolnick, P., and Paul, S. M. : Benzodiazepine receptor-mediated experimental "anxiety" in primates. Science 218:1332-1334, 1982.

Noyes, R., Anderson, D., Claney, J., Crowe, R., Slymen, D., Ghoneim, M., and Hinrichs, J. : Diazepam and propranolol in panic disorder and agoraphobia. Arch Gen Psychiatry 41:287-292, 1983.

O'Brien, G. T. : Clinical treatment of specific phobias. In: Phobia: Psychological and Pharmacological Treatment (Edited by M. Mavissakalian and D. H. Barlow). Guilford Press, New York, 1981, pp. 420-436.

Olsen, R. W. : GABA-benzodiazepine-barbiturate receptor interactions. J Neurochem 37:1-37, 1981.

Patel, J. B., and Malick, J. B. : Neuropharmacological profile of an anxiolytic. In: Anxiolytics: Neurochemical, Behavioral and Clinical Perspectives (Edited by J. B. Malick, S. J. Enna, and H. Yamamura). Raven Press, New York, 1983, pp. 86-153.

Paul, S. M., and Skolnick, P. : Comparative neuropharmacology of antianxiety drugs. Pharmacol Biochem Behav 17:37-41, 1982.

Phillis, J. W., Edstrom, J. P., Kostopoulos, G. K., and Kirkpatrick, J. R. : Effects of adenosine and adenine nucleotides on synaptic transmission in the cerebral cortex. Can J Physiol Pharmacol 57:1289-1312, 1979.

Polc, P., Ropert, N., and Wright, D. M. : Ethyl-β-carboline-3-carboxylate antagonizes the action of GABA and benzodiazepine in the hippocampus. Brain Res 217:216-220, 1981.

Redmond, D. E. : Alterations in the function of the nucleus locus coeruleus: a possible model for studies of anxiety. In: Animal Models in Psychiatry and Neurology (Edited by I. Hanin, and E. Usdin). Pergamon Press, New York, 1977.

Rees, L.: M.D. thesis Adenosine models in anxiety. University of London, 1970.

Roberts, E., Chase, T. W., and Tower, D. B.: GABA in Nervous System Function. Raven Press, New York, 1976.

Rodin, E. : Metrazol tolerance in a "normal" and volunteer population. EEG Clin Neurophysiol 10:433-446, 1958.

Rose, R. M., and Sachar, E.: Psychoendocrinology. In: Textbook of Endocrinology, 6th ed. (Edited by R. H. Williams). W. B. Saunders, Philadelphia, 1981, pp. 654-657.

Ross, R., Waszczak, B., Lee, E., and Walters, J.: Effects of benzodiazepines on single unit activity in the substantia nigra pars reticulata. Life Sci 31:1025-1035, 1982.

Sandler, M., Glover, V., Elsworth, J. D., and Clow, A.: Tribulin output in anxiety and panic. Presented at the 137th Annual Meeting of the American Psychiatric Association, Los Angeles, May 5-11, 1984.

Sanghera, M. K., McMillen, B. A., and German, D. C.: Buspirone, a non-benzodiazepine anxiolytic, increases locus coeruleus noradrenergic neuronal activity. Eur J Pharmacol 86:107-110, 1983.

Scheel-Kruger, J., and Petersen, F.: Anticonflict effects of the benzodiazepines mediated by a GABAergic mechanism in the amygdala. Eur J Pharmacol 82:115, 1982.

Seligman, M. E. P.: Helplessness. On Depression, Development and Death. W. H. Freeman, San Francisco, 1975.

Sheehan, D. V.: Current perspectives in the treatment of panic and phobic disorders. Drug Ther 12:179-193, 1982.

Skolnick, P., Moncada, V., Barker, J., and Paul, S. M.: Pentobarbital has dual actions to increase brain benzodiazepine receptor affinity. Science 211:1448-1450, 1981.

Skolnick, P., and Paul, S. M.: Molecular pharmacology of the benzodiazepines. Int Rev Neurobiol 23:103-140, 1982.

Snyder, S. H., and Sklar, P.: Behavioral and molecular actions of caffeine: focus on adenosine. (In press)

Squires, R. F., and Braestrup, C.: Benzodiazepine receptors in rat brain. Nature 266:732-734, 1977.

Study, R. E., and Barker, J. L.: Cellular mechanisms of benzodiazepine actions. JAMA 247:2147-2151, 1982.

Tenen, S. S., and Hirsch, J. D.: β-Carboline-3-carboxylic acid ethyl ester antagonizes diazepam activity. Nature 288:609-610, 1980.

Tallman, J., Thomas, J., and Gallager, D.: GABAergic modulation of benzodiazepine site sensitivity. Nature 274:383-385, 1978.

Tallman, J. F., Paul, S. M., Skolnick, P., and Gallager, D. W.: Receptors for the age of anxiety: pharmacology of the benzodiazepines. Science 207:274-281, 1980.

Uhde, T. W., Siever, L. J., and Post, R. M.: Clonidine: acute challenge and clinical trial paradigms for the investigation and treatment of anxiety disorders, affective illness, and pain syndromes. In: Neurobiology of Mood Disorders (Edited by R. M. Post and J. C. Ballenger). Williams & Wilkins, Baltimore, 1984, pp. 49-58.

Weir, R. L., and Hruska, R. E. : Interaction between methyl-xanthines and the benzodiazepine receptor. Arch Int Pharma-codyn 265:42-48, 1983.

Williamson, M. J., Paul, S. M., and Skolnick, P. : Labelling of benzodiazepine receptors in vivo. Nature 275:551-553, 1978.

Wurtz, R. H., and Goldberg, M. E. : Visual-motor function of the primate superior colliculas. Ann Rev Neurosci 3:189-226, 1980.

Young, W. S., and Kuhar, M. J.: Autoradiographic localization of benzodiazepine receptor in the brains of humans and animals. Nature 280:393-395, 1979.

Chapter 25

NEUROPHARMACOLOGY OF ANTIPSYCHOTIC AGENTS

Richard L. Hauger, M.D. and Steven M. Paul, M.D.

The discovery and development of antipsychotic agents approximately 30 years ago was a significant breakthrough in the treatment of major psychotic disorders. Prior to this important therapeutic advance schizophrenia was believed to be treatable only by long-term custodial hospitalization. Twenty years after antipsychotics were introduced into the mental health system of the United States, the resident populations of large mental hospitals had been reduced by two-thirds. Currently, antipsychotics are utilized not only for the treatment of schizophrenia but for organic psychoses and the manic phase of bipolar affective illness, as well as adjunctive agents in the treatment of psychotic depression.

The treatment of schizophrenia and other psychotic illnesses has a long history. The first antipsychotic treatment can be found in antiquity; the Rauwolfia serpentina root was used in native Hindu medicine as a treatment for insanity. Rauwolfia alkaloids such as reserpine briefly were used for the treatment of schizophrenia in the early 1950s. However, the relatively weak antipsychotic effect of this heterocyclic amine was outweighed by its potent monoamine-depleting properties which led to severe hypotension, excessive salivation, diarrhea, sedation, and depression. In 1949, chlorpromazine was synthesized in France for its presumed anesthetic-potentiating actions; however, a state termed "artificial hibernation" was observed whereby consciousness was maintained though the patient tended to sleep and be apathetic. This observation led the French psychiatrists Delay and Deniker to use chlorpromazine to treat successfully a patient with psychotic mania at Val-de-Grace Hospital in 1952; later these investigators treated patients suffering from other psychotic illnesses such as schizophrenia. Because Delay and Deniker had increased the doses of

chlorpromazine above those used by anesthesiologists until neurologic effects had appeared, they were the first to observe the
antischizophrenic effect of chlorpromazine.

Delay and Deniker believed that chlorpromazine was specifically antipsychotic. Subsequently, Lehmann and Hanrahan introduced chlorpromazine to the Western Hemisphere in 1954. In
the late 1950s another class of major tranquilizers was introduced when Janssen synthesized the butyrophenones while attempting to improve the analgesic agent normeperidine. More
recently, other classes of antipsychotic agents, including diben-
zoxazepines and diphenylbutylpiperidines, have been synthesized.

Delay and Deniker first coined the term neuroleptic for
these agents. The word neuroleptic refers to the ability of
chlorpromazine to diminish arousal of the central nervous system (CNS) without disinhibiting higher cortical centers. At therapeutic doses these medications were found to exert a specific
antipsychotic effect separate from their sedative properties.
This effect was contrasted with the effects of classical CNS depressants, i.e., general anesthetics, sedatives, and hypnotics.
Drugs used for the amelioration of psychoses will collectively
be referred to as antipsychotics throughout this chapter.

CHEMICAL STRUCTURES OF ANTIPSYCHOTIC AGENTS

The chemical structure of the phenothiazine class of antipsychotic agents is represented in Table 25-1. The tricyclic structure
consists of two benzene rings joined by sulfur and nitrogen
atoms. Substitution of electron-withdrawing groups at position
2 augments the clinical efficacy of phenothiazines. The three
carbon side-chain and the first amino nitrogen atom of the side-
chain is essential for antipsychotic activity; a two-carbon side-
chain results in an antihistaminic agent. Position 10 differentiates the various subclasses of phenothiazines. Currently, there
are more than 30 different phenothiazines. If an aliphatic group
is liked to the ring nitrogen at position 10, aliphatic phenothiazines such as chlorpromazine are synthesized. The aliphatic
phenothiazines are characterized by a low potency and a propensity to produce sedative, hypotensive, dermatologic, and anticholinergic side effects. Thioridazine, a chemically related
phenothiazine with similar low potency, has a piperidine group
at position 10. The most potent phenothiazines result from piperazine substitution at position 10 and are represented by trifluoperazine which induces significant neurologic symptoms but few
autonomic side effects.

The thioxanthenes, another class of phenothiazines, result

Table 25-1   Average Clinical Daily Dose for Antipsychotic Agents and in Vitro Potency at Striatal D2 Dopamine Receptors

Drug	Trade Name	Dose Equivalent (mg)[a]	Approximate Ratio to Chlorpromazine	Average Clinical Dosage (mg/day)[b]*		Clinical Structure
Phenothiazines						
Aliphatic						
Chlorpromazine	Thorazine	100	1:1	645 ± 22	25	Chlorpromazine
Piperidine						
Thioridazine	Mellaril	97.0 ± 7.0	1:1	615 ± 30	63	Thioridazine
Piperazine						
Perphenazine	Trilafon	9.0 ± 0.6	1:10	53 ± 4		
Fluphenazine	Prolixin, 5 mg	1.2 ± 0.1	1:50	12 ± 1	3.7	
Trifluoperazine	Stelazine	2.8 ± 0.4	1:20	27 ± 2	4.4	Trifluoperazine
Thioxanthenes						
Piperazine						
Thiothixene	Navane	4.4 ± 1.0	1:30	33 ± 2	4.5	Thiothixene
Aliphatic						
Chlorprothixene	Taractan	44.0 ± 8.0	1:2	341 ± 16		
Butyrophenones						
Haloperidol	Haldol	1.6 ± 0.5	1:50	12 ± 0.2	4.4	Haloperidol
Spiroperidol	Experimental			1.5	0.68	

Dibenzoxazepine Loxapine	Loxitane, Daxolin	8.7 + 0.1	1:10	82 + 9		Loxapine
Dibenzodiazepine Clozapine	Experimental	60		725	380	Molindone
Dihydroindolone Molindone	Moban, Lidone	6.0 + 0.9	1:10	51 + 6		
Diphenylbutylpiperidines Pimozide	Experimental	0.3 + 0.5		3 + 0.3	3.6	Pimozide
Penfluridol	Experimental	2 (1-week dose)d			7.8	Sulpiride
Benzamide Sulpiride	Experimental			300-600		
Rauwolfia alkaloids Reserpine	Serpasil	1.0 + 2.0		6 + 2		Reserpine

aDose equivalent is defined as the dose of the antipsychotic drug equal to 100 mg chlorpromazine (Davis and Garver, 1978). All the antipsychotics are reported to be equally effective in double-blind studies. Therefore, the "dose equivalents" listed are the number of milligrams of drug necessary to achieve what clinicians feel to be an optimal antipsychotic effect.

bAverage clinical dosages are averages of daily clinical dosages of antipsychotics found to be therapeutic in numerous sources, some of which vary. These numbers are only an approximate guide, and dosage for each patient must be established by clinical response. Others have reported that the average dose of chlorpromazine per day is 734 mg (Davis and Garver, 1978).

Table 25-1 (Continued)

cAffinities for the D_2 dopamine receptor site labeled by $[^3H]$ spiroperidol in the rat caudate (Peroutka and Snyder, 1980). The receptor affinity is expressed as K_i which is defined as follows:

$$K_i = \frac{IC50}{1 + \frac{C}{K_d}}$$

where C is the concentration of $[^3H]$ spiroperidol, K_d is its dissociation constant, and IC_{50} is the concentration of antipsychotic drug that inhibits $[^3H]$ spiroperidol binding by 50%. Therefore, the potency of antipsychotics at the striatal D_2 dopamine receptor increases as the K_i value becomes lower. Spiroperidol is the most potent antipsychotic at dopamine receptors labeled in this way.

dLong-lasting diphenylbutylpiperidines can be used once weekly; penfludridol can be used as 2% of a weekly dose of chlorpromazine (i.e., 40 mg/week can replace 2100 mg/week chlorpromazine).

*D_2 = Dopamine Receptor Affinity K_i^c (nM).

from a carbon replacing the nitrogen at position 10 with a double bond connecting the side chain. Likewise, the thioxanthenes can be subdivided on the basis of position 10 substitutions. Chlorprothixene, an aliphatic thioxanthene, has one-tenth the potency of cis-thiothixene, which has a piperazine substitution and a potency slightly less than fluphenazine and trifluoperazine.

The butyrophenone class of antipsychotic agents possess almost pure neuroleptic activity comparable or greater than the piperazine phenothiazines. Most of the butyrophenones are substituted piperidine compounds. Haloperidol and the recently developed experimental butyrophenone, spiroperidol, are very potent antipsychotics.

The diphenylbutypiperidines are related to the butyrophenones and appear quite promising. Pimozide, a remarkably potent antipsychotic, appears to be the most selective dopamine antagonist yet synthesized. Pimozide possesses an extraordinary potency and very long elimination half-life (approximately 50 hr) which would permit weekly oral dosage.

Other atypical antipsychotic agents are molindone, clozapine, and loxapine. Molindone, an indole compound, allegedly has very little appetite-stimulating properties which may differentiate this compound from other antipsychotic agents. Clozapine and loxapine, piperazine derivatives of dibenzazepine tricyclic molecules, resemble structurally the antidepressant imipramine. Clozapine has been reported to have virtually no neurologic side effects despite its antipsychotic efficacy. However, clozapine has been abandoned due to its association with agranulocytosis. Loxapine has recently been modified to produce the new antidepressant, amoxapine, which unfortunately may be associated with some of the same undesirable neurologic side effects produced by neuroleptics such as extrapyramidal symptoms and tardive dyskinesia. Sulpiride, a substituted benzamide, appears to have both antidepressant and antipsychotic activity with a low rate of adverse reactions.

PHARMACOKINETICS AND METABOLISM

Antipsychotics are highly lipophilic and can have a somewhat erratic absorption from the gastrointestinal tract. Rapid metabolism of chlorpromazine in the gut can lead to lack of clinical response. This gut inactivation can be circumvented by injecting chlorpromazine intramuscularly. Anticholinergic agents can also diminish the clinical efficacy of antipsychotics by slowing gut motility and permitting metabolism by bacterial flora.

Colloidal antacids also decrease absorption from the gut and thus decrease circulating levels of antipsychotics. Following absorption, antipsychotics are subjected to a marked first-pass effect. Approximately 90% of circulating antipsychotics are bound to plasma proteins, while the free form is believed to be biologically active. Because of this extensive binding to protein the levels of alpha-1-acid glycoprotein can become an important determinant of the circulating level of antipsychotics. Antipsychotics accumulate in body tissue with large blood supply and high lipid content, i.e., CNS, and can enter the fetal circulation and breast milk. Following long-term administration these agents also accumulate in keratin-containing tissues like skin, cornea, and lens and cannot be dialyzed out of the body. The elimination half-life of most antipsychotics is biphasic: a rapid phase of 2 hr followed by a slower phase of 30 hr. However, the biological effects of most antipsychotics are apparent for many hours following elimination from blood which most likely results from storage in high-lipid-content tissues such as brain and allows for the utility of single daily dosages.

The metabolism of the phenothiazines is quite complex, whereas the butyrophenones have a simple metabolism. Chlorpromazine, the prototypic phenothiazine, has been best studied. Eighty percent of chlorpromazine is metabolized by ring oxidation by hepatic microsomal enzymes to form phenolic derivatives at positions 3 and 7. There are at least 100 known metabolites of chlorpromazine, some of which are biologically active, i.e., 7-hydroxychlorpromazine and nor-chlorpromazine. These metabolites are subsequently conjugated to sulfate and glucuronide derivatives which increases their water solubility and renal excretion. In contrast, haloperidol undergoes a simple oxidative N-dealkylation, splitting the butyl moiety from the piperidine nitrogen. The metabolites of haloperidol appear to be inactive and are conjugated to glucuronic acid for renal excretion.

PLASMA LEVELS OF ANTIPSYCHOTICS

In contrast to the published correlations between plasma levels of imipramine and nortriptyline and clinical response, it has been quite difficult to establish whether any such correlation exists between plasma antipsychotic levels and clinical response. Initial studies suggested that plasma chlorpromazine levels were correlated with clinical response. However, several subsequent reports found at least a 10-fold variation in steady-state plasma levels after oral administration and failed to confirm these earlier findings. These inconsistencies may be explained by experimental designs in which the dosage of antipsychotic medication was not standardized, the complex metabolism of phenothiazines with the parent compound alone possibly not reflecting all therapeutic activity, and the use of less-sensitive gas-liquid chromatography methods to measure plasma drug levels.

The recent study of plasma butaperazine and haloperidol levels measured by very sensitive fluorometric or gas-liquid chromatography methods in chronic schizophrenic nonresponders and recently hospitalized schizophrenics on the same fixed dosage of antipsychotic medication has provided more consistent results. Acute and chronic nonresponsive schizophrenic patients had lower steady-state plasma and erythrocyte blood levels than responders. Another study demonstrated that high erythrocyte butaperazine levels corresponded to an increased incidence of dystonia. Additionally, this study suggested that a therapeutic window existed, for poor response was found at both low and very high red blood cell concentrations. The latter may be attributable to nonresponsive patients simply receiving higher dosages of antipsychotics, rather than the presence of a true therapeutic window.

Another recent report controlled for this confounding variable of nonresponding patients being given progressively higher doses of antipsychotics and developing higher plasma levels. A therapeutic window with poor drug response at both high and low blood haloperidol levels was observed. Consequently, it appears that during the acute treatment phase of schizophrenia haloperidol dosage should be adjusted to provide the midrange of plasma levels associated with therapeutic response. Patients with very high plasma haloperidol levels would do better if dose reduction allowed the level to fall into the optimum therapeutic range. Whether a therapeutic window exists for all antipsychotic agents remains to be determined.

Recently the "neuroleptic radioreceptor" assay has led to a further examination of this important issue. This assay is based on the competition by circulating neuroleptics (and metabolites) with a radiolabeled butyrophenone at usually specific presynaptic dopamine binding sites postsynaptic (D_2) in brain tissue. The assay was developed because of the good correlations between neuroleptic potency and relative affinity for the dopamine (D_2) receptor in brain (see below). The radioreceptor assay has the advantage of detecting all pharmacologically active metabolites, as well as parent compounds. Using the radioreceptor assay, two recent reports have confirmed a poor therapeutic response to a variety of antipsychotic agents at low plasma levels. Though these studies require further validation, antipsychotic levels measured by radioreceptor assay may be quite important in assessing clinical improvement in acutely psychotic patients. No studies yet have investigated the relationship between clinical remission and antipsychotic levels during maintenance therapy.

MECHANISM OF ACTION

Antipsychotic agents appear to be equally efficacious. However, the potency of individual agents varies considerably. The more potent antipsychotic agents achieve comparable clinical results as do the less-potent agents, but at far fewer milligrams per dose. Clinical potency expressed in terms of milligrams of orally administered drug equivalent to 100 mg chlorpromazine (see Table 25-1) ranges from pimozide (0.3-0.5 mg), the most potent, to thioridazine and chlorpromazine, which are the least potent. The dose equivalency of antipsychotic agents parallels the average clinical dosage (milligrams per day) administered to patients.

Dose equivalency of antipsychotics has recently been accounted for by the development of dopamine receptor binding assays. Dopamine "receptors" represent specific postsynaptic recognition sites that selectively bind dopamine or related agonists resulting in a subsequent biochemical event. The current major classes of dopamine receptors, D_1 and D_2, are delineated in Table 25-2. Early reports on dopamine metabolism during antipsychotic treatment indirectly revealed enhanced dopamine turnover. When direct methods of measuring postsynaptic dopamine receptors were established, it was determined that this increase in dopamine metabolites resulted from blockade of postsynaptic receptors. Initial studies centered upon the dopamine sensitive-adenylate cyclase associated with dopamine receptors. Unfortunately, the more potent butyrophenone antipsychotics were weak inhibitors of this enzyme compared to the pronounced inhibition exerted by phenothiazines. The dopamine-sensitive adenylate cyclase subsequently was found to be associated with only one class of dopamine receptors (D_1). A second class of dopamine receptors (D_2), which are preferentially labeled by butyrophenone antipsychotics [^{3}H] haloperidol and [^{3}H] spiroperidol, were soon discovered. An excellent correlation between the clinical potency of various antipsychotics and their affinity for blocking the D_2 receptor was subsequently found (Table 25-1). A lower D_2-receptor affinity (K_i) implies a greater blocking activity and higher clinical potency. Additionally, the best correlation for average clinical daily dose of antipsychotics is with their D_2-blocking activity (Fig. 25-1).

Table 25-2 Characteristics of Dopaminergic Receptors

	D_1	D_2
Agonist affinity		
Dopamine	Low (μM)	High (nM)
Apomorphine	Low (μM)	High$^-$ (nM)
Antagonist affinity		
Phenothiazines	High (nM)	High (nM)
Thioxanthenes	High (nM)	High (nM)
Butyrophenones	Low (M)	High (nM)
Substituted benzamides	Inactive	Low (M)
Adenylate cyclase association	Stimulatory	Inhibitory or unassociated
Guanine nucleotide sensitivity	++	++ or −
Striatal location	Intrinsic neurons	Intrinsic neurons and corticostriate afferents
Prototype receptor location	Parathyroid gland	Anterior and intermediate pituitary glands
Function	1. Parathyroid hormone release	1. Inhibition of pituitary hormone release
	2. Unknown function in corpus striatum	2. Dopamine-mediated behavioral responses and their antagonism by neuroleptics
Response to chronic antipsychotic administration	0	↑
Postmortem schizophrenic brain tissue	0	↑

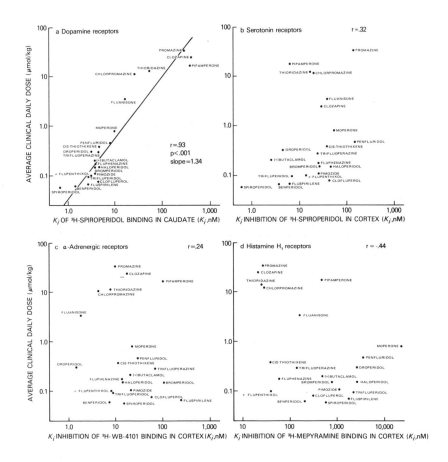

Figure 25-1   Correlation of average clinical dose with anti-psychotic affinity for dopamine receptors (a), serotonin receptors (b), alpha-adrenergic receptors (c), and histamine H1 receptors (d). Mean of each daily dose range listed for each drug was averaged and converted to micromoles per kilogram assuming a human body weight of 70 kg. Source Note: Adapted from Peroutka and Snyder (1980).

Consequently, antischizophrenic drugs are believed to act by blocking postsynaptic dopamine D_2 receptors.

Antipsychotic agents also bind to numerous other neurotransmitter receptors, including the serotonergic, histaminergic, and alpha-adrenergic receptors. However, no correlation between clinical potency and antipsychotic blocking activity at these receptors has been demonstrated (Fig. 25-1). Moreover, the relative affinities of many antipsychotics for these receptors may account for their common side effects, as will be discussed later.

Dopaminergic systems in the brain are organized into several distinct pathways. Currently, it is believed that medially situated dopamine neurons sending axons from the substantia nigra to the nucleus accumbens, portions of the frontal cortex, and limbic structures such as the central amygdaloid nucleus and olfactory tubercle (mesocortical and mesolimbic) represent the sites of antipsychotic drug action (the so-called A10 group of neurons). Antipsychotics also block dopaminergic receptors in the corpus striatum that receive the major dopaminergic projections via the substantia nigra (A9 group of neurons). Blockade of dopamine receptors in this pathway probably results in the parkinsonianlike and other extrapyramidal symptoms seen with antipsychotic agents. The greater propensity for striatal D_2-dopaminergic receptor blockade seen with the piperazine phenothiazines and butyrophenones results in a higher incidence of extrapyramidal side effects. However, certain neuroleptics, such as thioridazine, have a much lower incidence of extrapyramidal symptoms when given on an equimolar basis. This led to the formulation of the hypothesis that thioridazine exerts a site-specific blockade of limbic dopamine receptors while being several orders of magnitude less active in its action on striatal dopamine receptors. Unfortunately, this hypothesis has not been substantiated and it now appears that the anticholinergic properties of thioridazine may account for the rarity of extrapyramidal effects seen with this drug. The role of anticholinergic activity in preventing extrapyramidal symptoms will be discussed below.

Blockade of postsynaptic dopamine receptors by antipsychotics has become one of the cornerstones of the "dopamine hypothesis of schizophrenia." The demonstration that certain dopamine agonists, i. e. , L-DOPA (L-dihydroxyphenylalamine amine) and D-amphetamine, generally exacerbate schizophrenic symptoms or precipitate a schizophreniform psychosis in nonpsychotic individuals, also supports this theory. Furthermore, psychotic symptoms are improved by the reduction of intrasynaptic dopamine levels produced by apomorphine, alpha-methyl-paratyrosine, or reserpine.

Several recent reports, however, have raised questions about the general applicability of this theory. One objection to a "dopamine hypothesis" is the fact that dopamine receptor blockade by antipsychotics appears immediately, well before the onset of clinical efficacy which generally requires weeks of treatment. Additionally, current investigations suggest that acute dopamine receptor blockade in the corpus striatum may not be maintained during chronic treatment with antipsychotics. Tolerance appears to develop to the biochemical effects of initial dopamine receptor blockade. Subsequently, the density of striatal D_2 receptors is increased by chronic antipsychotic treatment and dopamine receptor supersensitivity emerges. The emergence of dopamine receptor supersensitivity also appears to occur in mesolimbic areas, but the evidence for mesocortical areas remains equivocal. Antipsychotics do not alter beta-adrenergic or serotonergic receptors. Since antipsychotics elicit generalized dopamine receptor supersensitivity, it becomes difficult to maintain that schizophrenia results from dopamine receptor overactivity.

Though these reports question whether hyperactive dopamine neurotransmission can be maintained as a hypothesis for schizophrenia, other recent reports provide support for the dopamine theory. A relationship between elevated plasma levels of the dopamine metabolite, homovanillic acid (HVA) in schizophrenic patients and a favorable response to antipsychotic treatment has been reported. While patients were treated with antipsychotics, the amelioration of schizophrenic symptoms was correlated with a time-dependent fall in plasma HVA levels. Consequently, these delayed effects of neuroleptic agents on presynaptic dopamine activity may more closely parallel their therapeutic actions than do their immediate effects in blocking postsynaptic dopamine receptors, and that a decrease in dopamine "turnover" may be responsible for their antipsychotic effects.

Additionally, recent electrophysiologic reports suggest that prolonged treatment with classical antipsychotic drugs decreases the number of spontaneously firing dopamine neurons in both nigrostriatal dopamine system (A9) and the mesolimbic and mesocortical dopamine system (A10). In fact, the time course of this decrease parallels the delayed onset of therapeutic effects during antipsychotic treatment of schizophrenic patients. These studies suggest that postsynaptic dopamine receptors are blocked clinically after administering antipsychotics, thereby decreasing the synaptic action of dopamine. Homeostatic mechanisms increase the firing rate of dopaminergic neurons with a consequent increase in the synaptic release of dopamine. The functional outcome of this will be to decrease the effective receptor block-ade by the neuroleptic and to reduce both its antipsychotic and extrapyramidal side effects. With time, however, dynamic changes take place. The homeostatic mechanisms fail as the dopaminergic neurons go into depolarization block and synaptic dopamine release is reduced. The effective blockade of post-synaptic dopamine receptors increases, maximizing the anti-psychotic effect of the drug and also its parkinsonian extrapyra-midal side effects. Since the atypical neuroleptics such as cloz-apine do not produce depolarization block of A9 neurons, dopa-mine is still released in the striatum, overcoming to some ex-tent the blockade of receptors there. Hence the atypical neuro-leptics do not produce the same degree of extrapyramidal side effects. However, these drugs effectively block activity in A10 neurons, giving rise to their antipsychotic activity.

Another related finding is the increase in the total number of dopamine D_2 binding sites observed in the caudate, nucleus accumbens, and olfactory tubercle of postmortem schizophrenic brains when compared to those of nonschizophrenic control sub-jects (Table 25-2). No elevation of D_1 receptors has been found; however, the significance of this finding remains unclear. It has been suggested, for example, that patients with type 2 schizo-phrenia characterized by the "negative" syndrome described by Kraepelin and Bleuler exhibit no increase in the density of D_2 sites. Type 2 schizophrenics exhibit a severe chronic illness with neurologic abnormalities such as enlarged cerebral ventri-cles and poor response to antipsychotics. It has been claimed they have a dopaminergic "underactivity" in contrast to the type 1 acute schizophrenics who show dopaminergic "overactivity" and an increase in CNS dopamine D_2 receptors. If these findings are verified, a high density of D_2 sites may be associated with responsiveness to antischizophrenic drugs. However, it is still not clear whether the increased numbers of D_2 receptors re-sults from prior treatment with antipsychotic medication.

Other hypotheses of schizophrenia implicate either norepin-ephrine or gamma-aminobutyric acid (GABA) as being critical to the development of psychotic symptoms. Increased levels of norepinephrine in cerebrospinal fluid and postmortem limbic forebrain have been found in patients with paranoid schizophren-ia. These alterations in brain norepinephrine are associated with lowered platelet monoamine oxidase activity in chronic schizophrenia. The GABA hypothesis suggests that the hypoac-tivity of GABAergic neurotransmission may play a role in the etiology of schizophrenia. This hypothesis has gained some re-cent support by the fact that high doses of diazepam improve the condition of antipsychotic-resistant chronic schizophrenic patients. Whether the action of antipsychotic drugs directly involves these neurotransmitter systems has not been resolved.

SIDE EFFECTS OF ANTIPSYCHOTIC AGENTS

ACUTE NEUROLOGIC SIDE EFFECTS

The most common acute neurologic side effects are pseudoparkinsonian reactions which are virtually indistinguishable from classical Parkinson's disease. These neurologic symptoms constitute a cephalic akinesia which spreads caudally and is manifested by masked facies, rigidity, stooped posture, unintentional tremor, and bradykinesia. Other acute neurologic side effects include dystonia, akathisia, and dyskinesia.

Acute dystonias are painful, sudden muscle spasms in the head and neck area (torticollis, retrocollis, opisthotonus, and oculogyric crises) occurring in the first several days of treatment, especially in young muscular men. All of these side effects result from blockade of striatal dopamine receptors. Normally, dopamine inhibits cholinergic interneurons in the striatum (Figure 25-2). According to the dopamine hypothesis, schizophrenia would be associated with excessive dopamine release, overstimulation of postsynaptic dopamine receptors, and diminution of acetylcholine release. During the initial phase of antipsychotic treatment, blockade of striatal dopamine receptors disinhibits the cholinergic interneurons and produces overstimulation of postsynaptic muscarinic cholinergic receptors. Comparable to the pathophysiology of Parkinson's disease, anticholinergic drugs will effectively reduce the excessive stimulation of muscarinic receptors. Generally, anticholinergic agents are given in low, divided doses until the alleviation of symptoms. After several months, these agents may be slowly withdrawn without any adverse effect. At this point dopaminergic blockade may be replaced by the development of striatal D_2 receptor supersensitivity. Recent reports have demonstrated that serum anticholinergic levels can vary considerably with a given dose. This finding, in conjunction with the possibility that anticholinergic drugs may lessen the improvement in schizophrenic symptoms produced by certain antipsychotics or that toxic confusional states may result from these agents, underscores the care with which they must be administered. Anticholinergic agents can also exacerbate angina or bladder outlet obstruction and are contraindicated in patients with narrow-angle glaucoma. Presently, prophylactic treatment is only recommended for patients with a previous history of extrapyramidal reactions to

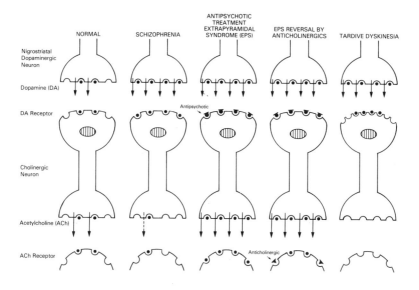

Figure 25-2   Function of the nigrostriatal dopaminergic system in the brain in schizophrenia. Dopaminergic nerve terminals provide an inhibitory innervation of cholinergic interneurons so that a normal release of dopamine (DA) provides a normal release of acetylcholine (ACh). It is postulated that the excessive DA release in schizophrenia inhibits ACh release to an abnormally low level. Antipsychotics block DA receptors and disinhibit the cholinergic interneuron. The classic anticholinergic drugs can reduce the excessive stimulation of muscarinic ACh receptors. Prolonged blockade of DA receptors by antipsychotics increases the number and sensitivity of striatal D_2 receptors, and may lead to tardive dyskinesia.

antipsychotics. Acute dystonic reactions often require immediate treatment with an intramuscular injection of 25-50 mg diphenhydramine which possesses both antihistaminic (sedating and anxiolytic effects) and anticholinergic properties.

The mechanisms underlying antipsychotic-induced akathisias is poorly understood. Akathisias generally do not respond to anticholinergics, but sometimes are ameliorated by benzodiazepines. Akathisias often mandate a change from a high-potency agent to a less-potent one.

It was previously mentioned that antischizophrenic and extrapyramidal effects of antipsychotics both result from dopamine receptor (D_2) blockade; the high-potency agents with greatest dopamine receptor affinities are associated with the highest incidence of extrapyramidal symptoms. However, extrapyramidal effects have been reported to be inversely proportional to the affinity of the antipsychotic agent for the muscarinic receptor. Consequently, the low incidence of extrapyramidal effects with thioridazine may be accounted for by its high affinity for the muscarinic cholinergic receptor. The butyrophenones have a high frequency of these neurologic side effects and very little affinity for the muscarinic receptor. Administration of antipsychotic medications may involve achieving a balance between dopamine receptor blockade and the presumed overactivity of the dopamine system in schizophrenia so that normal dopaminergic and cholinergic neurotransmission may occur.

TARDIVE DYSKINESIA

A not infrequent neurologic complication of long-term antipsychotic treatment is tardive dyskinesia. Tardive dyskinesia mainly consists of orofacial dyskinesias such as facial grimacing, lip smacking, and tongue and masticatory movements. These involuntary movements can become more extreme and widespread leading in some individuals to choreoathetotic movements. The incidence of tardive dyskinesia has been estimated to be as high as 40% in patients treated chronically for 6 months or more, however, in practice the percentage is probably far less. Numerous risk factors can be listed which include the following: length of treatment; total amount of antipsychotic medication administered; increased age of patient; preexisting organic brain pathology; and sex (i.e., being female). Tardive dyskinesia must be differentiated from other conditions, namely spontaneous orofacial dyskinesias, psychotic mannerisms, Huntington's chorea, and dyskinetic movements resulting from antihistaminic and antimuscarinic agents. Tardive dyskinesia must also be differentiated from the "rabbit syndrome." The "rabbit syndrome" is a perioral, involuntary, and extrapyramidal movement disturbance associated with prolonged use of antipsychotics and which is usually responsive to anticholinergic agents. Though some patients experience a resolution of their tardive movements after early discontinuation of antipsychotics, tardive dyskinesia appears to be relatively irreversible in the majority of patients. Currently, tardive dyskinesia appears to be best explained by the increased density of striatal dopamine (D_2) receptors which results from chronic antipsychotic treatment. The increased density of dopamine receptors in the basal ganglia leads to the development of "dopamine receptor supersensitivity" (Fig. 25-2). This situation is similar to denervation supersensitivity to dopamine which results from either anatomic or chemical lesions of the nigrostriatal dopamine pathway. The relevance of this hypothesis is supported by the previously mentioned increase of striatal dopamine receptors following chronic antipsychotic administration.

Additionally, electrophysiologic studies suggest that a time-dependent inactivation of nigrostriatal dopaminergic neurons (A9) occurs with prolonged administration of classical antipsychotic agents, which may be related to the delayed onset of tardive dyskinesia. Both behavioral and biochemical studies mentioned below suggest that chronic administration of classical antipsychotics increases the number of dopamine receptors (D_2) in the striatum producing a pharmacologic denervation "supersensitivity." The depolarization block of A9 neurons by such classical neuroleptics as haloperidol would certainly enhance the development of this "supersensitivity." Furthermore, there appears to be an increased number of dopamine neurons that demonstrate an unusual firing pattern after chronic neuroleptic administration in both the A9 and A10 areas. Perhaps the abnormal release of dopamine from these neurons, in conjunction with :supersensitive" receptors, could give rise to tardive dyskinesia. "Atypical" antipsychotics such as clozapine, which possess a low potential for causing extrapyramidal side effects and tardive dyskinesia, appear to inactivate mesolimbic and mesocortical dopaminergic neurons (A10) but do not inactivate nigrostriatal neurons (A9). Though clozapine currently is not administered to patients due to an association with agranulocytosis, these findings provide hope that novel antipsychotic agents that do not produce tardive dyskinesia will be found.

The "dopamine receptor supersensitivity" hypothesis can also explain the paradoxical exacerbation of tardive movements following the discontinuation of antipsychotics. Reduction in antipsychotic dose decreases dopamine blockade and permits dopamine to be more active at the "supersensitive" receptors.

Likewise, increasing the antipsychotic dose will transiently ameliorate symptoms by further blocking dopamine receptors. Unfortunately this may lead to a more severe tardive dyskinesia for the density of postsynaptic receptors will increase further. The use of anticholinergic drugs is also ill advised. Due to dopamine supersensitivity, striatal cholinergic function is impaired. Anticholinergic medications will further inhibit cholinergic neurotransmission, exacerbating the symptoms of tardive dyskinesia. Despite the evidence that tardive dyskinesia results from striatal "dopamine receptor supersensitivity," this hypothesis is not fully supported by current data. Chronic administration of antipsychotics increases dopamine receptor density probably in all patients but only a certain population develop tardive dyskinesia. One explanation for the age and duration of illness as factors in the development of tardive dyskinesia is that progressive age is associated with decreased brain cholinergic activity. Consequently, additional hypotheses have been proposed such as an imbalance between acetylcholine and dopamine or norepinephrine, and decreased intrastriatal GABA.

Since tardive dyskinesia, for the most part, is irreversible, the best treatment is to prevent its development. One possibility is to use the lowest dose of antipsychotic required. Since schizophrenia may be a syndrome of dopamine overstimulation, one should theoretically attempt to correct this overstimulation with a dose of antipsychotic that produces both normal dopamine and acetylcholine neurotransmission. As previously stated, some investigators separate schizophrenia into type 1 (acute, positive symptoms, dopaminergic overactivity) and type 2 (chronic, negative symptoms, dopaminergic underactivity). Type 1 and type 2 schizophrenics may carry different risks for tardive dyskinesia. Other investigators have suggested "drug holidays" as an attempt to prevent the development of tardive dyskinesia. However, striatal dopaminergic supersensitivity develops in laboratory animals treated both chronically and with "drug holidays."

No unequivocally effective treatment for tardive dyskinesia has been reported. In some patients the use of dopamine-depleting agents such as tetrabenazine have been modestly effective. GABA-mimetic agents such as baclofen have been reported to be beneficial while other investigators have used drugs that enhance cholinergic neurotransmission. Due to the very high "placebo effect" in the acute treatment of tardive dyskinesia it has been difficult to find an unequivocally effective drug for this condition.

NEUROLEPTIC MALIGNANT SYNDROME

The neuroleptic malignant syndrome is a life-threatening complication of antipsychotic treatment which seems to be a combination of extrapyramidal and autonomic effects. The syndrome
is characterized by the development of severe parkinsonian features (hypokinetic rigidity, gait disturbances, tremor) and subsequent alterations of autonomic function (hyperthermia,
marked tachycardia, labile blood pressure, profuse diaphoresis, dyspnea, and incontinence). This syndrome can even resemble the full clinical picture of catatonia. Neuroleptic malignant syndrome has some similarities with anesthetic-induced
malignant hyperthermia. Hyperthermia, the most serious symptom, may be aggravated by peripheral vasoconstriction or use
of anticholinergics, but the underlying etiology seems to be dopaminergic receptor blockade in the hypothalamus. This syndrome has an estimated mortality rate of 12% due to respiratory or renal failure, cardiovascular collapse, or arrhythmias.
Some recovered patients suffer from residual symptoms ranging
from decerebrate rigidity and paraplegia to pulmonary and renal
pathology. Treatment of neuroleptic malignant syndrome involves immediate cessation of all psychotropic medications and
supportive therapy. Recently it has been claimed that amanti-
dine, which may increase synaptic dopamine availability, or
bromocriptine, a dopamine agonist, may be beneficial.

GENERAL ANTICHOLINERGIC SIDE EFFECTS

Antipsychotic agents produce frequent autonomic side effects.
Common autonomic symptoms are anticholinergic side effects
such as xerostomia, blurred vision due to impaired accommo-
dation, skin flushing, constipation, and delayed micturition.
The incidence of anticholinergic side effects correlates well
with the affinity of various antipsychotic agents for the muscarinic cholinergic receptor. Consequently, aliphatic and piperidine
agents whibh have high anticholinergic activity elicit frequent
anticholinergic symptoms, whereas piperazine derivatives or
butyrophenones produce few of these side effects. At the beginning of treatment these side effects tend to be most pronounced
and usually diminish as treatment is continued.
More serious anticholinergic side effects are urinary retention, aggravation of narrow-angle glaucoma, intestinal dila-
tion due to paralytic ileus, impaired temperature regulation,
and mental confusion. Clozapine, which possesses the most anticholinergic activity, infrequently has led to an atropinelike delirium. Since central and peripheral anticholinergic blockade

Table 25-3 Relative Affinities of Antipsychotic Agents for Alpha-1-Adrenergic and H_1-Histaminergic Receptors

Drug	Alpha-Adrenergic Blocking Activity[a]	H_1-Histamine Receptor Affinity (nM) K_i[b]	Hypo-tension	Seda-tion
Haloperidol	8.4	2600	+	+
Loxapine			+	+
Fluphenazine	11	58	+	+
Trifluoperazine	22	135	+	+
Molindone			0	++
Perphenazine			+	++
Thiothixene	4.4	37	++	+ to ++
Thioridazine	0.4	25	++	+++
Chlorpromazine	0.5	28	++	+++
Clozapine	0.14	20	+++	+++

[a]"Alpha-1-adrenergic blocking activity" is defined as the ratio K_iWB:K_iHALO where K_i WB is the binding inhibitory potency of the antipsychotic drug for the displacement of [3H]WB-4101 binding in rat forebrain (alpha-1-adrenergic receptors) and K_i HALO is the binding inhibitory potency of the antipsychotic drug for the displacement of [3H] haloperidol binding in the calf corpus striatum (D_2-dopamine receptors). Antipsychotics are thought to exert their therapeutic antischizophrenic actions by blocking D_2-dopamine receptors in the brain. Clinical doses of antipsychotics are generally related inversely to their potencies in blocking D_2-dopamine receptors. Clinical sedative and hypotensive actions of these drugs are related to alpha-receptor blockade, and these side effects are predicted better by the ratio of potencies of these drugs on alpha-receptors and dopamine receptors and not simply by their absolute affinity for alpha-receptors. Consequently, lower alpha-1-adrenergic blocking activity corresponds to higher potency at the alpha-receptor and higher incidence of hypotension and sedation (Peroutka et al., 1977).

[b]K_i is defined as the binding inhibitory potency of the antipsychotic drug for the displacement of [3H] mepyramine binding to rat frontal cerebral cortex (H_1-histamine receptors). The highest affinity for H1-histamine receptors is represented by the lowest K_i value.

probably impairs the dissipation of body heat and leads to hyperthermia, the use of antiparkinsonian agents and antipsychotic agents with pronounced anticholinergic effects should be avoided in the elderly patient.

CARDIOVASCULAR SIDE EFFECTS

ORTHOSTATIC HYPOTENSION

Other common side effects of antipsychotic agents are autonomic sympatholytic effects such as orthostatic hypotension. Orthostatic hypotension results from blockade of alpha-adrenergic receptors which causes decreased vasomotor tone and peripheral vasodilatation leading to postural venous pooling. In general, aliphatic and piperidine phenothiazines such as chlorpromazine and thioridazine produce postural hypotension most frequently. The high incidence of postural hypotension with these agents correlates well with their pronounced alpha-adrenergic blocking activity (Table 25-3). Clozapine has the greatest tendency to elicit orthostatic hypotension and the highest alpha-1-receptor blocking activity. Thioxanthenes and butyrophenones tend to have a low incidence of orthostatic hypotension due to their weak alpha-1-blocking properties. Very rarely, catastrophic hypotension can occur with the use of antipsychotic agents possessing the higher alpha-1-blocking activities. Epinephrine should not be used to treat this emergency since stimulation of beta-adrenergic receptors results in further vasodilatation. Rather, severe hypotension and clinical shock should be treated with the vasoconstrictor norepinephrine. Strongly, alpha-blocking antipsychotic agents should be avoided in elderly patients.

Hypotensive side effects and central alpha-1-receptor potency also are related to clinical sedation. Higher alpha-blocking activity and incidence of orthostatic hypotension are associated with increased clinical sedation (Table 25-3). In general, the less-potent antipsychotic agents (aliphatic and piperidine phenothiazines) which have the highest affinity at the alpha-receptor, are the most sedative. Another receptor, which has relevance to clinical sedation may be the H_1-histaminergic receptor. For a long time it has been known that classical antihistaminic agents have sedative properties. High affinity for the central H_1-histaminergic receptor also has some correlation with clinical sedation (Table 25-3); however, the effects of antipsychotics at alpha-1-adrenergic receptors appear to have greater importance in the production of sedation.

CARDIAC SIDE EFFECTS

Antipsychotic agents produce several direct cardiac effects. Some antipsychotics like tricyclic antidepressants exhibit class 1-like antiarrhythmic membrane stabilization effects. Certain antipsychotic agents are associated with conduction defects on electrocardiograms such as prolonged QT intervals, depressed ST segments, flattened T waves, and the appearance of U waves. Increased susceptibility to arrhythmias may result from the hypotensive properties of antipsychotics. Risk factors such as hypokalemia, sudden exertion, high dosages of antipsychotics, preexisting coronary artery disease, and presence of other cardiotoxic drugs further increase the likelihood of cardiotoxicity. The rare instance of sudden death from phenothiazines also has been reported. Sudden death probably results from one of the following: aspiration with asphyxia, irreversible cardiac arrest, or catastrophic hypotension.

Thioridazine has one of the highest incidence of cardiovascular side effects among antipsychotic agents. In particular, thioridazine has been associated with numerous electrocardiographic abnormalities including QT prolongation, first-degree atrioventricular block, atrial flutter, premature ventricular beats, and ventricular tachycardia and fibrillation. A recent study has found that thioridazine is one of the most potent inhibitors among classical antipsychotics of [3H]nitrendipine binding to cardiac calcium channels. This peripheral calcium channel antagonism by thioridazine and its metabolite, mesoridazine, may explain these cardiovascular actions better than blockade of alpha-1-adrenergic or muscarinic cholinergic receptors.

ENDOCRINE SIDE EFFECTS

Long-term antipsychotic treatment is associated with a variety of endocrine effects. In general, patients receiving antipsychotics tend to gain weight and experience sexual dysfunction. Though these endocrine changes can occur in psychosis alone, the use of antipsychotics appears clearly to precipitate these symptoms. Weight gain can be extensive and patients need to be warned to limit their caloric intake. The mechanism of weight gain is unclear but probably involves hypothalamic dopamine receptor blockade which increases appetite and the reduction of motor activity. Antipsychotic therapy, particularly administration of chlorpromazine, also blunts the growth hormone response to releasing agents such as clonidine without altering basal levels of growth hormone.

The effect of antipsychotics on sexual functioning is complex.

In the male, erection is under parasympathetic central while ejaculation has an adrenergic mechanism. The antagonism of muscarinic cholinergic and alpha-adrenergic receptors has been related to impotency and delayed or retrograde ejaculation. Thioridazine is most frequently associated with sexual dysfunction, particularly impairment of ejaculation in the presence of normal erection. More recently it has also been proposed that peripheral calcium channel antagonism leading to blockade of smooth muscle contractions in sexual organs occurs at therapeutic plasma levels of thioridazine. Central dopamine antagonism may also play a role in sexual dysfunction by decreasing libido. Finally, antipsychotics have been reported to lower circulating gonadotropins and consistently increase serum prolactin concentrations. Both of these effects contribute to diminishing serum testosterone. Antipsychotics through similar mechanisms may decrease libido and sexual function in female patients.

Antipsychotic treatment exerts a marked effect on prolactin secretion. One of the major dopaminergic tracts in the CNS, the tuberoinfundibular system, sends neurons from cell bodies in the arcuate and periventricular nuclei to the median eminence which release dopamine into the pituitary sinusoids. Dopamine inhibits the release of prolactin by activating D_2 dopaminergic receptors on lactotrophs in the anterior pituitary. Antipsychotic agents by virtue of their dopamine receptor blocking activity release pituitary lactotrophs from this tonic inhibition, thus increasing prolactin secretion.

The release of prolactin occurs rapidly after antipsychotic administration and is greater in female patients due to the potentiating effect of estrogen on prolactin secretion. When antipsychotics are discontinued, prolactin levels return to normal in about 3-4 days. Several investigators have reported that a dose-response relationship exists between serum prolactin levels and the dose of antipsychotic until the dose is above 500-700 mg chlorpromazine/day. However, other investigators have found no ceiling on prolactin response. Likewise, a relationship has been found between plasma level of antipsychotic and serum prolactin levels. The incidence of extrapyramidal symptoms also may correlate with serum prolactin levels, but sulpiride, a drug which rarely produces extrapyramidal side effects, is most potent in causing prolactin release.

The finding of the prolactin stimulatory activity of antipsychotics led to the hope that serum prolactin levels would correlate with clinical response. However, no significant correlation has been found between plasma prolactin levels and clinical improvement. This lack of correlation seems to result from the extreme sensitivity of the dopamine receptors on the lactotroph such that clinically therapeutic doses of antipsychotics are much greater than the dose required for maximal stimulation of prolactin secretion. Recently, it has been shown that chronic schizophrenics with normal cerebral ventricles have low plasma prolactin levels and that there was an inverse relation between extent of psychotic symptoms and plasma prolactin levels. Such low prolactin levels would be predicted on the basis of the "dopamine hypothesis of schizophrenia." It may be that in such a group of patients, or in other subgroups of schizophrenics, plasma prolactin levels may have either a predictive or correlative relationship with clinical improvement on antipsychotics.

The relative prolactin-stimulating potencies of the various antipsychotic agents correlate highly with their clinical potencies and with their relative affinities to dopamine receptors. Unlike the chronic effects of antipsychotics on striatal dopamine receptors, supersensitivity of dopamine receptors in the tuberoinfundibular system does not appear to develop and antipsychotics seem to persistently elevate serum prolactin levels. Antipsychotic-induced hyperprolactinemia may interfere with sexual functioning, as well as producing menstrual disorders such as amenorrhea and oligomenorrhea. Additionally, gynecomastia and galactorrhea can result which led to fears that long-term antipsychotic treatment might be associated with breast cancer. However, epidemiologic studies to date have not revealed an increased risk of breast cancer in patients treated with antipsychotics, although chronic use of antipsychotics should be carefully considered in patients with hormone-sensitive breast cancers.

MISCELLANEOUS SIDE EFFECTS

Thioridazine, in doses in excess of 800 mg/day, is associated with a pigmentary retinopathy which can cause permanent retinal damage. The low-potency antipsychotics, particularly the aliphatic group represented by chlorpromazine, can cause skin coloration and photosensitivity reactions. All antipsychotics can elicit hypersensitivity or allergic reactions but chemically related antipsychotics can usually be substituted that will show no cross-sensitization. Phenothiazines, particularly chlorpromazine, have been associated with cholestatic jaundice but this is a rather rare side effect. Agranulocytosis occurs infrequently following the use of phenothiazines; this is presumably an allergic manifestation and is not dose-related. As previously mentioned, clozapine was highly associated with agranulocytosis leading to its withdrawal from use. Since agranulocytosis develops slowly, immediate discontinuation may prevent further aggravation. Aliphatic phenothiazines have some association with production of seizures, particularly in patients with a previous history of a convulsive disorder. Antipsychotics have not been shown to be teratogenic but their use should be avoided during the first trimester of pregnancy. Antipsychotics probably are secreted into breast milk as well and thus breast feeding is contraindicated in patients requiring antipsychotic treatment.

BIBLIOGRAPHY

Appleton, W. S., and Davis, J. M.: Practical Clinical Psychopharmacology, 2d ed. Williams & Wilkins, Baltimore, 1980.

Baldessarini, R. J.: Chemotherapy in Psychiatry. Harvard University Press, Boston, 1977.

Benes, F. M., Paskevich, P. A., and Domesick, V. B.: Haloperidol-induced plasticity of axon terminals in rat substantia nigra. Science 221:969-971, 1983.

Coyle, J. T.: The clinical use of antipsychotic medications. Med Clin N Am 66:993-1009, 1982.

Creese, J., Sibley, D. R., Hamblin, M. W., and Leff, S. E.: The classification of dopamine receptors: relationship to radioligand binding. Ann Rev Neurosci 6:43-71, 1983.

Davis, J. M., and Garver, D. L.: Neuroleptics: clinical use in psychiatry. In: Handbook of Psychopharmacology, Vol. 10 (Edited by L. L. Iverson, S. D. Iverson, and S. H. Snyder. Plenum Press, New York, 1978, pp. 406-421.

Gould, R. J., Murphy, K. M. M., Reynolds, I. J., and Snyder, S. H.: Calcium channel blockade: possible explanation for thioridazine's peripheral side effects. Am J Psychiatry 141:353-357, 1984.

Gruen, P. H., Sachar, E. J., Altman, N., Langer, G., Tabrizi, M. A., and Halpern, F. S.: Relation of plasma prolactin to clinical response in schizophrenic patients. Arch Gen Psychiatry 35:1222-1227, 1978.

Kruepelin, M.: Lehrbuch. Springer, Berlin, 1894.

Mavroidis, M. L., Kanter, D. R., Hirschowitz, J., and Garver, D. L.: Clinical response and plasma haloperidol levels in schizophrenia. Psychopharmacology 81:351-356, 1983.

Niemegeers, C. J. E., and Leysen, J. E.: The pharmacological and biochemical basis of neuroleptic treatment in schizophrenia. Pharmaceutisch Weekblad Scientific Edition 4:71-78, 1982.

Peroutka, S. J., and Snyder, S. H.: Relationship of neuroleptic drug effects at brain dopamine, serotonin, alpha-adrenergic, and histamine receptors to clinical potency. Am J Psychiatry 137:1518-1522, 1980.

Peroutka, S. J., U'Prichard, D. C., Greenberg, D. A., and Snyder, S. H.: Neuroleptic drug interactions with norepinephrine alpha receptor binding sites in rat brain. Neuropharmacology 16:549-556, 1977.

Rupniak, N. M. J., Jenner, P., and Marsden, C. C.: The effect of chronic neuroleptic administration on cerebral dopamine receptor function. Life Sci 32:2289-2311, 1983.

Simpson, F. M., Pi, E. H., and Sramek, J. J.: Adverse effects of antipsychotic agents. Drugs 21:138-151, 1981.

Smith, R. C., Crayton, J., Dekirmenjian, H., Klass, D., and Davis, J. M.: Blood levels of neuroleptic drugs in nonresponding chronic schizophrenic patients. Arch Gen Psychiatry 36:579-584, 1979.

Snyder, S., Greenberg, D., and Yamamura, H. I.: Antischizophrenic drugs and brain cholinergic receptors. Arch Gen Psychiatry 31:58-61, 1974.

Snyder, S.: Schizophrenia. Lancet 2:970-974, 1982.

Tardive Dyskinesia: Summary of a Task Force Report of the American Psychiatric Association. Am J Psychiatry 137:1163-1172, 1980.

Tune, L. E., Creese, I., Depaulo, J. R., Slavney, P. R., Coyle, J. T., and Snyder, S. H.: Clinical state and serum neuroleptic levels measured by radioreceptor assay in schizophrenia. Am J Psychiatry 137:187-190, 1980.

van Praag, H. M.: Psychotropic Drugs. Brunner/Mazel, New York, 1978.

White, F. J., and Wang, R. Y.: Differential effects of classical and atypical antipsychotic drugs on A9 and A1 0 dopamine neurons. Science 221:1054-1057, 1983.

Chapter 26

SYMPATHOMIMETICS

Mark S. Gold, M.D. and Cary L. Hamlin, M.D.

The term <u>sympathomimetics</u> denotes a set of chemical compounds that mimic the effects of stimulation of the sympathetic
ganglia in the peripheral nervous system. These effects are
mediated by postsynaptic stimulation of alpha- and beta-adrenergic receptors on visceral cells. For example, beta-adrenergic stimulation of the sinoatrial node accelerates heart rate
while stimulation of the heart muscle produces a shifting of cardiac function curves to the left. Alpha-1-adrenergic stimulation
of the arterioles in the skin causes constriction, whereas beta-
adrenergic stimulation of arterioles in striated muscle opposes
that constriction. Sympathetic stimulation of the iris of the eye
is responsible for mydriasis. Sympathetic stimulation of the
gut produces constipation, stimulation of the salvatory and lac-
rimal glands produces dry mouth and eyes, stimulation of the
bladder produces distensibility and inhibited micturition, and
stimulation of the kidney produces release of renin. Sympathomimetics activate the peripheral catecholamines and produce the
autonomic state which is seen associated with the mood of anxiety or with environments containing the threat of noxious exposure.
    Sympathomimetics which will be discussed here are a sub-
set of catecholamine-mimetic drugs: D-amphetamine, cocaine,
and methylphenidate.

MECHANISTICS OF SYMPATHOMIMETIC ACTION

In 1940, Mann and Wuastel (see Carlsson, 1970) observed that
oxidative deamination of catecholamines by chopped animal
brain was inhibited by D-amphetamine. Rutledge subjected this
observation to an elegant dissection and observed the following:

(1) incubated brain cortical slices have a dose-related inhibition of oxidative deamination when superfused with D-amphetamine solution; (2) synaptosomal incubates also have an inhibited oxidative deamination when superfused with D-amphetamine; and (3) lysis of synaptosomes results in elimination of this amphetamine-induced MAO inhibition, except at 10 μM concentration. Rutledge concluded that observed MAO inhibition from 1 μM D-amphetamine is not caused by direct action on mitochondrial outer-membrane monoamine oxidase (MAO).

In 1962, Axelrod (see Copper, et al., 1974) noted that D-amphetamine caused increased noradrenaline release from peripheral nerves. In 1971, Farnebo observed that D-amphetamine in central and peripheral nervous tissues which had been prelabeled by incubation with radioactive dopamine or noradrenaline caused (in 10^{-7} M concentration) increased net release of dopamine and noradrenaline. Furthermore, these D-amphetamine concentrations potentiated stimulation-induced catecholamine release. The increased catecholamine release is not secondary to dopamine or noradrenaline transporter blockade because pretreatment by D-amphetamine in high concentration fails to block intraneuronal uptake of radioactive intraventricularly injected dopamine or noradrenaline. In contrast, cocaine does act to block the uptake pumps. The releasing action of D-amphetamine probably is by action of the drug on the plasma membrane itself. This effect occurs both in peripheral and central catecholaminergic neurons. Methylphenidate is like D-amphetamine but is more lipid-soluble which allows more rapid brain penetration and fewer peripheral sympathetic effects.

Carlsson noted in 1959 that D-amphetamine affected neither noradrenaline level nor normetanephrine level in brain. However, the reserpine- and nialamide-induced decline in noradrenaline and increase in normetanephrine (catechol-o-methyltransferase's extraneuronal catabolite of noradrenaline) was potentiated by D-amphetamine. This led Carlsson to postulate that noradrenaline release is from the cytoplasmic pool. He then demonstrated with subcellular fractionation studies that D-amphetamine primarily depletes catecholamines in the cytoplasmic pool unless the vesicular storage is disrupted by reserpine. Then D-amphetamine depletes both vesicular and cytoplasmic catecholamine pools. Glowinski, using a different paradigm, noted just D-amphetamine causes about a 33% decrease in brain noradrenaline content and about a 250% increase in normetanephrine content. D-Amphetamine acutely increases the turnover of noradrenaline and dopamine in catecholaminergic neurons. See Chapter 4 for a description of the anatomy of catecholaminergic systems.

SYMPATHOMIMETICS AND ANIMAL BEHAVIOR

As noted in the introductory section of this chapter, sympathomimetics mimic the effects of peripheral sympathetic adrenergic arousal, a state that can be associated with fear. However,
the aversive subjective effects of cocaine, amphetamine, and
methylphenidate are obviously not responsible for the fact that
venous self-injecting animals, intraventricular self-injecting
animals, and nucleus accumbens self-injecting animals will
abandon reinforcers like food and sex and will just keep pushing
the bar. At low doses sympathomimetics cause an increase in
locomotor activity, and animals increase their rate of investigation of the environment. At higher doses, this activity becomes
frenetic and has a driven quality. Rats sniff the same object or
no object repeatedly and do the same in effective motor excur-
sions stereotypically. If prodded with a pencil, the rats are
more likely to bite it. One rat that had been given a large dose
of amphetamine just sat in the cage grinding its teeth. When
prodded, the rat jumped almost a foot in the air, vocalizing
loudly, and then ran numerous times around the cage. A resemblance to catatonic stupor-excitement was remarkable.

Randrup and Munkvad discovered that the tyrosine hydroxylase inhibitor alpha-methyl-paratyrosine, which can totally deplete the brain of its catecholamines, blocks locomotor activation and stereotypes caused by amphetamine. These behavioral
responses can be restored by L-DOPA. The findings are not
due to Parkinsonian akinesia. They reflect the fact that catecholamines are necessary to the behavioral actions of sympathomimetics.

Amphetamine alone can accelerate noradrenaline turnover
in brain by about 100%. However, the addition of a nociceptive
stimulus potentiates this increase to about 300%. A role for amphetamine in attenuating conditioned anxiety is suggested by the
experiment of Cappell and coworkers. Rats were trained to
press a bar for milk and were conditioned to expect an impending foot shock upon hearing a click. Pressing the bar was suppressed by presentation of the click. However, pretreatment
with amphetamine blocked the suppression of bar pressing which
was caused by the click. Thus no amphetamine-induced competing responses could explain this result. Amphetamine, and presumably catecholamines, inhibit anxiety and increase tolerance
to physiologic stressors.

Various attempts have been made to dissect apart the roles
of noradrenergic and dopaminergic neuron systems in the excitatory response to sympathomimetics. As reading Chapter 2
reveals, the same catecholamines at different sites may produce

opposite effects (e.g., amphetamine in paraventricular hypothalamus versus perifornical hypothalamus). Some investigators try to associate locomotor activation with noradrenergic potentiation and stereotypic behavior with dopaminergic potentiation. However, Carlsson (1970) demonstrated that FLA-63, at doses that completely inhibited dopamine beta-hydroxylase, failed to block amphetamine's locomotor response. These attempts have thus far not been successful.

SYMPATHOMIMETICS AND HUMAN BEHAVIOR

The current epidemic of cocaine abuse, in spite of its being illegal and expensive, is a testimony to the rewarding motivational properties of sympathomimetics in humans. The average cocaine-dependent person spends about $50,000/year on the drug. The cocaine user often buys cocaine instead of paying the rent. Often what brings the cocaine abuser to treatment is financial ruin which doesn't permit continued use and exposes the patient to cocaine withdrawal.

Given the obvious importance of understanding the motivational basis of sympathomimetics abuse, it is a sad commentary that most evidence about this question is anecdotal and few systematic studies have been done. Fischman and colleagues investigated the effects of intravenous cocaine and D-amphetamine upon cardiovascular variables and mood state in cocaine addicts. They noted that both drugs produced a dose-dependent increase in heart rate from normal levels which peaked about 15 min after administration. Thirty milligrams of cocaine produced an average peak heart rate of 112 beats/min. Systolic blood pressure increased to a peak about 20% above baseline at the same time. Mole per mole, cocaine and D-amphetamine were approximately equally potent to produce these cardiovascular changes. However, the duration of effect was somewhat longer for amphetamine. The effect of sympathomimetics upon mood was to produce euphoria and hostility. The subjects experienced a sense of increased energy and vigor. The dose-response curve of these changes had an inverted "U" shape, and peak effects were seen after an average dose of about 24 mg of intravenous cocaine.

The effect of withdrawal of amphetamine upon adrenergic turnover and mood state in dependent patients taking 50-400 mg amphetamine/day was investigated by Schildkraut and associates. On admission to the study, subjects' daily 3-methoxy-4-hydroxyphenylylycol (MHPG) excretion level was about 3300 μg, and patients were clinically "hypomanic." Upon withdrawal from

Table 26-1   Chronic Medical Complications of Intravenous
                     Cocaine Use

Hepatic
   Hepatitis B
   Hepatitis A
   Non-A, non-B hepatitis
   Epstein-Barr virus hepatitis
   Delta-agent hepatitis
Infections
   Skin
   SBE
   Septic pulmonary emboli
   Pneumonia
   Brain abscess
   Ophthalmologic
Granulomas
   Pulmonary
   Hepatic
   CNS
   Ophthalmologic
Polyarteritis nodosa
AIDS

Abbreviations: AIDS, acquired immune deficiency syndrome;
CNS, central nervous system; SBE, subacute bacterial endo-
carditis.

amphetamine, patients experienced a rebound of depressed
mood associated with a decline of MHPG excretion of 900 g.
Patients' mood remained depressed and daily MHPG excretion
remained suppressed below normal for about 5 days until a eu-
thymic mood and $2000 \mu g/day$ MHPG excretion were observed.
Thus, as euphoric and anergic moods were followed by anxious
and guilty ones there was a change of adrenergic turnover from
hyper- to hyponormal. These findings are consistent with the
existence of a sympathomimetic withdrawal syndrome.

The resemblance of sympathomimetic intoxication to the
manic phase of bipolar affective disorder suggests that lithium
carbonate treatment of sympathomimetic-dependent patients
may be useful in blocking the emotional changes wrought by
those drugs. Empirical evidence suggests that lithium may indeed partially block the behavioral and emotive changes that are
produced by sympathomimetic intoxication. Neuroleptics seem
somewhat less useful in this regard.

The pattern of cocaine ingestion varies with experience of
the drug. Most users start by nasal administration (i.e.,

Table 26-2   Chronic Medical Complications of Intranasal
Cocaine Use

Rhinorrhea
Hoarseness
Frontal sinusitis
Nasal perforation

"snorting"). This mode of administration is followed by intravenous or inhalation methods which get more of the drug to the
brain faster. Each route has its own attendant risks. These
are reviewed in Tables 26-2 through 26-3. Nasal administration
can result in erosion of the cribiform plate caused by chronic
inflammation and vasoconstriction. Frontal lobe abscess can
result. Intravenous administration can result in hepatitis, en-
docarditis, and embolism just as intravenous administration of
opiates does. Inhalation of "free base" (i.e., cocaine purified
with ether) can produce bronchitis, and using ether in close
quarters can be very dangerous. There is a danger that cocaine
or amphetamine can produce ventricular arrhythmias and death.

The chronic high-dose administration of D-amphetamine or
cocaine can cause a condition which resembles paranoid mania
or even schizophrenia or psychotic major depression right down
to the hearing of derogatory voices and the presence of delusional guilt. This type of administration in animals is associated
with depletion of catecholamine stores and denervation supersensitivity. The possibility that this psychosis in fact is the result of too little and not too much catecholamine turnover has
not been addressed. Studies of daily MHPG excretion and daily
homovanillic acid excretion may be helpful in addressing what
happens to catecholamines in chronic sympathomimetic psychosis.

Cocaine addiction appears to occur, and a variety of detoxification protocols have been proposed from methylphenidate
administration to our procedure of giving tyrosine (100 mg/kg)
in divided (tid) doses with vitamine B_6 1500-2000 mg/day and
vitamin C 5-6 mg/day for 14 days. This protocol is particularly
helpful in reversing cocaine withdrawal-related dysphoria, irritability, aggression, and drug craving.

Table 26-3   Chronic Medical Complications of Chronic "Free
Base" Cocaine Use

Explosions
Burns
Increased carbon monoxide in blood
Diffusing capacity

BIBLIOGRAPHY

Cappell, H., Ginsberg, R., and Webster, C.: Amphetamine and conditioned "anxiety." Br J Pharmacol 45:525-531, 1972.

Carlsson, A.: Amphetamine and brain catecholamines. In: Amphetamines and Related Compounds (Edited by E. Costa and S. Garattini). Raven Press, New York, 1970, pp. 289-300.

Copper, J., Bloom, F., and Roth, R.: The Biochemical Basis of Neuropharmacology. Oxford University Press, Toronto, 1974, pp. 90-174.

Ellinwood, E.: Amphetamine psychosis: I. Description of the individuals and process. J Nerv Ment Dis 144(4):273-284, 1967.

Farnebo, L. O.: Effect of d-amphetamine on spontaneous and stimulation induced release of catecholamines. Acta Physiol Scand Suppl 72:371, 1971.

Fischman, M., Schuster, C., and Resmekov, L.: Cardiovascular and subjective effects of intravenous cocaine administration in humans. Arch Gen Psychiatry 33:983-989, 1979.

Griffith, J., Cavanaugh, J., Hled, J., and Oates, J.: Experimental psychosis induced by the administration of d-amphetamine. In: Amphetamines and Related Compounds (Edited by E. Costa and S. Garrattini). Raven Press, New York, 1970, pp. 897-904.

Randrup, A., and Munkvad, I.: Role of catecholamines in the amphetamine excitatory response. Nature 211:540, 1966.

Rutledge, W.: The mechanism by which amphetamine inhibits oxidative deamination of norepinephrine in brain. J Pharmacol Exp Ther 17(2):386-398, 1970.

Schildkraut, J., Watson, R., Draskoczry, D., and Hartman, E.: Amphetamine withdrawal: depression and MHPG excretion. Lancet I 284:485-486, 1971.

Ungerstedt, U.: Striatal dopamine release after amphetamine and nerve degeneration revealed by rotational behavior. Acta Physiol Scand Suppl 367:49-93, 1971.

Chapter 27

CLONIDINE AND BETA-BLOCKERS IN PSYCHIATRY

James R. Merikangas, M.D., Kathleen R. Merikangas, Ph.D.,
and Henry R. Black, M.D.

The discovery of the antipsychotic drugs and the fact that their
antipsychotic potency is proportional to their efficiency in
blocking dopamine receptors has been the paradigm for studies
of the effect of other neurotransmitter systems in psychiatry.
Since the discovery that norepinephrine-depleting drugs (e.g.,
reserpine) may cause depression, and norepinephrine-enhancing
drugs (e.g., amphetamine) may cause euphoria or mania, there
has been much focus on the noradrenergic system in mood regulation.

Norepinephrine is derived from the amino acid, tyrosine,
which is then converted to dihydroxyphenylalanine, or dopa.
Dopa is decarboxylated to form dopamine, which may then be
converted to norepinephrine by beta-hydroxylase. The largest
clusters of central noradrenergic neurons are found in the locus
coeruleus, which is located in the anterior pons.

There are two primary types of adrenergic receptors: the
alpha-adrenergic-receptors, which are stimulated by agonists
in the following order of potency: epinephrine > norepinephrine
>>isoproterenol; and the beta-adrenergic-receptors, which re-
spond to agonists in the order of isoproterenol > epinephrine ≥
norepinephrine. Epinephrine acts upon both alpha- and beta-receptors in the periphery, a phenomenon that led to much pharmacologic confusion before the receptor concept was clarified.
Pharmacologic and radioligand studies have resulted in further
subdivision of the alpha- and beta-receptors.

Alpha-adrenergic receptors are subdivided into alpha-1-
receptors, which are stimulated by phenylephrine or methoxa-
mine and are primarily postsynaptic, and alpha-2-receptors,
which respond to the agonist clonidine and may be either presynaptic or postsynaptic in the brain. Depending on the peripheral

tissue, the postsynaptic receptor population may consist of alpha-1-receptors, alpha-2-receptors, or a mixture of both types.

Beta-adrenergic receptors are divided into beta-1-receptors, with a response potency of norepinephrine = epinephrine > isoproterenol, and beta-2-receptors, with a response potency of isoproterenol > >epinephrine > norepinephrine. Activation of a beta-1-receptor will stimulate the heart, and activation of a beta-2-receptor will dilate the bronchioles and the blood vessels in skeletal muscle. Some of the beta-adrenergic antagonists show relative specificity for beta-1 or beta-2 response. In contrast to the alpha-receptors, no selective radioligands exist for the two types of beta-adrenergic receptors.

The assessment of the role of noradrenergic systems in psychopathology has primarily involved either indirect measures of the products of noradrenergic function or pharmacologic challenges that enhance or diminish noradrenergic activity. It has been difficult to attribute the response to such challenges to specific actions, however, because most psychopharmacologic agents simultaneously influence several neurotransmitter systems. The advent of drugs with selective action on a specific neurotransmitter system such as clonidine, an alpha-2-adrenergic agonist, and propranolol, a beta-adrenergic antagonist, has enabled investigators to observe specific effects of these agents and to develop hypotheses about the mechanisms of the pathophysiology of psychiatric disorders.

CLONIDINE

Clonidine hydrochloride has been used since 1966 primarily for the treatment of hypertension. The drug's antihypertensive effect is probably mediated by the central action of clonidine and the side effects of this drug suggest a psychotropic effect. The neurochemical effects of clonidine and its major side effects in man are shown in Table 27-1. The alpha-2-adrenergic receptor, which is usually located on the sympathetic presynaptic nerve ending, functions as a negative feedback on the norepinephrine system. Stimulation of the norepinephrine system in the locus coeruleus of experimental animals produces a response that is indistinguishable from the fear response. Yohimbine and piperoxane increase norepinephrine flow and turnover through an alpha-2-adrenergic agonist effect, and with clonidine, can therefore be used to manipulate central norepinephrine for the study of fear, anxiety, and other norepinephrine-mediated responses in psychiatric illness. A summary of the use of clonidine in psychiatric conditions is presented in Table 27-2.

Table 27-1   Neurochemical Effects and Common Side Effects
            of Clonidine

Neurochemical effects

Low doses
      Stimulation of alpha-2-adrenergic receptors (usually pre-
      synaptic)
      Decreases norepinephrine content in brain
      Decreases norepinephrine flow and turnover in locus co-
      eruleus
      Inhibits serotonergic system
      Decreases MHPG concentration in brain and plasma
High doses
      Stimulation of alpha-1-adrenergic receptors (postsynaptic)
      Stimulation of platelet aggregation
      Stimulation of growth hormone release
      Induction of prostanglandin E synthesis

Common side effects

      Drowsiness, tiredness, sedation
      Dry mouth
      Dizziness, vertigo
      Insomnia, sleep reversal

Abbreviation: MHPG, 3-methoxy-4-hydroxyphenylglycol.

WITHDRAWAL SYNDROMES

Alcohol Withdrawal

Bjorkqvist first reported of the use of clonidine for alcohol
withdrawal in a double-blind study which compared clonidine
and placebo. Improvement of withdrawal symptoms was more
rapid in the clonidine group than in the placebo group. This
finding was replicated by Walinder and associates, who reported
that clonidine treatment seemed to be at least as effective in
suppression and management of the alcohol withdrawal syndrome
as other routinely used withdrawal regimens.

Opiate Withdrawal Syndrome

Clinical studies have shown the efficacy of clonidine in eliminat-
ing the symptoms of opiate addicts undergoing voluntary withdrawal. Because animal studies have suggested that opiate

Table 27-2   Summary of Studies of Clonidine in Psychiatric
                     Conditions

	Double-Blind Studies	Dosage (mg/day)	Beneficial[b] Drug Effect
Affective disorders			
Mania	Yes[a]	0.45	—
Depression or mania	Yes[a]	0.26 - 1.0	?
Anxiety disorders	Yes	0.2 - 0.5	?
Attention deficit disorder	Yes[a]	0.07 - 0.25	Yes
Drug withdrawal			
Alcohol	Yes	0.45	Yes
Opiates	Yes	0.3 - 1.9	Yes
Schizophrenia	Yes[a]	0.2 - 0.9	
Tardive dyskinesia + psychosis	No	0.3 - 0.7	—
Gilles de la Tourette syndrome	No	0.2 - 2.0	—
Wernicke-Korsakoff syndrome	Yes[a]	0.3	Yes

[a]Small numbers of subjects.
[b]In controlled or double-blind studies.

withdrawal symptoms result from excessive noradrenergic activity in the locus coeruleus, the effect of clonidine on withdrawal symptoms may result from its stimulatory action at presynaptic alpha-adrenergic receptors of the locus coeruleus, thereby reducing noradrenergic activity. Double-blind studies conducted by Gold and colleagues have demonstrated that clonidine reversed both the affective and physiologic symptoms and signs of withdrawal from methadone and other opiates. These effects permitted abrupt discontinuance of chronic methadone treatment without severe physiologic or affective disturbance. Because of excessive sedation and hypotensive effects, however, clonidine has limited utility in outpatient programs. Lofexidine, an analog of clonidine which lacks the above side effects, appears to be preferable to clonidine in outpatient detoxification.

ANXIETY DISORDERS

Because of the possible anxiolytic effect of clonidine suggested in numerous animal studies, clonidine has been used in clinical studies of anxious patients. The majority of the patients in these studies had agoraphobia with panic as defined by the Diagnostic and Statistical Manual of Mental Disorders, 3d ed. (DSM-III) criteria. Overall, the results have failed to confirm the efficacy of clonidine in this condition.

In the largest study of clonidine for anxiety, Hoehn-Saric and coworkers reported that in a 4-week double-blind study, only 21% of the patients improved significantly more on clonidine than on placebo. Furthermore, there was a very high frequency of side effects such as irritability, restlessness, and sedation which dissipated somewhat over time. In an open 2-week trial of clonidine (0.15-0.225 mg) in 14 patients with severe anxiety, Siever and colleagues reported that significant anxiety reduction occurred in less than half of the patients. The negative results were attributed to concurrent depression in 75% of the clonidine nonresponders. Similar results were obtained by Ko and associates in a double-blind crossover study comparing clonidine and imipramine in six subjects with agoraphobia and panic. Although clonidine was somewhat more effective than imipramine in treating symptoms of panic, only one-third of the patients chose to continue clonidine treatment at the end of the study. Liebowitz and colleagues reported that in an open trial of 12 patients with panic disorder, sustained improvement was observed in only one-third of the patients.

PSYCHOSIS

Psychosis has been reported to occur both at the initiation of clonidine therapy for hypertension in nonpsychiatric patients and after withdrawal of clonidine in schizophrenic and manic patients. In the latter group, resumption of clonidine failed to reverse the psychotic symptoms.

In the few studies of clonidine as a treatment for schizophrenia, clonidine was found to either increase psychopathology or to have a transitory beneficial effect. Because of the absence of controlled studies in well-defined groups of patients, the efficacy of clonidine in treating symptoms of schizophrenia has not been established. Based on the few studies available, the use of clonidine in schizophrenic patients appears to be more informative in studying alpha-adrenergic receptor function than in treatment of the condition itself.

WERNICKE-KORSAKOFF SYNDROME

Clonidine has also been found by McEntee and Mair to be an effective treatment for the memory deficit of patients with Korsakoff syndrome. The effect of clonidine in this condition was interpreted as being consistent with the hypothesis that damage to ascending norepinephrine-containing neurons in the brain stem and diencephalon may be the basis of the amnesia of Korsakoff's psychosis.

GILLES DE LA TOURETTE SYNDROME

The efficacy of clonidine in the amelioration of symptoms of Tourette syndrome was reported by Cohen and colleagues in an open study of 25 patients. Subsequent case reports about the use of clonidine in this syndrome have had conflicting results. In an open trial comparing clonidine and neuroleptics in treating Gilles de la Tourette syndrome patients, Shapiro and associates found that neuroleptics were more effective than clonidine in a larger number of patients across a broad range of symptoms. There was a small subgroup of patients who appeared to benefit from clonidine. Carefully controlled clinical trials are necessary to resolve these divergent results.

AFFECTIVE DISORDERS

Mania

The antimanic properties of clonidine were reported by Jouvent and associates in eight patients, six of whom improved on clonidine. Others have reported that hypomania or exacerbation of mania have occurred after cessation of clonidine treatment.

Depression

Because it has been suggested that there is an abnormality of the alpha-adrenergic receptor system in depression, the effects of clonidine have been studied in the treatment of depressed patients. In a review of the antidepressant activity of clonidine, Malick concluded that clonidine does not appear to be an effective antidepressant in animals, and that its effects appear to be contradictory in humans. That is, while it has been reported to be an effective antidepressant in some patients, it appears to precipitate depression in others. As in several other psychiatric conditions described above, both the antimanic and antidepressant properties of clonidine await clinical trials before its role in affective disorders can be established.

OTHER USES

Clonidine has also been used in the treatment of attention deficit disorder and tardive dyskinesia, although the latter use has been in conjunction with treatment of psychosis.

BETA-BLOCKERS

Since their introduction in 1964, the beta-adrenergic blocking agents have been used in the treatment of a variety of psychiatric syndromes and symptoms (Table 27-3). Originally marketed for the treatment of cardiac arrhythmias, angina pectoris, hypertrophic obstructive cardiomyopathy, and pheochromocytoma, studies have demonstrated the efficacy of the beta-blockers in treating numerous other conditions including hypertension, migraine headaches, thyrotoxicosis, and prevention of reinfarction and sudden death in patients who have had acute myocardial infarctions.

The beta-blockers are pharmacologically heterogeneous, with varying degrees of membrane-stabilizing activity, beta-receptor selectivity, intrinsic sympathomimetic activity, and central nervous system penetration. Although both animal and human studies suggest some degree of central action of propranolol, other studies suggest the primarily peripheral site of action of beta-blockers.

ANXIETY DISORDERS

The most widely studied psychiatric indication for the beta-blocking drugs is in the treatment of anxiety states. Summaries of evidence in previous reviews have shown that beta-blockers are generally efficacious in treating patients with anxiety states.

Most of the double-blind crossover studies of beta-blockers in anxiety states have shown the beta-blocker to be superior to placebo in anxiety reduction, particularly in reduction of somatic symptoms. Only two controlled studies have demonstrated a significant response of the psychic as well as somatic manifestation of anxiety. Tanna and colleagues demonstrated a dose effect of propranolol in treating panic disorder. Whereas 120 mg propranolol/day was efficacious in anxiety reduction, a dosage of 40 mg/day was not effective. The results of a few controlled studies suggest that there is no beneficial behavioral or subjective effect of beta-blockers in treating simple phobias, such as fear of snakes or spiders.

Published clinical studies of beta-blockers in the treatment of large numbers of anxious patients have shown that the drug

Table 27-3   Summary of Studies of Beta-Blockers in Psychiatry

	Double-Blind Studies	Drug/Dosage (mg/day)	Beneficial Drug Effect[a]
Affective disorders			
Depression			
Delusional	No	Pindolol 7.5-45	—
Nondelusional	No		—
Mania (psychosis)	Yes	Propranolol 500-3000	Yes
Anxiety disorders			
Panic, general anxiety	Yes	Oxprenolol 240	Yes
		Practolol 400	
		Propranolol 80-240	
		Sotalol 80-400	
Phobia (agoraphobia or simple)	Yes	Propranolol 40	No
		Tolamol 200	
Neurocirculatory states	Yes	Alprenolol 120-400	Yes
		Propranolol 40-240	
Stress-induced	Yes	Atenolol 100	Yes
		Oxprenolol 40-200	
		Propranolol 40-120	
Drug abuse			
Alcohol (as antagonist)	Yes	Propranolol 40-160	No
Opiates (as antagonist)	Yes	Propranolol 10-160	No

Drug withdrawal/toxicity			
Alcohol	Yes	Oxprenolol 160 Propranolol 80–160	Yes
Amphetamine	Yes	Oxprenolol 160	Yes
Antidepressant (tricyclic)	No	Propranolol 40	—
Benzodiazepine	Yes	Propranolol 60–120	Yes
Cocaine	No	Propranolol 1 mg/min IV 8 mg max.	—
LSD	No	Propranolol 30	—
Opiate	Yes	Propranolol 30–160	No
Lithium tremor	Yes	Oxprenolol 160–320 Propranolol 30–240	Yes
Rage and violence	No	Propranolol 60–960	—
Schizophrenia	Yes	Propranolol 500–3000	No
Tardive dyskinesia	Yes	Propranolol 20–800	Equivocal

aIn controlled or double-blind studies.

dosage found to produce clinical response was considerably higher than that employed in controlled trials, with a median daily dose of 160 mg propranolol. Furthermore, prolonged treatment (i. e. , about 6 weeks) was necessary before improvement in psychic anxiety was observed. Indeed, the median duration of controlled studies of propranolol was less than 2 weeks. Suzman reported that in his 12-year follow-up study of propranolol treatment of 725 patients with anxiety neurosis, 88% relapsed when placebo was substituted for active drug in a single-blind manner. Whereas propranolol produced immediate resolution of cardiac and somatic symptoms, there was a delayed resolution of psychic anxiety.

Studies of the comparative efficacy of beta-blockers and other anxiolytic agents generally show that the benzodiazepines and beta-blockers are approximately equally efficacious in reduction of somatic anxiety. In patients with primarily psychic anxiety, benzodiazepines were superior in most studies. The combination of diazepam (22.5 mg) and propranolol (180 mg) has been found to have a greater antianxiety effect than either drug alone or placebo. To date, there are no published comparative trials of beta-blockers and other standard treatments for patients with anxiety disorders, such as monoamine oxidase inhibitors or tricyclic antidepressants.

Only one study to date has compared two beta-blocking agents in the treatment of anxiety. In a double-blind study comparing propranolol with oxprenolol, Becker demonstrated equal efficacy of the two drugs, but oxprenolol appeared to be better tolerated than propranolol. The antianxiety effects of the beta-blockers do not appear to depend on their ability to cross the blood-brain barrier. Bonn and Turner demonstrated that D-propranolol, which readily passes the blood-brain barrier but has no beta-blocking ability, was no different from placebo in reducing anxiety. This suggests that the beta-blockade itself rather than another mode of action is responsible for the anti-anxiety effect of propranolol.

The comparability and interpretation of the results of the studies of beta-blockers in anxiety states are limited by the variable definitions of anxiety states, small numbers of patients, relatively low doses of drugs, variability of outcome criteria, and brief duration of drug treatment. Because many of these studies were conducted prior to the introduction of standardized systems of diagnostic criteria, a heterogeneous group of patients with anxiety syndromes including neurotoxic anxiety, thyrotoxic anxiety, anxiety neurosis, generalized anxiety disorder, panic disorder, agoraphobia, and various neurocirculatory disorders with cardiac symptoms and anxiety as prominent features have been examined.

Anxiety and Cardiovascular Disorders

The beta-blocking drugs have been extensively used in the treatment of autonomically mediated cardiovascular disorders. The original syndrome, DaCosta's syndrome, was characterized by dyspnea, palpitations, exhaustion, precordial pain, nervousness, dizziness, decreased work capacity, tachycardia, headache, sweating, and syncope. In a review of the literature on propranolol treatment of the neurocirculatory disorders, Marsden found that there were more than 200 cases in which propranolol was used in the treatment of these disorders. Propranolol was found to be effective in suppressing the cardiac symptoms, but the evidence was insufficient to determine whether propranolol was effective in the control of anxiety itself.

Stress-Induced Anxiety

Beta-blockers have also been widely used in the treatment of situational or stress-induced anxiety, such as that found in individuals with stage fright or "exam nerves." Several double-blind placebo-controlled studies of the efficacy of beta-blockers in ameliorating symptoms of stage fright among musicians or public speakers have demonstrated the superiority of beta-blocking agents over placebo in alleviating such symptoms. As in the treatment of pathologic anxiety states, the major action of the drug appears to be peripheral rather than central. The subjects on beta-blockers do not generally report a decrease in anticipatory anxiety, but a decrease in both reported and actual somatic symptoms of anxiety is observed. External ratings of performance show a significant difference between the subjects on beta-blockers and those on placebo, with improved performance among the former group. The initial level of anxiety should be considered in prescribing beta-blocking agents, however, for their performance may actually be somewhat impaired in subjects with low initial anxiety levels. Beneficial effects of beta-blockers have also been reported for stress responses to civil unrest, ski jumping, race car driving, and dental surgery. When beta-blockers are administered to normal subjects in situations of experimentally-induced stress, the results tend to support the peripheral mode of action of propranolol in anxiety reduction. Cleghorn and colleagues demonstrated that beta-adrenergic blockade had no inhibiting effects on psychological anxiety in healthy subjects in whom somatic symptoms were absent. Thus, in the laboratory situation in which the stress induced by electric shocks, stressful interviews, or hypnotic suggestion appears to be centrally mediated, the beta-blockers are not generally efficacious in anxiety reduction.

Taken together, the studies of patients with anxiety disorders and subjects with stress-induced anxiety demonstrate that the beta-blockers are effective in reducing the somatic manifestations of anxiety and in some situations, the psychic manifestations of anxiety as well. However, the lack of efficacy in reducing artificially induced stress in normal subjects suggests that different underlying mechanisms may be involved in normal and pathologic anxiety states. The results of these studies recall the debate of James (1930) who postulated that psychic anxiety was a response to perception of peripheral anxiety, and Cannon (1977) who showed that somatic symptoms were under central control. It is probable that both theories were correct with central mechanisms of anxiety leading to somatic manifestations, which in turn provide secondary reinforcement of the psychic anxiety. Patients with pathologic anxiety may either have a disturbance in central mechanisms or a disturbance in factors underlying somatic mechanisms, or both. Pathologic anxiety states with predominant somatic symptoms appear to be more likely to be ameliorated by beta-blockers than those with predominant cognitive symptoms.

PSYCHOSIS

Schizophrenia

Numerous studies have reported the efficacy of high-dose propranolol in the treatment of schizophrenia. The majority of studies have been uncontrolled, employed small numbers of subjects, and have not been conducted in a double-blind or randomized fashion. The results of these studies have been equivocal. Although some controlled studies in which propranolol was compared to placebo in conjunction with neuroleptic treatment have shown that propranolol plus neuroleptic was superior to neuroleptic alone, others have had negative results. Peet and colleagues demonstrated that this effect was attributable to the pharmacokinetic interaction between chlorpromazine and propranolol such that the plasma levels of chlorpromazine and its active metabolites were increased markedly when propranolol was added. The enhancement of the therapeutic effect of propranolol is due to increased plasma levels of the neuroleptic, rather than to a specific antipsychotic effect of propranolol.

Double-blind comparisons of propranolol alone, neuroleptics alone, and placebo in a relatively large number of chronic schizophrenic patients have found no consistent advantage of high-dose propranolol (range 640-1920 mg/day) over placebo in the treatment of schizophrenic inpatients. Yorkston and colleagues conducted the only controlled study of propranolol in the treatment of acute schizophrenic patients and found chlorpromazine treatment to be somewhat superior. In summary, the current data do not support the use of propranolol in the treatment of either acute or chronic schizophrenia.

Mania

A recent double-blind placebo-controlled study of propranolol (1000-2000 mg/day) found slight to marked improvement in six patients with manic psychosis. Antimanic activity was found with both DL-propranolol and D-propranolol (which is devoid of beta-blocking properties), but larger doses of D-propranolol were necessary to achieve the same effect. The authors concluded that the mechanism of antimanic action of propranolol was not central beta-blockade. However, there is some evidence that D-propranolol has beta-blocking activity at very high doses. This finding is of greater theoretical than practical interest because of the high incidence of side effects and the need to monitor bodily functions at such high doses.

RAGE AND VIOLENCE

A relatively new therapeutic possibility that merits further study is the use of propranolol in the treatment of rage and violence. Effective use of propranolol for this indication has now been reported in 17 cases. These reports have described patients who are serious management problems because of episodic dyscontrol manifested by belligerence, rage, and violence. To date, there are no controlled trials of propranolol treatment for rage and violence.

DRUG WITHDRAWAL

Propranolol has been reported to be successfully used to treat anxiety states related to lysergic acid diethylamide (LSD), cocaine toxicity, benzodiazepine withdrawal, and anxiety states related to alcoholism. The only double-blind controlled study of drug-induced anxiety was that of Tyrer and colleagues, who compared propranolol (60-120 mg/day) with placebo in 40 patients withdrawing from lorazepam or diazepam. Although it did not affect the dropout rate, propranolol was related to a significant reduction in the severity of withdrawal symptoms. The findings of propranolol treatment of alcohol-related anxiety and tension are inconclusive.

OTHER USES

Successful beta-blocker treatment has also been reported for the following conditions: tardive dyskinesia, narcolepsy, lithium tremor, antidepressant toxicity, migraine, phantom limb, stuttering, menopausal symptoms, and action tremor.

SIDE EFFECTS OF BETA-BLOCKING AGENTS

The major adverse reactions which have been reported to occur with beta-blocker treatment include asthma, heart failure, hypoglycemia, heart block, bronchospasm, bradycardia, claudication, Raynaud's phenomenon, and a withdrawal syndrome following abrupt cessation of beta-blocker therapy. Central nervous system effects include vivid dreams, hallucinations, and insomnia. Severe depression has been reported, especially with lipid-soluble agents (e. g. , propranolol) in patients receiving large doses over long periods of time. No marked sedation has been detected for propranolol, sotalol, oxprenolol, or atenolol. Most of the side effects have been reported for propranolol, but the occurrence of side effects may differ for other beta-blocking agents according to the degree of cardioselectivity, intrinsic sympathomimetic activity, and lipid solubility. Several recent studies have shown that side effects are much less frequent in the beta-blockers that are primarily water-soluble and do not enter the brain in large concentration such as nadolol and atenolol. Most of the studies that have examined functional impairment i. e., eye-hand coordination, serial subtraction, reaction time, critical flicker frequency, percentage fast activity in the electroencephalogram (EEG) have not demonstrated significant levels of impaired performance in subjects on beta-blockers.

SUMMARY

Clonidine has been most extensively used in psychiatry for the treatment of acute withdrawal syndromes. In general, the non-specific sedative effect of clonidine appears to be responsible for its efficacy in numerous psychiatric conditions. Research evidence supports the use of clonidine in treating opiate withdrawal symptoms in inpatient settings and possibly in outpatients as well. The efficacy of clonidine in the treatment of Gilles de la Tourette syndrome, mania, depression, and tardive dyskinesia remains to be established by double-blind studies employing larger numbers of subjects than those of current studies and case reports. Conditions for which clonidine has been found to be less effective than traditional agents include anxiety disorders and psychosis. However, despite the lack of evidence for widespread applicability of clonidine in psychiatric conditions, the application of clonidine in the treatment of such conditions has been valuable in suggesting hypotheses for possible pathophysiologic mechanisms involved in various psychiatric disorders.

Current evidence on the use of beta-blockers for psychiatric symptoms and conditions suggests that they are most efficacious in alleviating the somatic manifestations of anxiety in the following conditions: generalized anxiety disorder, panic disorder, stress-induced anxiety, and cardiovascular conditions with associated anxiety. Psychic manifestations of anxiety do not consistently appear to be ameliorated by treatment with beta-blockers. However, further studies that employ higher doses of beta-blockers over longer periods are necessary to fully evaluate the efficacy of beta-blockers in the treatment of psychic anxiety. Beta-blockers may be preferable to benzodiazepines for anxiety because of their lack of sedation, lack of addictive potential, and lack of impairment of performance. The beta-blockers are more effective in patients with pathologic anxiety rather than in those with "normal" levels of anxiety. The relative efficacy of the various classes of beta-blockers, and that of beta-blockers used in conjunction with standard treatments other than benzodiazepines for treatment of panic and other anxiety and depression appear to be less likely to respond to beta-blockers than to benzodiazepines.

Two potential major applications of beta-blockers that are suggestive in the literature are in the treatment of the side effects of psychotropic medications such as lithium-induced tremor and tardive dyskinesia, and in the treatment of agitation and anxiety related to organic states and drug withdrawal. Current evidence does not support the use of high-dose beta-blockers alone in the treatment of either acute or chronic schizophrenia.

Methodologic factors that limit the interpretability of numerous studies include: lack of application of standardized criteria for psychiatric diagnoses, inadequate dosage of medication, diagnostic heterogeneity of the study sample, small numbers of subjects, failure to examine the role of affective disorders in response to treatment and side effects, and variability of outcome criteria. The latter problem was particularly notable, since some studies employed solely psychophysiologic measures, others used external rater criteria, while others used subjective rating scales. Numerous studies failed to consider the subjective response of the patient in determining drug response.

Perhaps the most important contribution of the use of beta-blockers and clonidine in psychiatry is in their potential role for understanding the pathophysiology and treatment of disorders in the anxiety and depression spectrum.

BIBLIOGRAPHY

Abernathy, D. R., Greenblatt, D. J., and Shader, R. I.: Treatment of diazepam withdrawal syndrome with propranolol. Ann Intern Med 94:354-355, 1981.

American Psychiatric Association: Diagnostic and Statistical Manual of Mental Disorders, 3d ed. American Psychiatric Association, Washington, D.C., 1980.

Becker, A. L.: Oxprenolol and propranolol in anxiety states. S Afr Med J 50:627-629, 1976.

Bernadt, M. W., Silverstone, T., and Singleton, W.: Behavioral and subjective effects of beta-adrenergic blockade in phobic subjects. Br J Psychiatry 137:452-457, 1980.

Bjorkqvist, S. E.: Clonidine in alcohol withdrawal. Acta Psychiatr Scand 52:256-263, 1975.

Bonn, J. A., and Turner, P.: D-Propranolol and anxiety. Lancet 1:1355-1356, 1971.

Brantigan, C. O., Brantigan, T. A., and Joseph, N.: Effect of beta blockade and beta stimulation on stage fright. Am J Med 72:88-94, 1982.

Cannon, W. B.: The James-Lange theory of emotions: a critical examination and an alternative theory. Am J Psychol 39: 106-124, 1927.

Carlsson, C., and Bengt-Goran, F.: A comparison of the effects of propranolol and diazepam in alcoholics. Br J Addict 71:321-326, 1976.

Cleghorn, J. M., Peterfly, G., Pinter, E. J., and Pattee, C. J.: Verbal anxiety and the beta adrenergic receptors: a facilitating mechanism? J Nerv Ment Dis 151:266-272, 1970.

Cohen, D. J., Detlor, J., Young, G., and Shaywitz, B.: Clonidine ameliorates Gilles de la Tourette syndrome. Arch Gen Psychiatry 37:1350-1357, 1980.

Cole, J. O., Altesman, R. I., and Weingarten, C. H.: Beta blocking drugs in psychiatry. In: Psychopharmacology Update (Edited by J. O. Cole). Collamore, Lexington, MA, 1980, pp. 43-68.

Editorial: Hazards of non-practolol beta blockers. Br Med J, 221:529-530, 1977.

Elizur, A., and Liberson, Z.: An acute psychotic episode at the beginning of clonidine therapy. Prog Neuropsychopharmacol 4:211-213, 1980.

Fielding, S., and Lal, H.: Clonidine: new research in psychotropic drug pharmacology. Med Res Rev 1:97-123, 1981.

Freedman, R., Bell, J., and Kirch, D.: Clonidine therapy for coexisting psychosis and tardive dyskinesia. Am J Psychiatry 137:629-631, 1980.

Frishman, W. H. (editor): Clinical pharmacology of the beta-adrenoceptor blocking drugs. Appleton-Century-Crofts, New York, 1980.

Gallant, D. M., Swanson, W. C., and Guerrero-Figueroa, R.: A controlled evaluation of propranolol in chronic alcoholic patients presenting with symptomatology of anxiety and tension. J Clin Pharmacol 13:41-43, 1973.

Giannini, A. J., Extein, I., Gold, M. S., Pottash, A. L. C., and Castellani, S.: Clonidine in mania. Drug Dev Res 3:101-104, 1983.

Gold, M. S., Pottash, A. C., and Sweeney, D. R.: Opiate withdrawal using clonidine. JAMA 243:343-346, 1980.

Gottschalk, L. A., Stone, W. N., and Glesser, G. C.: Peripheral versus central mechanisms accounting for antianxiety effects of propranolol. Psychosom Med 36:47-56, 1974.

Hallstrom, C., Treasaden, I., Edwards, J., Guy, T., and Lader, M.: Diazepam, propranolol and their combination in the management of chronic anxiety. Br J Psychiatry 139:417-421, 1981.

Hartley, L. R., Ungapen, S., Davie, I., and Spencer, D. J.: The effect of beta adrenergic blocking drugs on speakers' performance and memory. Br J Psychiatry 142:512-517, 1983.

Hoehn-Saric, R., Merchant, A., Keyser, M., and Smith, V.: Effects of clonidine on anxiety disorders. Arch Gen Psychiatry 38:1278-1282, 1981.

Int Drug Ther Newsletter. 16:19-20, 1981.

James, W.: Principles of Psychology, Holt, Rinehart and Winston, New York, 1930.

Jefferson, J. W.: Beta adrenergic receptor blocking drugs in psychiatry. Arch Gen Psychiatry 31:681-691, 1974.

Jimerson, D. C., Post, R. M., Stoddard, F. J., Gillin, J. C., and Bunney, W. E.: Preliminary trial of the noradrenergic agonist clonidine in psychiatric patients. Biol Psychiatry 15:45-57, 1980.

Johnson, G., Singh, B., and Leeman, M.: Controlled evaluation of the beta adrenoceptor blocking·drug oxprenolol in anxiety. Med J Aust 1:909-912, 1976.

Jouvent, R., Lecrubier, Y., Puech, A. J., Simon, P., and Widlocher, D.: Antimanic effect of clonidine. Am J Psychiatry 137:1275-1276, 1980.

Kathol, R., Noyes, R., Slymen, D. J., Crowe, R. R., Clancy, J., and Kerber, R. E.: Propranolol in chronic anxiety disorders: a controlled study. Arch Gen Psychiatry 37:1361-1367, 1980.

Ko, G. N., Elsworth, J. D., Roth, R. H., Rifkin, B. G., Leigh, H., and Redmond, D. E.: Panic-induced elevation of plasma MHPG levels in phobic-anxious patients. Arch Gen Psychiatry 40:425-430, 1983.

Lechin, F., Van der Dija, B., Gomez, F., and Lechin, E.: On the use of clonidine and levodopa in minimal brain dysfunction syndrome. Schizophr Bull (in press).

Lefkowitz, R. J.: Beta-adrenergic receptors: recognition and regulation. N Engl J Med 295:323-328, 1976.

Liden, S., and Gottfries, C. G.: Beta blocking agents in the treatment of catecholamine-induced symptoms in musicians. Lancet 2:529, 1974.

Liebowitz, M. R., Fyer, A. H., McGrath, P., and Klein, D. F.: Clonidine treatment of panic disorder. Psychopharmacol Bull (in press).

Malick, J. B.: Clonidine: antidepressant potential. In: Psychopharmacology of Clonidine (Edited by J. B. Malick). Alan R. Liss, Inc., New York, 1981, pp. 165-175.

Marsden, C. W.: Propranolol in neurocirculatory asthenia and anxiety. Postgrad Med 47(Suppl):100-103, 1971.

McEntee, W., and Mair, R.: Memory enhancement in Korsakoff's psychosis by clonidine: further evidence for a nonadrenergic deficit. Ann Neurol 7:466-470, 1980.

Med Lett. 17:45-46, 1975.

Motulsky, H., and Insel, P.: Adrenergic receptors in man. N Engl J Med 307:18-29, 1982.

Myers, D. H., Campbell, P. L., Cocks, N. M., Flowerdew, J. A., and Muir, A.: A trial of propranolol in chronic schizophrenia. Br J Psychiatry 139:118-121, 1981.

Noyes, R., Kathol, R., Clancy, J., and Crowe, R. R.: Antianxiety effects of propranolol: a review of clinical studies. In: Anxiety: New Research and Changing Concepts (Edited by D. F. Klein and J. Rabkin). Raven Press, New York, 1981, pp. 81-93.

Peet, M., and Yates, R. A.: Beta blockers in the treatment of neurologic and psychiatric disorders. J Clin Hosp Pharmacol 6:155-171, 1981.

Peet, M., Bethell, M. S., Coates, A., Khamnee, A. K., Hall, P., Cooper, S. J., King, D. J., and Yates, R. A.: Propranolol in schizophrenia. II. Clinical and biochemical aspects of combining propranolol and chlorpromazine. Br J Psychiatry 138:105-111, 1981.

Pitts, F. N., and Allen, R. : Beta adrenergic blocking agents in the treatment of anxiety. In: Phenomenology and Treatment of Anxiety (Edited by W. E. Fann, I. Karucan, A. D. Porkorny, and R. L. Williams). SP Scientific Books, Jamaica, NY, 1979, pp. 337-350.

Rappolt, R. T., Gay, G. Inaba, D. S., and Rappolt, N. R. : Propranolol in cocaine toxicity. Lancet 2:640-641, 1976.

Shader, R. I., Good, M. I., and Greenblatt, D. J. : Anxiety states and beta adrenergic blockade. In: Progress in Psychiatric Drug Treatment (Edited by D. F. Klein and R. Gittelman-Klein). Brunner/Mazel, New York, 1976, pp. 509-528.

Shand, D. G. : Drug therapy: propranolol. N Engl J Med 293: 280-285, 1976.

Shapiro, A. K., Shapiro, E., and Eisenkraft, G. J. : Treatment of Gilles de la Tourette's syndrome with clonidine and neuroleptics. Arch Gen Psychiatry 40:1235-1240, 1983.

Siever, L., Insel, T., and Uhde, T. : Noradrenergic challenges in affective disorders. J Clin Psychopharmacol 1:193-206, 1981.

Suzman, M. M. : Propranolol in the treatment of anxiety. Postgrad Med 52(Suppl):168-174, 1976.

Taggart, P., Caruthers, M., and Somerville, W. : Electrocardiogram, plasma catecholamines, and lipids, and their modification by oxprenolol when speaking before an audience. Lancet 2:341-346, 1973.

Tanna, V. T., Penningroth, R. P., and Woolson, R. F. : Propranolol in the treatment of anxiety neurosis. Comp Psychiatry 18:319-326, 1977.

Turner, P. : Clinical and experimental studies on the effects of propranolol in anxiety. Adv Clin Pharmacol 12:61-62, 1976.

Tyrer, P., Rutherford, D., and Haggett, T. : Benzodiazepine withdrawal symptoms and propranolol. Lancet 1:520-521, 1981.

Tyrer, P. J. : Use of B-blocking drugs in psychiatry and neurology. Drugs 20:300-308, 1980.

Tyrer, P. J., and Lader, M. H.: Physiological and psychological effects of +/- propranolol, + propranolol and diazepam in induced anxiety. Br J Clin Pharmacol 1:379-385, 1974.

Von Zerssen, D., and Emrich, H.: New drugs for mania? Br J Psychiatry 142:532-533, 1983.

Walinder, J., Balldin, J., Bokstrom, K., Karlsson, I., Lundstrom, B., and Svensson, T.: Clonidine suppression of the alcohol withdrawal syndrome. Drug Alcohol Depend 8:345-348, 1981.

Washton, A., and Resnick, R.: Outpatient opiate detoxification with clonidine. J Clin Psychiatry 43:39-41, 1982.

Washton, A. M., Resnick, R. B., and Rawson, R. A.: Clonidine hydrochloride: a nonopiate treatment for opiate withdrawal. Psychopharmacol Bull 16:50-52, 1980.

Yorkston, N. J., Zaki, S. A., Weller, M. P., Gruzelier, J. H., and Hirsch, S. R.: DL-Propranolol and chlorpromazine following admission for schizophrenia. Acta Psychiatr Scand 63:13-27, 1981.

Chapter 28

OPIATE ADDICTION

A. James Giannini, M.D. and William A. Price, M.D.

It is the inhibitory interaction of opiates with catecholamines that creates the pleasure of opiate abuse, the tragedy of opiate addiction, and the pain of opiate withdrawal. There are three major groups of exogenous opiates. Those that derive from opium including morphine and heroin are the "true" opiates. Dilaudid and meperidine are "synthetic" opiates. Methadone and propoxyphene do not chemically resemble the true opiates but stereochemically there is much congruence.

The action of true opiates such as morphine is similar to the endorphine and enkephalins. Morphine acts directly on the postsynaptic neuron to deactivate it by at least two means. A direct interaction between this drug and the mu-receptor (using the mu-kappa-sigma classification system) results in the deactivation of the cyclic nucleotide cyclic GMP (cGMP) and possibly of cyclic AMP (cAMP). In addition, sodium ion permeability is decreased by another direct action, this time of the channel protein. Chronic use of morphine is associated with increased sensitivity of mu-receptors while their number is unchanged. This is thought to be due to a progressive change in receptor conformation throughout the course of the addiction.

The phenomenon of opiate addiction is also involved with the opiate receptors' intimate association with other neurotransmitters. The most important of these are acetylcholine, histamine, and norepinephrine. Acetylcholine levels throughout the cerebral cortex are increased by opiate addiction. This is caused by imposed restraints on release, synthesis, and turnover rate. Morphine-inhibited release has been demonstrated in the cortex and striatum while uptake decrements have been found in the occipital cortex though not in the striatum. Acetylcholine appears to act with the opiates to produce analgesia. Morphine-induced analgesia is augmented by administration of

either acetylcholine or anticholinesterase. This finding has
been replicated by administration of these agents either sys-
temically or interventricularly to bring about enhancement of
the analgesia. It may be that the conjoint action of acetylcholine
and opioids/opiates is mediated by serotonin.

Injection of morphine and heroin causes a massive release
of histamine from the mast cells. It may be that this effect accounts for emesis, hypotension, and tachypnea reported by
heroin abusers. In overdoses H-1-antagonists restore consciousness but do not appear to affect analgesia, euphoria, or
respiratory depression.

The most important neurotransmitter is norepinephrine. It
will be discussed later in this chapter along with the various
treatment strategies for addiction.

Overdose with morphine is due to an increased level in the
number of receptor-transmitter interactions as well as an increase in the receptors affected. Systemic effects appear to be
due to modulation of the neurotransmitters discussed above as
well as substance P and gamma-aminobutyric acid (GABA).

The opiate antagonist, naloxone, can displace morphine
from mu-receptors by changes in receptor conformation. It is
associated with an increase in postsynaptic sodium permeability. A history of addiction increases the case of naloxone displacement presumably due to previously caused alterations in
the receptor glycoprotein. Naloxone also reverses GABA inhibition.

The treatment of opiate addiction is a much more complicated process than treatment for opiate overdose. One treatment possibility is the continuance of the patient's addiction with
a similar compound. A second direct approach is the use of a
long-acting antagonist. A third treatment strategy involves acting upon collateral neurotransmitter systems to eradicate withdrawal symptoms.

The first approach is the most studied and the most utilized.
Methadone acts in a similar manner at the cellular level as does
morphine. Its physiologic advantages are its lack of euphoriant
effects and its resistance to gastrointestinal degradation. Methadone withdrawal is also less severe than that of the opium derivatives.

Naloxone and naltrexone are used with some success to
maintain an addict in a nonabusive state. Changes in the receptor conformation as well as receptor blockade and increased
sodium permeability produce the desired effect. Any injected
opiate in a naloxone- or naltrexone-maintained patient will have
absolutely no effect. There will be literally no place for it to
work.

A final approach is the use of clonidine to detoxify the patient. This is a quite exciting strategy since it acts on a system other than the opiate peptides. This assures that there will be absolutely no abuse potential.

The noradrenergic system accounts for most of the symptoms of withdrawal. Within the pons is located a major source of brain norepinephrine, a 5000-cell cluster termed the locus coeruleus. This nucleus projects to the cortex and the limbic system including the hypothalamus. Neurons in this area contain a large number of endorphin receptors. When these are activated by opiates or opioids, norepinephrine levels are decreased and noradrenergic activity is diminished. The sudden decrease in available opiates as experienced during abstinence causes a massive overactivity of the locus coeruleus. It is this increased noradrenergic activity that then produces the objective and subjective symptoms of withdrawal.

Since morphine and similar agents switch off the locus coeruleus and their withdrawal switches it back on with a vengeance, the goal of any detoxification strategy would be to switch off again the norepinephrine overactivity. One marginally successful approach has been the use of a postsynaptic blockade. Propranolol, a beta-2-antagonist, blocks the actions of norepinephrine release from the locus coeruleus. Unfortunately, other effects not mediated by beta-2 sites are untouched. A more fruitful approach acts directly on the presynaptic neurons. Alpha-2-agonists reduce the rate of norepinephrine release and decrease norepinephrine turnover. An agent such as clonidine does, in fact, decrease the release of norepinephrine from the locus coeruleus. Since an alpha-2-antagonist, piperoxane, reverses this effect, it may be assumed that its clonidine-like detoxifying effect is strictly related to its alpha-2 agonist activity.

BIBLIOGRAPHY

Aghajanian, G. K.: Tolerance of locus coeruleus neurons to morphine and suppression of withdrawal response by clonidine. Nature 276:186, 1978.

Albanese, A., and Butcher, L. L.: Locus coeruleus somata contain both acetylcholinesterase and norepinephrine. Neurosci Lett 14:101, 1979.

Bergstrom, L., and Terenius, L. L.: Enkephalin levels decrease in rat striatum during morphine abstinence. Eur J Pharmacol 60:349, 1979.

Bird, S. J., and Kihar, M. J. : Iontophoretic application of opiates to the locus coeruleus. Brain Res 122:523, 1977.

Calderini, G., Morselli, P. L., and Garattini, S. : Effect of amphetamines on brain noradrenaline and MOPEG-S04. Eur J Pharmacol 34:345, 1979.

Cedarbaum, J. M., and Aghajanian, G. K. : Catecholamine receptors on the locus coeruleus. Brain Res 112:413, 1976.

Giannini, A. J., Slaby, A. E., and Giannini, M. C. : Emergency Guide to Overdose Detoxification. Medical Examination Publishing, New Hyde Park, NY, 1983.

Gold, M. S., Byck, R., and Sweeney, D. R. : Endorphin locus coeruleus connection mediates opiate action and withdrawal. Biomedicine 30:1, 1979.

Gold, M. S., Donabedian, R. K., and Dillard, M. : Antipsychotic effect on opiate agonists. Lancet 2:348, 1977.

Gold, M. S., Pottash, A. L. C., and Annitto, W. J. : Lofexidine: a clonidine analog effective in opiate withdrawal. Lancet 1(8227)992, 1981.

Gold, M. S., Redmond, D. E., and Kleber, H. D. : Clonidine in opiate withdrawal. Lancet 1(8070):929, 1978.

Gold, M. S., Pottash, A. L. C., Sweeney, D. R., and Kleher, H. D. : Clonidine detoxification. Am J Psychiatry 136:982, 1979.

Kuhar, M. J., and Atweh, S. F. : Autoradiographic localization of opiate receptors in rat brain. Brain Res 129:1, 1977.

LaCorte, W. S., Jain, A. K., and Ryan, J. R. : Comparative efficacy and tolerability of lofexidine and clonidine. Clin Pharmacol Ther 29:259, 1981.

O'Brien, C. P., and Testa, T. : Conditioned narcotic withdrawal in humans. Science 195:1000, 1977.

Petrocelli, L. V., and Cipriano, M. C. : Clonidine in methadone withdrawal. Drug Abuse Rep 2:112, 1982.

Riordan, C. E., and Kleher, H. D. : Rapid opiate detoxification with clonidine and naloxone. Lancet 1 (8177):1079, 1980.

Rothman, M., Riegle, T., and Orsulak, P. : Further studies of the effects of MHPG in rat brain. Neuropharmacology 18: 483, 1979.

Tennat, F. S., Russell, B. A., and Casas, S. K. : Heroin detoxification. JAMA 232:1019, 1975.

Terenius. L. : Characteristics of the receptor for narcotic analgesics in synaptic plasma membrane fraction from rat brain. Acta Pharmacol Toxicol 33:377, 1978.

Chapter 29

NOOTROPICS: TOWARD THE MIND

William A. Price, M.D. and A. James Giannini, M.D.

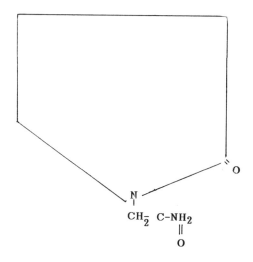

Figure 29-1   Structural formula of piracetam (2-oxo-1-pyrrolidine acetamide).

Piracetam (2-oxo-1-pyrrolidine acetamide; see Figure 29-1 for its structural formula) is an intriguing new compound and the first representative of a new class of drugs, the nootropics (noos = mind; tropein = toward) which are presumed to exert their influence upon telencephalic plasticity and upon the integrative activity of the brain.

Piracetam is a cyclic derivative of gamma-aminobutyric acid (GABA) which appears to work upon the cerebral cortex and related telencephalic structures. Piracetam has been used extensively in the study of learning and memory and has been

315

recently introduced in Europe as a nonstimulant, nonsedative drug for the treatment of reduced alertness and impaired memory function in elderly patients.

Experimental work with animals suggest that piracetam protects the brain from the effects of electroconvulsive stimulation and delays hypoxic amnesia. Piracetam does not affect motor behavior in animals, but has been shown to facilitate maze learning. Acquisition of new behavior was also enhanced by the drug through its effects on registration mechanism. In other animal studies piracetam has been shown to increase the threshold of central nystagmus excitability. More importantly it has been shown to increase the amplitude of the transcallosal-evoked potential as well as providing increased transfer of interhemispheric visual information. Evidence of callosal facilitation has also been obtained for man. This information supports its theoretical mechanism of action, namely, the enhancement of associative cortical functioning and the interhemispheric transfer of information. Researchers have discovered that piracetam exerts varied control over other functions of the body, e.g., increasing adenosinetriphosphate (ATP) formation in liver mitochondrion and increasing the polyribosome content of brain cells. It has also been suggested that the drug might selectively improve the adenosinetriphosphate:adenosinediphosphate (ATP:ADP) ratio in the telencephalon. Thus it appears as though the drug exerts its action upon learning and memory through enhancing protein synthesis and energy supply.

In the area of cognitive functioning in man, an investigation on a population of chronic alcoholics revealed improvement in the coordination of behavior when patients treated with piracetam were studied. Positive clinical effects have been reported in cognitively impaired elderly patients with mild to moderate impairment, but not in those with severe dementia. Piracetam has also been shown to counteract the impairment of mental functions induced in patients with pacemakers by lowering their pulse rate. When used on healthy young college students, those individuals receiving the nootropic, piracetam, daily performed significantly better on a verbal memorization test than did the control subjects who received a placebo. In normally aging individuals, piracetam improved performance on a reaction time test, as well as improving critical flicker fusion threshold and visual acuity without any indication of sedation or central stimulation. Piracetam has also been shown to diminish significantly the postoperative confusion of patients who have undergone brain surgery. Dyslexics receiving piracetam significantly increased their verbal learning rate by 15.0%, and students increased their level of verbal learning by 8.6% over and above the increase shown by individuals taking placebos. Piracetam has been studied for use in treating chronic schizophrenia since it is believed that in schizophrenia there are failures in the transfer between the two hemispheres. However, the results suggest some cognitive improvement, but little if any change in the disease state of the patient.

Not all the reports are as promising. The drug was not superior to placebo in protecting depressed patients from the retrograde amnesia that follows electroconvulsive therapy. Conflicting results have been reported on the usefulness of piracetam on improving mental functions in patients with cognitive impairment. These results seem to indicate that piracetam did not significantly improve mental functions in geriatric patients with organic dementia. Further research will be needed to evaluate the possible usefulness of piracetam and other nootropics in increasing cognitive capabilities in human beings.

Piracetam, and the other nootropic drugs that possess similar properties, are unique in that although they possess definite central nervous system (CNS) effects they are free of any peripheral effects. Piracetam differs from other pharmacologic agents used to treat cognitive decline in the aged in that it exhibits no sedative, tranquilizing, stimulant, or analgesic properties. It is also important to note that piracetam does not effect regional cerebral blood flow like the vasodilators used to treat senile dementia. However, piracetam has been reported to possess anxiolytic properties, and this finding has been proposed as a possible explanation for the drug's effect on cognitive ability. Piracetam does not appear to have any antihistaminic, anticholinergic, or antiserotonergic properties. The drug appears to work very quickly if it is going to work at all. It has been suggested that if the effects of piracetam do not become apparent within the first 2-4 weeks, they will not become apparent at all. In summary, piracetam and the other drugs belonging to the class of compounds bearing the name "nootropic" are unique in their central effects, their lack of peripheral effects, and their lack of toxicity.

Further investigation on the effects of piracetam on brain levels of catecholamines and catecholamine metabolites have revealed some interesting results. Piracetam, at 5 g/kg, increased the levels of dihydroxyphenylacetic acid (DOPAC), homovanillic acid (HVA), and 3-methoxy-4-hydroxyphenylethylene glycol (3, 4-MHPG), whereas levels of 5-hydroxyindoleacetic acid (5-HIAA) were unaffected. The level of dopamine in dopamine-rich brain regions was unchanged following the administration of piracetam. The drug has also been shown to increase the level of serum prolactin, a sensitive index of central dopamine receptor blockade. The results would seem to indicate that piracetam accelerates the turnover of brain catecholamines via a blockade of catecholamine receptors in a manner similar to that suggested for neuroleptic drugs. This is in contrast to the mode of functioning of central stimulants which decrease the levels of catecholamines by releasing the transmitters and inhibiting their reuptake, and GABAnergic drugs which inhibit the activity of dopamine neurons in which the transmitter accumulates due to decreased release. Thus it seems possible that piracetam possesses neuroleptic metabolic effects at high doses whereas at low doses the drug affects learning processes unrelated to catecholamine metabolism.

Piracetam is a fascinating and unique pharmacologic compound which is the forerunner of a new set of drugs, the nootropics. There is some evidence to suggest that piracetam may be useful in improving the cognitive ability of patients with mild to moderate dementia, but not in those with severe impairment. More research is needed to answer the many questions surrounding this interesting class of compounds. Once their pharmacologic properties are elucidated, the nootropics may play an important role in the treatment of cognitive impairment in the elderly.

BIBLIOGRAPHY

Buresova, O., and Bures, J.: Piracetam-induced facilitation of interhemispheric transfer of visual information in rats. Psychopharmacologia 46:93-102, 1976.

Burnotte, R. E., Gobert, J. G., and Temmerman, J. J.: Piracetam (2-pyrrolidinone acetamide) induced modifications of the brain polyribosome pattern in aging rats. Biochem Pharmacol 22:811-814, 1973.

Dimond, S. J.: Drugs to improve learning in man. In: The Neuropsychology of Learning Disorders (Edited by R. M. Knights and D. J. Bakker). New York, Raven Press (In Press).

Giurgea, C.: The nootropic approach to the pharmacology of the integrative action of the brain. Conditional Reflex 8:108-115, 1973.

Giurgea, C.: The pharmacology of piracetam (UCB 6215): nootropic drug. Report UCB-Pharmacology Division. Brussels,
DDRM, 1971.

Giurgea, C., and Mouravieff-Lesuisse, F.: Effect facilitateur
du piracetam sur un apprentissage repetitif chez le rat. J
Pharmacol 3:17-30, 1972.

Giurgea, C., and Moyersoons, F.: Differential pharmacological reactivity of three types of cortical evoked potentials. Arch
Int Pharmacodyn Ther 188:401-404, 1970.

Giurgea, C., and Moyersoons, F.: On the pharmacology of
cortical evoked potentials. Arch Int Pharmacodyn Ther 199:67-
68, 1972.

Giurgea, C., Lefevre, D., Lescrener, C., and David-Renacle,
M.: Pharmacological protection against hypoxia induced amnesia in rats. Psychopharmacology (Berlin) 20:160-168, 1971.

Pede, J. P., Schimpfessel, I., and Crokaert, R.: The action
of piracetam on the oxidative phosphorylation. Arch Int Physiol
Biochem 79:1036-1037, 1971.

Piracetam: Basic Scientific and Clinical Data. Report B-1060.
UCB Pharmaceutical Division, Brussels.

Sara, S. J., and Lafevre, D.: Hypoxia-induced amnesia in
one-trial learning and pharmacological protection by piracam.
Psychopharmacology (Berlin) 25:32-40, 1972.

Wolthuis, O. L.: Experiments with UCB 6215, a drug which
enhances acquisition in rats: its effects compared with those of
metamphetamine. Eur J Pharmacol 16:283-297, 1971.

Chapter 30

MARIJUANA

Karl Verebey, Ph. D.

INTRODUCTION

Marijuana smoking represents an unprecedented level of illegal drug use in the United States. Nearly one-quarter of the total American population has used marijuana, representing a thirty-fold increase from 1960 to 1980. Nearly half of those who try marijuana once continue its use and the age at which marijuana use starts has been steadily going down over the past decade. Daily use of marijuana involved more than 1 in 10 high school seniors. These alarming statistics motivated significant research efforts toward the elucidation of marijuana's acute effects and the consequences of its chronic use. This chapter reviews our current knowledge of marijuana's pharmacologic, physiologic, and behavioral effects.

THE CHEMISTRY OF MARIJUANA

NAMES OF THE NATURAL SUBSTANCES

Cannabis, marijuana, hashish, charas, bhang, ganja, and dagga. Cannabis plant material when used in a cigarette as an intoxicant is called marijuana.

NAME OF THE PRESUMED PSYCHOACTIVE SUBSTANCES

Delta-9-tetrahydrocannabinol (THC) and other less-active cannabinoids. The chemical structure of THC is shown in Figure 30-1.

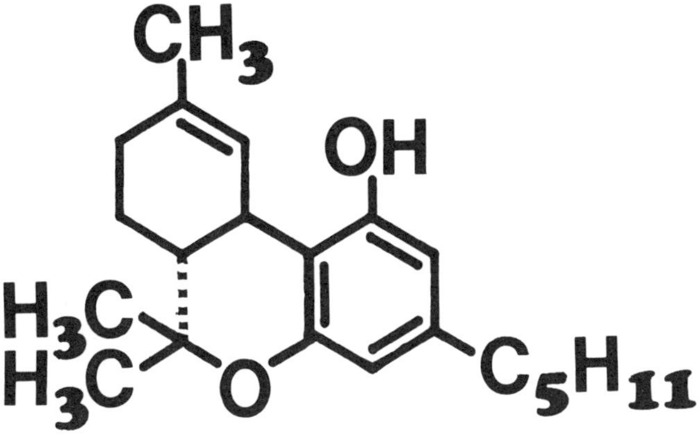

Figure 30-1   Tetrahydrocannabinol (delta-9-THC).

CHEMISTRY OF THC

An interesting feature that separates THC from most pharmacologically active substances is the absence of an amino nitrogen in its structure, which is thought to be the active principle
in many drugs. THC is very lipid-soluble. High lipid solubility
is important in helping drugs quickly penetrate biological or
neuronal membranes and get to their site of action. It is generally observed that substances with high lipid solubility have
quick, intense, and often brief pharmacologic action. This is
also true for THC. Its behavioral effects last only a couple of
hours, yet it is detected for in the urine as long as 30 days after the last exposure to marijuana smoking. The high lipid solubility is responsible for THC's persistence in adipose tissue
and consequently, its slow elimination from the body.

CHEMISTRY OF THE NATURAL SUBSTANCES

More than 400 potentially active chemicals have been identified
in the crude plant material. Of these chemicals more than 60
cannabinoid compounds have been identified. Furthermore,
during the smoking process, due to the very high temperature,
pyrolysis occurs. Many chemicals breakdown or react with
each other, producing even more new chemicals in the inhaled
smoke. About 150 compounds have been identified in the smoke
itself. Benzopyrene, a carcinogenic substance, was 70% more

abundant in marijuana than in tobacco smoke. Also, more tar was found in marijuana than in tobacco smoke. Thus the potential variation in qualitative and quantitative pharmacologic ingredients of the plant material make it difficult to study uniform and expected effects of marijuana. The converse issue is that studies conducted with pure THC preparations do not represent the effects of the crude mixture of numerous chemicals in the plant material, which is the substance commonly used. Thus the results of studies should be scrutinized for their true applicability to the ever-changing "real life" situation which depends on the active constituents of marijuana. Despite all these adversities there are useful data available for the limited understanding of THC pharmacology. THC is thought to be the primary psychoactive substance in marijuana.

SOURCE OF THE PSYCHOACTIVE SUBSTANCES

The most commonly used substances are prepared from the three varieties of cannabis. C. sativa, C. indica, and C. americana. The resinous exudate of the tops of the female plants are the most plentiful source of THC. Smaller amounts are found in the dried leaves of the female plant. Potency of the natural substances are evaluated by analysis of their percent THC content. In confiscated marijuana THC concentration increased from 0.5-3.0% from 1974 to 1982.

BIOAVAILABILITY

Marijuana is almost exclusively administered by smoking. One question is, how much THC is available in a given plant material, and another is, how much gets into the blood stream? Answers to these questions are available from studies utilizing smoking machines. The results indicate that 20 to 70% (an average of 35%) of the available THC is delivered to the lungs. The wide range of estimation results from the variation in depth and rate of puffing. Studies in human subjects utilizing THC blood levels as measures of bioavailability estimated an average of 17.5% (8-24%) THC delivery, which is half of the estimated 35% THC delivered to the lung in the smoke phase.

As described earlier natural marijuana contains a large number of active chemical ingredients. Their metabolism and disposition would be extremely difficult to follow individually. Even when THC metabolism was studied exclusively a large number of hydroxylated and carboxylated metabolites were isolated. Many of these metabolites are further conjugated by glucuronidation to increase water solubility and thus promote excretion. Estimated psychoactivity of the hydroxylated metabolites were 4-10% of THC while the carboxy metabolites were almost totally inactive.

In human studies THC and its metabolites excretion was followed in urine and feces. Eighty to 90% of the THC dose was recovered in 5 days. Fecal excretion was the major route, amounting to 65%, while urinary excretion was 23%. Early pharmacokinetic studies found wide variation among individuals for the half-life of THC in blood. In naive subjects the terminal half-life was as long as 56 hr, while in chronic users it was 28 hr. This reduction of half-life in chronic users indicates that metabolic tolerance develops after chronic marijuana use. The long half-life values also document the fact that THC and its metabolites are cleared from the body significantly more slowly than other psychoactive drugs.

BEHAVIORAL EFFECTS AND CENTRAL NERVOUS SYSTEM SITES OF THC ACTION IN RELATION TO EFFECTS ON NEUROCHEMICALS

Behavioral effects of drugs are significantly influenced by their physiological effects. Table 30-1 shows some of the physiologic effects of marijuana and/or THC. The magnitude of effects are dependent on the size of the THC dose. The cardiovascular effects appear to be the result of THC interference with the reuptake of adrenergic neurotransmitters in the acute phase of intoxication (Table 30-2). In chronic users there is a decrease in the adrenergic tone due to depletion of adrenergic transmitters. This may contribute to the loss of energy in chronic users. Dryness of mouth and throat, nausea, and vomiting appear to be THC's anticholinergic effect. While increase in appetite is possibly related to increased serotonergic stimulation of the lateral

Table 30-1 Physiologic Actions of THC	
Blood pressure	Increase
Pulse rate	Increase
Vascular congestion	Excessive
Blood sugar	Increase
Micturation	Increase
Dryness of mouth and throat	Present
Nausea and vomiting	Present
Diarrhea	Present
Hunger and appetite	Increase

Table 30-2   THC Effects on Neurotransmitters

Dopamine (DA)	Initial increase than depletion by blocking reuptake
Norepinephrine (NE)	- - 11 - - 11 - - 11 - -
Serotonin (5-HT)	Increase in serotonergic tone
Acetylcholine (Ach)	Decreased Ach activity, an anticholinergic effect
Gamma-aminobutyric acid (GABA)	Increased GABAnergic tone

hypothalamus; serotonin is known to influence feeding behavior.
Also it is possible that THC releases endorphins which are
known for their euphoric effects and also known to increase appetite. It is difficult to explain every physiologic or behavioral
effect of THC specifically by changes in concentration of single
neurotransmitters or neurohormones because there are many
checks and balances and multiple backup systems modulating
the numerous central nervous system (CNS) events. The com-
posite effect of THC on the total neurochemistry appears to be
significant in producing the particular behavioral effects that
are observed (Table 30-3).   The dreamy, sedated state often experienced after THC consumption is likely due to the THC's effect of increasing serotonergic and gamma-aminobutyric acid
(GABA)nergic tone and lowering of the adrenergic tone, especially in chronic users. The major difficulty in connecting the
effects of THC with specific anatomic sites, neurohormones,
and neurotransmitters is that currently available studies report
the measurement of only one or two transmitters. Thus, one
cannot see the whole dynamic state of the rest of the neurochemicals which likely influence the observed marijuana-related behavior. It is believed, however, that THC influences
hypothalamic-pituitary function through its effect on the various
neurotransmitters at the level of the hypothalamus. Table 31-4
shows how adrenocorticotropin (ACTH), thyroid-releasing hormone (TRH), and prolactin release are regulated by various
neurotransmitters. This information may be interpolated with
the information in Table 30-2 which shows how THC affects the
various neurotransmitters. Again, the combination of this information may or may not lead to explanation of THC's observed
effects, because other control mechanisms of known or unknown
neurochemicals may also be involved. Virtually all drugs that

Table 30-3   Behavioral Effects of THC

Dreamy state (increased sexual pleasure)	Vivid hallucinations (related to user's personality, not to specific THC effect)
Altered consciousness (ideas disconnected, uncontrollable, and free-floating)	Extreme euphoria (inner joyousness, referred to as a "high")
Long-forgotten things remembered (and well-known ones can't be recalled)	Exaltation, excitement
Time perception altered (minutes seem like hours)	Uncontrollable laughter (and hilarity at minimal stimuli)
Space perception altered (near objects may appear far)	Depression (is prominent especially when individuals use marijuana alone)

Larger doses
Panic states
Fear of death
Distorted body image
(head often feels swollen and extremities heavy)
Illusions
(manifested in dual personality

aTHC effects depend on dose, drug experience, personality, and psychological state of the user.

Table 30-4   Neurotransmitter Effects on Neurohormone Release

ACTH release	
Alpha-adrenergic agonists	Increase
Beta-adrenergic agonists	Decrease
5-HT	Decrease
Ach	Increase
TRH release	
NE	Increase
(DA ineffective without NE)	
5-HT	Decrease
Ach	No effect
Prolactin release	
DA (by inhibiting prolactin intribitory factor)	Decrease
5-HT (by stimulating prolactin-releasing factor)	Increase
EOP (naloxone reverses EOP effects)	Increase

Abbreviation: EOP, endogenous opioids; other abbreviations as in text and Table 30-2.

inhibit the release of luteinizing hormone (LH) and follicle-stimulating hormone (FSH) are releasers of prolactin. THC is an exception in this regard because it blocks the release of all three neurohormones.

In future research, with the improvement of analytical methodology it is likely that a clearer understanding will result from the monitoring of all known neurochemicals which maybe involved in the psychotropic effects of THC and other drugs.

ROLE OF LABORATORY TESTING

It is often useful to test biofluids of subjects who are in psychological council for their use of illicit drugs or found impaired while operating a motor vehicle. THC and its metabolites in chronic users may remain in the body for as long as 3-4 weeks (detected by urine analysis). Yet psychoactivity is observed only for a couple of hours after use. Thus detection of THC or its metabolites in blood or urine cannot be used as proof of impairment since it is not known when marijuana was smoked. THC and its metabolites are not secreted into saliva as indicated by the absence of radioactivity in saliva after intravenous administration of radiolabeled THC. Interestingly, when the saliva of subjects who had smoked marijuana-containing cigarettes was tested by radioimmunoassay (RIA), THC was found in high concentrations: over 50 ng/ml up to 2 hr after smoking and measurable levels of over 10 ng/ml up to 6 hr after smoking. These salivary levels of THC are likely related to surface attachment of THC to the oral mucosa during smoking. THC occurrence in saliva has little relationship to THC blood levels, bioavailability, or behavioral effects. Nevertheless, it may be useful to narrow down the time frame of marijuana use from weeks to hours. Urine analysis alone simply confirms use or exposure to marijuana at anytime between an hour to 3-4 weeks. Positive salivary levels of THC confirm use within a 12-hr period.

CONCLUDING REMARKS

The effects of alcohol and marijuana are often compared and it is questioned which is less dangerous. From the pharmacologic and medical point of view both agents have potentially long-term toxic effects. Due to the much larger number of chronic alcoholics the devastating toll in human life and health is acutely seen in the disease. Alcoholism interferes with productivity, produces cardiovascular and hepatic decreases, and leads to

untimely death in chronic users. The effect of chronic marijuana use at present is not as clear as it is with alcohol because
its illegal status keeps the number of chronic marijuana users
compared to the number of alcoholics relatively low. In general,
marijuana use has not been identified with serious medical
problems. But, based on the manner of intake, specifically the
smoking process, it is possible that in chronic use, pulmonary
complications develop, similar to the situation as in cigarette
smokers. Although long-term genetic defects are implicated
from animal studies their real danger has not been observed or
proven in humans. Similarly a direct relationship between marijuana and a motivational syndrome observed in daily users is
not clear. Marijuana use is widespread despite its illegal status
and there are numerous chronic users. In time the real chronic
effects of marijuana on human health will be revealed by the
experience of the self-experimenting pioneers. However, the
value of knowing the safety or dangers of marijuana or any other
drug use may be only academic. Few alcoholics, heavy smokers
and chronic coffee drinkers listen to warnings offered by the
Surgeon General that their health is in danger. Once dependence
on any substance is established, breaking the dependence is the
major problem; reversal of the user to the abstinent state is the
challenge of the future.

BIBLIOGRAPHY

Harris, L. S., Dewey, N. L., and Razdan, R. K.: Cannabis.
Its chemistry, pharmacology, and toxicology. In: Drug Addiction, Vol. 2. Amphetamine, Psychotogen and Marijuana Dependence, Springer-Verlag, New York, 1977, pp. 371-429.

Hawks, R. L.: The constituents of Cannabis and disposition and
metabolism of cannabinoids. In: The Analysis of Cannabinoids,
in Biological Fluids (Edited by R. L. Hawks). NIDA Research
Monograph 42. National Institute on Drug Abuse, 1982, pp. 125-
137.

Hollister, L. E., Gillespie, H. K., Olson, A., Lindgren, J.
E., Wahlen, A., and Agurell, S.: Do plasma concentration of
delta-9-tetrahydrocannabinol reflect the degree of intoxication?
J Clin Pharmacol 21:1715-1775, 1981.

Jaffe, J. H.: Cannabinoids (marijuana). In: Goodman and Gilman's The Pharmacological Basis of Therapeutics (Edited by A. G. Gilman, L. S. Goodman, and A. Gilman). Macmillan, New York, 1980, pp. 560-563.

Jones, R. T.: Human effects: An overview. In: Marijuana Research Findings 1980 (Edited by R. C. Petersen). NIDA Research Monograph 31. National Institute on Drug Abuse, 1980, pp. 54-80.

Kanter, S. L., Hollister, L. E., and Zamora, J. U.: Marijuana metabolites in urine of man XI. Detection of conjugated and unconjugated delta-9-THC-11-oic acid by thin layer chromatography. J Chromatogr 235:597-612, 1982.

Marijuana and Health. Ninth Report to the U.S. Congress from the Secretary of Health and Human Services, Department of Health and Human Services (DHHS) Publication No. (ADM) 82-1216, 1982, p. 5.

Olson, A., Lindgren, J. E., Wahlen, A., Aqurell, S., Hollister, L. E., and Gillespie, H. K.: Plasma delta-9-THC concentrations and clinical effects after oral and intravenous administration and smoking. Clin Pharmacol Ther 28:409-413, 1980.

Peterson, R. C.: Marijuana and health, In: Marijuana Research Findings: 1980 (Edited by R. C. Peterson). NIDA Research Monograph 31. National Institute on Drug Abuse, 1980, pp. 1-53.

Smith, C. G.: Effects of marijuana on neuroendocrine function. In: Marijuana Research Findings: 1980. NIDA Research Monograph 31. National Institute on Drug Abuse, 1980, pp. 120-136.

Turner, C. T., Elsohly, M. A., and Boeren, E. G.: Constituents of Cannabis Sativa L. XVII. A review of the natural constituents. J Nat Prod 43:169-234, 1980.

Wall, M. E., Brine, D. R., and Perez-Reyes, M.: Metabolism of cannabinoids in man. In: The Pharmacology of Marijuana, Vol. 1 (Edited by M. C. Braude and S. Szyra). Raven Press, New York, 1976, pp. 93-116.

Chapter 31

ALCOHOLISM

Ronald J. Leinen, Ph. D.

The term "alcoholism" denotes various clinical entities with
different etiologies and symptoms. Ethanol abuse may be socio-
cultural and circumstantial in origin or a self-medication for a
psychopathologic condition. Individuals with such secondary alcoholism may or may not show signs of physiologic addiction.

On the other hand, physiologic addiction can develop in
persons who may not have manifested significant premorbid
psychopathology. It is characterized by: (1) increased tissue
tolerance, in which a higher local level of ethanol is needed to
produce the same effects as in a naive subject; (2) altered cellular metabolism; (3) typical withdrawal symptoms; and (4) the
ambiguous sign of "craving. "

The effects are mainly psychomotor, along with intellectual
and emotional impairment. Withdrawal which, it must be emphasized, begins when blood ethanol levels are merely reduced,
generates tremor, convulsions, and disorders of thought, perception, and reasoning. These effects are in contrast to the
largely autonomic effects produced by the opiates during both
intoxication and withdrawal. This distinction is important for
evaluating current research on the existence of a possible
ethanol-opiate linkage.

In addition to this linkage hypothesis, many other explanations have been offered. Does ethanol affect cell membranes?
Does it alter neurotransmitter metabolism or function? What is
its role in relation to cotransmitters? What, if any, is the genetic liability produced by ethanol abuse?

Whatever the merits of particular hypotheses, the causes
of physiologic addiction disturb neurochemical homeostasis. If
at the same time, ethanol suppresses a dysphoria resulting
from the disturbance, one would expect: (1) withdrawal symptoms even in the presence of substantial, though suboptimal,

blood ethanol concentration; (2) persistence, and possibly increase, of craving at a low level of intake; and (3) progression of impairment and the inability of moderate doses of ethanol to alleviate the resulting dysphoria. These phenomena occur, supporting the notion that addiction progresses because ethanol has both a toxic and imperfect palliative effect on the central nervous system (CNS).

In regard to cellular metabolism, chronic ethanol decreases brain glucose. This effect may be compensated by the shunting of gamma-aminobutyric acid (GABA) to succinate to supply energy. Decreased GABA inhibition may explain tremor and seizures.

Acute ethanol lowers the temperature for the transition of phospholipids from the gel to the liquid crystalline state. Moreover, dopaminergic, beta-adrenergic, and peripheral-type benzodiazepine (BZ) agonists acting at their receptors promote methylation of cephalins and thus enhance membrane fluidity. It has been suggested that ethanol or its derivatives may act on such receptors (see below). On the other hand, chronic ethanol interferes with incorporation of unsaturated lipids and increases the cholesterol:phospholipid ratio, thus counteracting the fluidizing effect of acute ethanol. Some investigators believe that genetic complement or dietary or other epigenetic influences in infancy or in utero may also render membranes more resistent to a gel-liquid transition. Finally, chronic ethanol suppresses Na^+-K^+- adenosinetriphosphatase (ATPase) as well as Na^+ and K^+ transport, affecting the excitability of the neural membrane.

The most prominent area of research during recent years has been that concerned with opiatelike substances formed by Pictet-Spengler condensation of acetaldehyde (and other aldehydes) with neuroamines to form tetrahydroisoquinolines (TIQs) from dopamine (DA) or norepinephrine (NE), and beta-carbolines from serotonin (5-HT) and other indolealkylamines. The reaction occurs spontaneously in aqueous media at pH 7 and has been shown to occur in vivo. The formation of salsolinol (SAL) from DA and acetaldehyde and tetrahydropapaveroline (THP) from DA and 3, 4-dihydroxyphenylacetaldehyde have received particular attention.

The fact that THP is a natural precursor of morphine in Papaver somniferum, that TIQs interfere with high-affinity Ca-binding as does morphine, that naloxone can diminish the interference with Ca-binding and abolish some effects of ethanol intoxication, and the general similarity in structure of opiates and some TIQs has suggested the functional link between ethanol and opiate addiction already indicated, in spite of differences in symptoms. However, the affinity of both SAL and THP for opiate

receptors of either the enkephalin or morphine type is relatively weak. It has been suggested that these TIQs may have proper
receptors, but this has not been established.

In regard to other receptors, all TIQs tested inhibit specific binding of alpha-2-adrenergic ligands, but have little effect
at alpha-1-adrenergic sites. THP shows high affinity and is a
potent agonist at beta-1-adrenergic receptors. Other TIQs, in
general, show low affinity at such sites.

Salsolinol readily displaces apomorphine, a DA agonist and
acts as a weak antagonist; norsalsolinol shows weak agonist action, and THP is a high-affinity antagonist at these receptors.
The THP derivatives, tetrahydroberberine and boldine (the latter an aporphine) displace spiroperidol, a DA antagonist, at
low molar concentrations.

The displacement capability of THP at 5-HT receptors is
weak, though THP derivatives are more active. SAL has no effect.

No TIQ shows activity at muscarinic cholinergic or BZ receptor sites in displacing other ligands. Overall, a clear pattern of TIQ action at a variety of receptors has not emerged
from these studies.

THP can influence behavior. Injection into the cerebrolat-
eral ventricles of the rat or monkey during 12-14 days has been
shown to induce a preference for ethanol which persisted for
many weeks following cessation of the THP infusion. More precisely placed injections showed that limbic structures were especially responsive to a range of THP concentrations within upper and lower bounds. Preference was also induced with some
other TIQs and tryptoline (1, 2, 3, 4-tetrahydro-beta-carboline).
On the other hand, 5-hydroxymethtryptoline has been reported
to reduce ethanol consumption in the rat. Moreover, ingestion
of ethanol does not create preference, though it does generate
acetaldehyde adducts. Clarification of their role awaits more
precise qualitative and quantitative assay of these substances at
particular brain sites.

Ethanol or its derivatives may influence the metabolism or
function of naturally occurring or native opioid substances.
There is evidence that ethanol triggers the release of beta-endorphin and could conceivably place excessive demands upon the
endorphinergic system. Moreover, acetaldehyde forms imidazo-
lidinone derivatives with both enkephalins and beta-endorphin;
these adducts are not active in inhibiting electrically stimulated
contractions in the guinea pig ileum as do the parent opioids.

Alcohols themselves also selectively reduce the binding
capacity of delta- (enkephalin-related) receptors but not of mu-
(opiate-related) receptors. It has been suggested that

delta-receptors may be more important in the production of
sedation and some convulsive and behavioral effects. If, as has
been proposed, neuropeptides including enkephalins and endorphins act as cotransmitters with main neurotransmitter systems, modulating the "gain" at the synapse, ethanol or its derivatives may act on these systems by way of influencing the
endorphinergic or enkephalinergic components. The above observations have given rise to the hypothesis that ethanol addiction results from endorphinergic dysfunction, whether innate or
consequent to ethanol abuse.

A special role for NE has been suggested by some studies,
indicating a high correlation between bipolar disorder and ethanol abuse, a familial relation between depression and alcoholism,
and a reduction of ethanol consumption on a regime of lithium
salts. Various interpretations have been proposed.

In regard to 5-HT-ethanol interactions, it is of historical
interest that the first monoamine-acetaldehyde adduct studied
was the beta-carboline derivative, 10-methoxyharmalan, a potent 5-HT antagonist and monoamine oxidase inhibitor (a property shared by a number of TIQs and beta-carbolines). There is
some evidence that ethanol and 5-HT mutually potentiate a soporific effect. Nevertheless, reports of the actions of chronic
ethanol on 5-HT metabolism are contradictory and, on the whole,
the interactions of the substances have not been clearly demonstrated.

Recent studies of the action of beta-carbolines at BZ receptors have given research yet another direction. Those beta-
carboline compounds that are substituted in the C-3 position
with an esterified carboxylic group have a high affinity for BZ
receptors and can displace BZs, acting as antagonists of the
anxiolytic, anticonvulsant, and sedative-hypnotic properties of
these drugs. If there exist native BZ ligand(s), they may be
beta-carboline-like agonist(s). Ethanol-derived beta-carbolines
could displace these native agonist(s) with antagonist or partial
agonist ligand(s), or even agonist(s).

Such action could explain some likenesses between barbiturate and ethanol addiction. Both BZ and barbiturate receptors
are near GABA receptors and potentiate GABA-activated inhibition in the CNS. The similarities of action of barbiturates and
ethanol include not only intoxication with its associated sedation,
impairment of mental ability, increased emotional instability,
confusion, and ataxia, but also parallels in the development of
tolerance and abstinence syndromes. In both cases, tolerance
develops only after use at appreciably elevated levels, and withdrawal symptoms appear in a like sequence. The cross-tolerance
of these substances is well established. Alteration of GABAnergic

function via BZ receptors may, therefore, mediate the effects of ethanol and explain cross-tolerance with barbiturates.

The avenue of speculation is complicated by the ability of GABA, barbiturates, and halogen anions to increase BZ receptor affinity for agonists but not for antagonists, though relief of ethanol withdrawal symptoms by barbiturates is compatible with this finding, particularly if barbiturates favor binding of the hypothetical native BZ agonist(s). However, at the present time, there is no unequivocal demonstration of a naturally occurring BZ ligand, nor is it certain that the ethanol-generated beta-carboline compounds that have been reported to occur in vivo are not, at least in part, artifacts of technique.

By way of a clinical corollary to the above, it may be noted that there is one form of psychogenic alcoholism, which may or may not lead to physiologic addiction, for which triazolobenzodiazepines have proved particularly effective. There is evidence that the underlying disease, an endogenous anxiety disorder, results from a genetic vulnerability not yet specifically defined. Persons with this illness experience panic attacks and even phobic symptoms. They may turn to ethanol to find transient relief. Alprazolam (Xanax) relieves the cause of the abuse of ethanol, though psychotherapy is indicated for long-term maintenance. In any case, the patient is well advised to practice abstinence from ethanol.

Other avenues of research, involving other substances and mechanisms too numerous to discuss in this summary presentation, are being explored. The diversity of contemporary investigations may prove in the end to be less competitive than contributive to a synthesis. Even from a circumscribed psychobiological perspective, physiologic addiction to ethanol may well really constitute a family of illnesses differing in their precise constellations of abnormal neuroamine, receptor, or systems activities, and similar in that the resultant loss of homeostasis and abuse of ethanol as a palliative leads to similar clinical symptoms.

BIBLIOGRAPHY

Bloom, F. E.: Beta-carbolines and Tetrahydroisoquinolines. Alan R. Liss, Inc. (ed.), New York, 1982.

Giannini, A. J., Slaby, A. E., and Giannini, M. C.: Handbook of Overdose and Detoxification Emergencies. Medical Examination Publishing, New Hyde Park, NY, 1982, p. 170.

Goodwin, D. W. , and Erickson, C. K. : Alcoholism and Affective Disorders. Spectrum Publications, Jamaica, New York, 1979.

Hamilton, M. G. , and Hirst, M. : Alcohol-related tetrahydroisoquinolines: pharmacology and identification. Substance Alcohol Actions Misuse 1:121-144, 1980.

Lehninger, A. L. , McKusick, V. A. , and Santora, P. B. : Proceedings of the conference on genetic and biochemical variability in response to alcohol. Alcohol Clin Exp Res 5:435-468, 1981.

Majchrowicz, E. E. , and Noble, E. P. (editors): Biochemistry and Pharmacology of Ethanol, Vol. 2. Plenum Press, New York, 1979.

Messiha, F. S. , and Tyner, G. S. (editors): Alcoholism: a Perspective. PJD Publications, Westbury, New York, 1980.

Rigter, J. , and Crabbe, J. C. (editors): Alcohol Tolerance and Dependence. Elsevier/North-Holland Biomedical Press, New York, 1980.

Sandler, M. (editor): Psychopharmacology of Alcohol. Raven Press, New York, 1980.

Chapter 32

CAFFEINISM

Andrew E. Slaby, M.D., Ph.D., M.P.H.

Caffeine (1,3,7-trimethylxanthine) is probably the most commonly used psychoactive drug in the United States and Canada. The white, bitter, odorless, aqueous extract of a plant alkaloid is consumed in coffee, tea, cocoa, and some soft drinks and is found in chocolate and over-the-counter cold preparations, painkillers, and stimulants. It is a powerful stimulant of the central nervous system in addition to the fact it produces diuresis, relaxes smooth muscle, stimulates cardiac muscle, and increases gastric secretion.

Widespread advertising promotion of instant coffee and soft drinks has led to a dramatic increase in their consumption in recent years. It is estimated that Americans consume as much as 2.7 billion pounds of coffee per year. In the Province of Ontario (Canada) 90% of adults drink a caffeine-containing beverage daily. Caffeine consumption has increased among younger people in recent years. Alcoholics with a coexisting psychiatric disorder have been found to consume more than psychiatric patients without a history of alcoholism. General hospital patients are provided with pharmacologic doses of caffeine daily in a number of foods, complicating the clinical presentation of a number of medical, surgical, and psychiatric illnesses. Interestingly, while total annual volume of caffeine consumption has increased over the years, per capita daily intake has not. This has been attributed to the fact that the quantity of caffeine in a soft drink is about the same or less in the instance of diet beverages.

HISTORY

The coffee bean is reported to have been discovered in Arabia.

The coco bean, the kola nut, and the tea leaf were first used medicinally in Mexico, West Africa, and China, respectively. Despite medical warnings and efforts to suppress coffee use because of its purported intoxicating properties, consumption of the beverage spread rapidly from Arabia and Turkey to Ethiopia and from there to North Africa, the Near East, and eventually to Europe and North and South America.

SOURCES

Common sources of caffeine are presented in Table 32-1. The amount of caffeine in a cup of coffee, the most popular source, depends on the size of the cup, the measurement of ingredients, the blend used, and the method of brewing. Because many non-cola drinks (particularly those of citrus flavor) contain caffeine, individuals who are particularly sensitive to the drug should be encouraged to read the label. Both theophylline and caffeine are contained in chocolate with the average bar containing approximately 25 mg of the latter. The restriction of amphetamine marketing by the Food and Drug Administration (FDA) has led to the development and promotion of a large number of over-the-counter caffeine-containing preparations for weight reduction. Caffeine is used in cola drinks, some baked goods, frozen dairy products, soft candies, puddings, and gelatins. As little as three cups of coffee, one cola drink, and two headache tablets can provide a total intake of over 500 mg of caffeine.

ABSORPTION AND DISTRIBUTION

Caffeine is readily absorbed from the gastrointestinal tract following oral ingestion and is rapidly distributed throughout all tissues and organs. Peak plasma levels are obtained in 30-60 min. The type of caffeine-containing substances consumed affects absorption rate. Caffeine is absorbed more slowly from cola drinks than from either tea or coffee. The amount of caffeine reaching the brain and other organs is proportional to their water content. Tissue response is directly proportional to the amount of caffeine absorbed.

Caffeine is completely and rapidly metabolized in the liver. It is excreted by the kidneys as the methylxanthine derivative. Patients with liver failure exhibit a markedly decreased rate of elimination. Plasma half-life of caffeine has been reported between 2.5 and 4.5 hr (mean 3.5 hr, 15% metabolized/hr) in healthy adults. There is some question as to whether there is

Table 32-1   Common Sources of Caffeine

Beverages	Caffeine Content
Brewed coffee	29-176 mg/cup (85 mg/5 oz)
Instant coffee	60 mg/5 oz)
Decaffeinated coffee	3 mg/5 oz
Cocoa	6-142 mg/5 oz
Cola drinks	32-65 mg/12 oz
Brewed green tea	30 mg/5 oz
Brewed black tea	50 mg/5 oz
Instant tea	30 mg/5 oz
Milk chocolate	3 mg/oz
Diet colas	32-33 mg/12 oz

Prescription Medications	Caffeine per Tablet
APCs (aspirin, phenacetin, caffeine)	32
Darvon compound	32
Fiorinal	40
Cafergat	100
Migral	50

Nonprescription Medications	Caffeine per Tablet (mg)
Excedrin	60
Anacin	32
Midol	32
Aspirin compound	32
Cope	32
Vanquish	32
No-Doz tablets	100
Pre-Mens	66
Empirin compound	32
Dristan	30
Easy-Mens	32
Sinarest	30
Bromo-Seltzer	32.5
Capron	32
Stanback tablets	16
Trigesic	30
Dolor	30
Many cold preparations	30
Many stimulants	100

day-to-day accumulation of caffeine, theophylline, and theobromine in the blood stream. At least one investigator has reported that it takes up to 7 days to completely decaffeinate the blood of those who habitually drink coffee heavily.

Caffeine storage rates vary among regular and occasional users. The half-life of caffeine is significantly shorter in smokers than in nonsmokers. This is believed related to the increased liver aryl hydrocarbon activity in smokers. The fact that smokers drink more coffee than nonsmokers suggests that some of the symptoms commonly ascribed to nicotine withdrawal may be attributed to caffeine overload.

Caffeine's absorption in the stomach is directly related to gastric pH. Despite the tannin content of tea, rates of absorption of tea and caffeine are similar when determined by blood levels. The low pH of most cola drinks is deemed responsible for the delayed absorption of the caffeine they contain.

Absorption after oral administration of caffeine is delayed in preterm infants such that maximum levels do not occur until 4 or 5 hr has elapsed. This probably relates both to the variability in gastric acidity and slow gastric emptying time (approximately 6-8 hr) of the neonate.

One-half of an intravenously administered dose of caffeine passes into the tissues approximately 1.5 min following injection. The ratio of urine:plasma caffeine concentration in man is about 1:4 under normal conditions.

When caffeine is given as coffee with meals, there is no resultant delay in the caffeine reaching peak plasma levels, suggesting that food does not delay absorption.

METABOLISM

Caffeine and its related compounds, theophylline which is found in tea and theobromine which is found in cocoa and chocolate, are methylated xanthines structurally similar to purine and uric acid. This similarity in structure facilitates use within the body. The first step in the metabolism in the human of caffeine 3-N-demethylation yielding paraxanthine (1, 7-dimethylxanthine). Subsequent 7-N-demethylation of paraxanthine followed by 8-oxidation results in 1-methyluric acid, the principal product of caffeine in the urine. The paraxanthine pathway for the first demethylation of caffeine has been confirmed by recent investigations that have demonstrated, in addition, that nearly one-half of the urinary metabolites are 1-methylxanthine and its derivatives. Only 3-6% of ingested caffeine appears unchanged in the urine.

Methylxanthines stimulate cellular oxygen consumption, increase muscle lactate acid, and cause muscle twitches and contractures in high concentration. Caffeine potentiates normal thermal responses and increases oxygen consumption. This suggests that caffeine, by virtue of its thermogenic properties and negligible energy value, could be of value in weight reduction. Ingestion of moderate amounts of caffeine significantly increases urinary catecholamine excretion. Theoohylline, the active ingredient in tea, exerts its greatest action on the cardiovascular and musculoskeletal systems, specifically relaxing bronchioles. Metabolic and physiologic effects of methylxanthines are felt to be due in part to the fact that they inhibit phosphodiesterase breakdown of cyclic 3':5" adenosine monophosphate, thereby prolonging its metabolic-stimulating action in the cells. Mackenzie and coworkers (1981) have found a reduction in the isoproterenol stimulation 3 days after withdrawal of coffee and other caffeine-containing substances, without a reduction in prostaglandin-mediated cyclic AMP production. This suggests that the phenomenon is specific to the beta-adrenergic system and does not involve more general mediators of cyclic AMP metabolism. The mechanism is not clear but it is felt this may represent a biochemical correlate of the caffeine withdrawal syndrome.

Caffeine metabolism has been studied in groups of athletes, obese individuals, and normal-weight people. Caffeine increased endurance among athletes due to enhanced fat oxidation (lipolysis) and exerts a positive influence on nerve impulse transmission. It increased the metabolic rate of both the normal-weight and obese individuals but increased fat oxidation only in normal-weight subjects.

The metabolism and pharmacodynamics of caffeine in non-human species differs from that of humans, making interspecies comparisons difficult.

PHYSIOLOGIC EFFECTS

CARDIOVASCULAR EFFECTS

The effects of caffeine on the cardiovascular system are varied and provide a partial physiologic explanation for some of the symptoms comprising the syndrome known as caffeinism. Stimulation of beta-adrenergic sites results in palpitations, tachycardia, increased cardiac contractibility, and change in duration of the action potential. Habituation occurs and low consumers of caffeine are more likely to report cardiac symptoms than habitual users. Caffeine has the least potent effect of the methyl-xanthines on the circulatory system, but cardiac muscle is strongly stimulated which increases heart rate, force of contraction, and cardiac output. The effect is somewhat masked by the fact that caffeine also stimulates the medullary vagal nuclei which acts to slow heart rate. As a result, bradycardia, tachycardia, or no change in heart rate may be seen at low levels. Large doses of the drug cause tachycardia.

Pulmonary, cardiac, and general systemic blood vessels are dilated by caffeine, relaxing the smooth muscle in the vessel walls. The effect on the cerebral circulation is the opposite. Xanthines constrict blood vessels in the brain and cause a decrease in cerebral blood flow.

The relationship among coffee drinking, coronary heart disease, and myocardial infarction is unclear. Some reports implicate coffee drinking in the development of myocardial infarctions.

In one study of healthy volunteers, it was found that mean blood vessel pressure rose by 14/10 mmHg and plasma epinephrine levels increased over 200% one hour following ingestion of 250 mg caffeine. Other investigators do not find coffee a risk factor in the development of cardiovascular disease. The risk, if any, appears to be small.

The fact that caffeine decreases blood flow to the brain is the basis of using it to obtain relief from hypertension headaches and certain types of migraine headaches.

CENTRAL NERVOUS SYSTEM EFFECTS

Caffeine is a potent stimulant of the central nervous system, and has effects impacting on cortical and medullary functioning. Tachypnea experienced by caffeine-sensitive individuals is the result of direct stimulation of the medullary respiratory center. Low doses (50-200 mg) result in increased alertness, lessened fatigue, and decreased drowsiness. Higher doses (200-500 mg) cause hyperesthesia, headache, nervousness, irritability, and tremors. Caffeine's effect on objectively measured performance appears minimal, if any, despite the fact that some users report feeling more physically active and alert. Abstainers are more sensitive to the central nervous system's effect than heavy users.

The sympathomimetic effects are considered a result of the inhibition of phosphodiesterase, an enzyme that degrades the beta-adrenergic messenger, cyclic AMP. Some of the symptoms seen are the result of the increase in circulating catechols increasing adrenoceptor sensitivity from enhanced adrenomedullary secretion.

Caffeine appears to increase norepinephrine output more when it is consumed at times of stress than under more peaceful circumstances. The drug may accentuate the neurotransmitter response cycle, enhancing symptoms already present at a time of stress.

GASTROINTESTINAL EFFECTS

Gastric secretion is stimulated by caffeine. The effect is transient in normal subjects but sustained in those with active ulcer disease. The latter supports the hypothesis that excessive use of caffeine-containing beverages contributes to the pathogenesis of ulcers and should be avoided by those so prone. This effect is attributed to stimulation of gastric myenteric and submucal nerve networks and central nervous system stimulation by cholinergic nerves. Hydrogen ion secretion by the gastric mucosa is increased by the increase in cyclic AMP. Decaffeinated coffee and nondecaffeinated coffee are equally potent in stimulating gastric acid secretion.

Diarrhea results from stimulation of phasic contraction of smooth muscle in the lower part of the gastrointestinal tract, inhibition of synthesis of protein and RNA in the indigenous bacteria Escherichia coli, and local irritation from oils contained in caffeinated drinks.

SERUM GLUCOSE

Caffeine has been reported to be a hyperglycemic agent, although not all studies have confirmed this observation. Release of pancreatic insulin is reduced and glucose tolerance diminished following a large dose of glucose.

On caffeine withdrawal, serum glucose drops slightly and does not return to prewithdrawal levels.

RENAL EFFECTS

Diuresis results from caffeine's effects on the renal system and synergism between the increased levels of cyclic AMP and antidiuretic hormone.

PSYCHOLOGICAL EFFECTS

The psychological symptoms experienced with the use of caffeine and other methylxanthines represent: (1) an awareness of physiologic changes induced by caffeine use that are similar to somatic correlates of anxiety and depression when the subject is in a drug-free state, and (2) a defense against alterations in the individual's psyche. As an individual defends himself against external psychological and physical assault, his awareness or perceived-awareness of potential assault, seen with dementia, is increased by the caffeine. Psychological symptoms are influenced by dosage and duration of caffeine use, by concurrent use of other drugs, and by other physical and psychiatric illnesses the individual may have.

Ingestion of 50-200 mg caffeine (the content of an average cup of coffee) decreases fatigue and drowsiness and increases alertness, although response time and coordination have been found to be lowered significantly.

Caffeine's effect on response time appears greatest in individuals working under adverse conditions such as after use of alcohol or with decreased amount of light. Of the xanthines, caffeine has the greatest effect on the central nervous system. Theobromine has nearly no effect on the central nervous system. Theophylline's greatest influence is on the cardiovascular and muscoloskeletal system.

The depression reported with excess caffeine use is incompletely understood. Individuals may be first depressed and use coffee and other xanthine-containing compounds for self-medication, thereby modifying the clinical picture of affective illness. Depressive symptomatology may also result from the modification of catecholamine levels, the inhibition of phosphodiesterase breakdown of cyclic AMP in the central nervous system, and the sensitization of central catecholamine receptors, particularly those for dopamine.

EFFECT ON SLEEP

Caffeine taken before retiring interferes with both quantity and quality of sleep. Although impact is greater on abstainers and light users, even heavy users report sounder sleep on caffeine-free nights.

Increased sleep latency and number of awakenings is reported, along with decreased sleep time and decreased amount of deep sleep as indicated by electroencephalography.

In addition, more small body movements are reported during sleep following caffeine use in sensitive individuals.

CAFFEINISM

The term caffeinism has been used to refer both to the symptoms associated with habitual heavy use of caffeine as well as to the symptoms associated with caffeine withdrawal. Caffeine withdrawal will be discussed separately in this chapter.

Caffeinism is defined as the syndrome produced by acute or chronic excessive use of caffeine with subsequent pharmacologic toxicity. All symptoms discussed in the previous sections may be seen including psychomotor agitation, anxiety, insomnia, increased heart rate, irritability, and other symptoms that make the syndrome indistinguishable from an anxiety neurosis. Higher doses cause delirium. The panoply of symptoms that are experienced leads to excess use of other drugs such as sedative/hypnotics, minor tranquilizers, alcohol, and cigarettes, thus further complicating the clinical picture. The fact that the picture is so multifaceted had led some authors to conclude that caffeinism does not exist as a clinical phenomena but rather represents a variable clinical syndrome consisting of a mixture of anxiety and depressive symptoms. Although sensitivity varies, it is felt that an average intake of 18 cups or more than 1000 mg/day of caffeine is needed to produce the symptom complex which includes anorexia, low-grade fever, and irritability. (See Table 32-2).

The fact that the first description of the "restless leg syndrome" ("anxietas tibiarum") was written by Thomas Willis in 1685 (see Bickerstaff, 1790) at the time tea and coffee first reached England from Venice, has had some investigators to conclude that the introduction of caffeine may have been a major etiologic factor in the causation of this syndrome. The increased nervous system arousal as well as direct contractile effect on striated muscle seen in "restless leg syndrome" leads to myclonus, myokomia, and heightened proprioceptive awareness.

CAFFEINE WITHDRAWAL

The symptoms of caffeine withdrawal are comparable to those accompanying excessive use. Headache, depression, and anxiety are commonly seen. Withdrawal symptoms, such as irritability, lethargy, yawning, and rhinorrhea may accompany the headache. Headaches increase on weekends for individuals who consume large amounts of coffee at work but abstain or reduce intake at home and are also seen in the morning before the first cup of coffee is taken. Headache-prone caffeine users report a

Table 32-2   Signs and Symptoms of Caffeinism

Anorexia	Low-grade fever
Anxiety	Malaise
Arrhythmias	Muscle twitching
Delirium	Nausea
Depression	Nervousness
Diarrhea	Palpitations
Diuresis	Psychomotor agitation
Dizziness	Psychosis
Fatigue	Restlessness
Feeling "blue"	Sensory disturbances
Feeling like crying	Tachycardia
Feeling upset	Tachypnea
Flushing	Tension
Gastrointestinal disturbances	Tremulousness
Headache	Vomiting
Insomnia	
Irritability	

*Abelson and Fishburne, 1976; Damrau and Damrau, 1963; Dreisbach and Pfeffer, 1643; Editorial, 1975; Gilliland and Andrews, 1981; Goldstein, et al. , 1965, 1969; Goldstein and Kaizer, 1969; Greden, 1974; Greden, et al. , 1978, 1979; Henry and Oused, 1969, and Lukash, 1975; Kletson, 1978; Molde, 1975; McManam, Schube, 1967; Molde, 1975; Neil, et al. , 1978; Peters, 1972; Reimann, 1967; Roth, et al. , 1944; Speilberger, Stephenson, 1977; Stillner, et al. , 1978; Victor, et al. , Winstead, 1976.

cerebral "fullness" about 18 hr after discontinuation of use that develops with time into a painful, throbbing diffuse headache exacerbated by exercise. Discomfort peaks in 3-4 hr but the headache itself may last as long as 7 days. About one-fourth of persons undergoing caffeine withdrawal report "upset stomach" or nausea. Ingestion of caffeine temporarily reduces symptoms creating a vicious circle. Individuals who experience withdrawal headaches tend to have consumed greater than 600 mg/day of the drug but even moderate and light users have reported headaches.

Individuals susceptible to headache generally report more symptoms of depression and anxiety on psychometric examination and consume more antianxiety agents.

REPRODUCTION AND TERATOGENICITY

There is considerable disagreement over the mutagenic potential of coffee. Research in the area is complicated by the fact that there are no suitable animal models available for the study of chromosomal damage.

Caffeine crosses both the blood-testicular and fetal-placental barriers but does not diffuse freely into breast milk. Maternal serum caffeine levels are considerably higher than those in breast milk. The rate of metabolism of caffeine in women during pregnancy and in premature and full term infants is decreased. Neonates do not have the enzymes for oxidizing methylated xanthines. Infants do not attain serum levels of these enzymes comparable to those of adults until 4-8 months of age. As a result, caffeine remains in an infant's serum longer. Plasma half-life of caffeine is 4 days in the neonate compared to about 4 hr in the adult. The observation that uterine muscle contraction is inhibited by methylxanthines in normal dose ranges has led to the use of caffeine in the management of premature labor and threatened abortion.

The evaluation of potential teratogenicity is difficult and complicated by factors such as dose selection, species appropriateness, and maternal toxicity. High-dose studies of the effect of caffeine on animal populations have raised questions about its teratogenic nature and impact on birth weight and neonatal performance.

These findings have not been corroborated by human studies involving at least 14, 000 mothers.

At least one investigator feels caffeine may be an important factor in infertility as the maturational process of the gamete in males may be affected by increased levels of cyclic nucleotides maintained by heavy caffeine consumption. It is recommended that pregnant women avoid or limit caffeine consumption.

CARCINOGENICITY

Caffeine has never been unequivocally implicated as a risk factor in the development of cancer despite a number of suggestive clinical reports.

Cyclic nucleotide levels have been found to be increased in tissue obtained at biopsy of women with fibrocystic disease and fibroadenoma, suggesting possible involvement of caffeine and other methylxanthines in the development of breast masses. Elimination of all methylxanthines from the diet has led to resolution of the lumps in at least one study of women with benign breast disease.

The absence of an ideal animal model for the prediction of the effects of caffeine on humans makes infrahuman studies of potential mutagenic effects difficult.

ALLERGY

Caffeine allergies, in some cases so severe as to incapacitate the individual, have been reported.

In some instances, symptoms resisted all forms of drug treatment used.

EPILEPTOGENICITY AND NARCOLEPSY

Local application of caffeine, theophylline, and aminophylline to the cerebral cortex has produced epileptiform discharge. The effect on humans from ingestion, however, varies and some patients report relief from seizures. Prior to the advent of ephedrine sulfate in 1930 and amphetamine in 1935 for narcolepsy, caffeine was a recommended therapeutic agent.

INTERACTION WITH OTHER DRUGS

The interaction of caffeine with a number of drugs has been studied. Phenobarbital, an effective hypnotic when taken alone, is no more efficacious than placebo when taken in combination with caffeine. Caffeine antagonizes clinically the effect of the monoamine oxidase inhibitors and is a competitive inhibitor of diazepam (Valium) bonding to the brain receptor sites specific for benzodiazepines. The latter finding suggests that competitive interference with endogenous benzodiazepine ligands may explain the anxietogenic effect of caffeine. In such instances, obviously caffeine ingestion should be reduced rather than the dose of anxiolytic increased. There is some evidence from liver microsomal enzymes, that suggests that caffeine increases the metabolic breakdown of other drugs. This fact is of particular importance in heavy caffeine consumption by patients taking medications with a narrow therapeutic index.

OVERDOSE

At least eight cases of fatalities from excess caffeine use have been reported in the English-language literature. The minimal lethal dose is estimated to be 10 g (or 170 mg/kg body weight) taken over a brief period of time giving an indicated plasma serum level of 79-158.5 $\mu g/ml$.

The low incidence of death from overdose or excessive use is explained in part by the fact that gastric irritability and vomiting occur before absorption of toxic amounts can occur.

The high levels of circulatory catecholamines induced by high doses of caffeine explain the metabolic acidosis (from generation of lactate), ketosis, hyperglycemia, and sinus tachycardia. Caffeine-induced hyperventilation and sustained beta-adrenergic stimulation explain the development of hypokalemia seen with overdose. Caffeine poisoning is included together with salicylate poisoning and diabetes in the differential diagnosis of hyperglycemia, hyperventilation, and metabolic acidosis associated with behavioral abnormalities.

EFFECTS ON THE NEONATE

The therapeutic effects of methylxanthine at appropriate doses and methylxanthine's use in monitoring the newborn with apnea is felt to outweigh the fact that adverse effects may occur.

As mentioned earlier, the plasma half-life of caffeine in the neonate is greater than the adult and ranges from 32 to 149 hr.

More than 95% of caffeine ingested is excreted unchanged in the urine of a 1-month-old infant. The ratio of unchanged caffeine to urinary metabolites does not reach adult levels until about 6-8 months.

The use of caffeine as a respiratory stimulant in the asphyxiated infant is not as supported as use in treatment of apnea of prematurity. Signs and symptoms of caffeine overdose in the neonate include tremor of extremities, tachypnea, opisthotonus, nonpurposeful jaw and lip movements, and tonic-clonic movements.

EFFECT ON CHILDREN

Heavy consumption of caffeine-containing soft drinks and coffee can alter a child's behavior. One can of a soft drink and a chocolate candy bar ingested by a small child may be equivalent to an adult drinking four cups of instant coffee.

EFFECT ON OLDER PEOPLE

Although there appears to be decreased tolerance to caffeine with age and increased sleep disruption in older people taking caffeine at bedtime, it has been suggested that older persons take morning coffee as an energizer. Older people with organic mental syndromes secondary to atherosclerosis may benefit from the phosphodiesterase-inhibiting action of caffeine, which prolongs the metabolic stimulating-action of cyclic AMP in the brain.

EFFECT ON PSYCHIATRICALLY ILL PATIENTS

Heavy tea, coffee, and cola drink consumption by psychiatrically ill patients may enhance symptoms and confuse the clinical picture. Anticholinergic drugs increase thirst and patients seek to alleviate boredom and reduce drug- or depression-induced lethargy by drinking beverages and consuming food. Caffeine intake has been associated with increased agitation, anxiety, sleep disturbances, and rebound depression and delirium in patients with a variety of psychiatric diagnoses. Caffeine withdrawal has also been associated with precipitation of psychotic episodes.

Prolonged sleep latency and sleep interruption lead to prescription of soporific agents that confuse both the clinical psychiatric picture and the clinical picture of caffeinism or caffeine withdrawal. Consumers of large quantities of caffeine consumption of alcohol, cigarettes, minor tranquilizers, and sedative/hypnotics than low users.

Clinicians should be cautious not to suggest the use of caffeine to reduce drowsiness experienced with psychiatric medications as is sometimes recommended.

There is some evidence suggesting enhanced toxicity from the interaction of high-dose caffeine with tricyclic antidepressants, monoamine oxidase inhibitors, and lithium. This is believed to reflect the synergistic effects of these substances on amine turnover.

MINIMAL BRAIN DAMAGE

Children with minimal brain damage are known to respond paradoxically to central nervous system stimulants such as methylphenidate in providing impulse control and attention. Caffeine has been found to be as effective as methylphenidate in controlling the behavior of hyperkinetic children. Children who respond to the latter substance do not necessarily also respond to the former.

MANAGEMENT OF CAFFEINE-INDUCED SYMPTOMS

Management of caffeine-induced symptoms and the clinical syndrome of caffeinism is accomplished by elimination of caffeine-containing beverages, food, and medications from the diet. Minor tranquilizers, because of their sedative and muscle-relaxing effects, provide temporary relief of the symptoms of both caffeine excess and withdrawal. Analgesics may be needed for symptomatic relief of caffeine withdrawal-related headaches.

BIBLIOGRAPHY

Acheson, K. J.: Caffeine and coffee: their influence on metabolic rate and substrate utilization in normal weight and obese individuals. Am J Clin Nutr 33:989-997, 1980.

Aldridge, A., Aranda, J. V., and Neims, A. H.: Caffeine metabolism in the newborn. Clin Pharmacol Ther 25:447, 1979.

Aranda, J. V.: Maturation of caffeine elimination in infancy. Arch Dis Child 54:946-949, 1979.

Axelrod, J., and Reichenthal, J.: The fate of caffeine in man and a method for its estimation in biological material. J Pharmacol Exp Ther 107:519, 1953.

Battel, H., and Mielczarek, J.: Teratogenic effect of caffeine on the development of extremities in mice. Ginekol Pol 44:507-513, 1973.

Bickerstaff, I.: The Tutler, Vol. 2. Rivington, Marshall and Bye, London, 1790, p. 109.

Bonk, S., and Stocksmeier, U.: Bestehen zusamenhange zwischen kaffeegenuss and herzinfarkt. Munch Med Wochenschr 116:2013, 1974.

Bren, A. S., Martin, H., and Stern, L.: Toxicity from tea ingestion in an infant: a computer simulation analysis. Clin Biochem 10:148-150, 1977.

Caffeine and pregnancy. FDA Drug Bull 10:19-20, 1980.

Christensen, H. D., Whitsett, T. L., and Manion, C. V.: The assessment of caffeine kinetics for linearity by superposition. Fed Proc (abstr) 39:613, 1980.

Cook, C. E., Tallent, C. R., Amerson, E. W., Myers, M. W., Kepler, J. A., Taylor, G. F., and Christensen, H. D.: Caffeine in plasma and saliva by a radioimmunoassay procedure. Pharmacol Exp Ther 199:679, 1977.

DiMaio, V. J. M., and Garriott, J. C.: Lethal caffeine poisoning in a child. Forensic Sci 3:275-278, 1974.

Farago, A.: Lethal caffeine poisoning in a child. Forensic Sci 3:275-278, 1974.

Galant, S. P. , Lakshmi, D. , Underwood, S. , and Insel, P. A. : Decreased beta-adrenergic receptors on polymorphonuclear leukocytes after adrenergic therapy. N Engl J Med 299:933-936, 1978.

Georgian, L. , Moraru, I. , and Comisel, V. : Caffeine effects on the chromosomal aberrations induced in vivo by sarcolysine and methotrexate. Rev Roum Morphol Embryol Physiol 26:179-183, 1980.

Gessa, G. L. , Krishna, G. , Forn, J. , Tagliamonte, A. , and Brodie, B. B. : Behavioral and vegetative effects produced by dibutyl cyclic AMP injected into different areas of the brain. Adv Biochem Psychopharmacol 3:371-381, 1970.

Gilliland, R. S. , and Andress, D. : Ad lib caffeine consumption, symptoms of caffeinism, and academic performance. Am J Psychiatry 138:512-514, 1981.

Greden, J. F. : Anxiety or caffeinism: a diagnostic dilemma. Am J Psychiatry 131:1089-1092, 1974.

Gross, R. A. , and Ferrendelli, J. A. : Effects of reserpine, propranolol, and aminophylline on seizure activity and CNS cyclic nucleotides. Ann Neurol 6:296-301, 1979.

Horning, M. G. , Harvey, D. J. , Nawlin, J. , Stillwell, W. G. , and Hill, R. M. : The use of gas chromatography-mass spectrometry method in perinatal pharmacology. Adv Biochem Psychopharmacol 7:113, 1973.

Horrobin, D. F. , Manku, M. S. , Franks, D. J. , and Dehy, D. R. : Methylxanthine phosphodiesterase inhibitors behave as prostaglandin antagonists in a perfused rate mesenteric artery preparation. Prostaglandins 13:33-40, 1977.

Johansson, S. : Cardiovascular lesions in Sprague-Dawley rats induced by long-term treatment with caffeine. Acta Pathol Microbiol Scand 89:185-191, 1981.

Lentini, S. , Pirro, C. , and DiVeroli, C. : Effetti metabolici della caffeina: ruolo del sistema nervoso centrale e dell' AMP ciclico. Arch Sci Med 131:38, 1974.

Linn, D. G. , and Orsini, I. : Decreased spermatogenesis induced by high caffeine consumption. Int J Reprod Sci 17:281, 1982.

Mackenzie, T. B., Popkin, M. K., Dziubinski, J., et al.: Effects of caffeine withdrawal on isoproterenol-stimulated cyclic adenosine minophosphate. Clin Pharmacol Ther 30:436-438, 1981.

Mitoma, C., Sorich, T. J., and Neubauer, S. E.: The effect of caffeine on drug metabolism. Life Sci 7:145, 1968.

Robertson, D., Frolich, J. C., Carr, R. K., Watson, J. T., Hollifield, J. W., Shand, D. G., and Oates, J. A.: Effects of caffeine on plasma renin activity, catecholamines and blood pressure. N Engl J Med 298:181-186, 1978.

Sant'Ambrogio, G., Mognomi, P., and Ventrella, L.: Plasma levels of caffeine after oral, intramuscular and intravenous administrative. Arch Int Pharmacodyn Ther 150:259, 1964.

Slaby, A. E., Lieb, J., and Tancredi, L. R.: Handbook of Psychiatric Emergencies, 2d ed. Medical Examination Publishing Company, New Hyde Park, New York, 1981.

Speilberger, C. D., Gorsuch, R. L., and Lushene, R. E.: Strait-Trait Anxiety Inventory Manual. Consulting Psychologists Press, Palo Alto, CA, 1970.

Sullivan, J. L.: Caffeine poisoning in an infant. J Pediatr 90: 1022-1023, 1977.

Tyrala, E. E., and Dodson, W. E.: Caffeine secretion into breast milk. Arch Dis Child 54:787-800, 1979.

Viola, P.: Gli effetti biofarmacologici del caffe. Sintesi conclusiva. Arch Sci Med 131:52, 1974.

Volkheimner, G., Schulz, F. H., Hofer, E., and Schicht, J.: Effetto della caffeine sull'indice di << persorbimento >>. Arch Sci Med 129:17, 1972.

Chapter 33

PHENCYCLIDINE AND THE DISSOCIATIVES

A. James Giannini, M.D.

INTRODUCTION

Phencyclidine (PCP) is the prototypical member of a small
group of mind-altering drugs known as the dissociatives. Phencyclidine is the generic term for 1-(1-phenylcyclohexyl)piperi-
dine hydrochloride. It was first synthesized by Parke Davis
Laboratories in 1957 and marketed the following year under the
name of Sernyl. Though it was released as a nonbarbiturate,
nonnarcotic anesthetic, it produced postanesthetic dysphoria,
agitation, and delirium. By 1967 it was a popular drug of abuse
because of its unique combination of excitation, sedation, hal-
lucination, anesthesia, and amnesia. In the 1970s it accounted
for 25% of all "psychedelic" drug use. Today one American in
16 in the 12- to 17-year age group has abused PCP at least
once and nearly 12% of all Americans in the 18- to 25-year
group have used this drug. Since phencyclidine can be taken by
numerous routes (snorting, inhalation, injection, ingestion,
douching, smoking, rectal suppository) and produces a variety
of results, it is often sold in disguised form. Nearly 25% of all
PCP used is sold illicitly as another drug. In both disguised and
nondisguised forms, PCP accounts for 30% of all drug abuse in
the United States. After marijuana it is America's most abused
drug.

CHEMICAL STRUCTURE

Phencyclidine hydrochloride is a member of the chemical group
known as the arylcyclohexylamines. This group is pharmacologically and psychologically distinct from all other classes of
psychoactive compounds. As a pure base it is highly insoluble

in water so it is usually prepared as the readily soluble hydrochloride salt. Phencyclidine hydrochloride is soluble in propor-
tions of 1:6 water, 1:7 of alcohol, and 1:2 of chloroform. It is
insoluble in ether. Phencyclidine hydrochloride is a white,
odorless crystalline powder with a melting point of approximately 228ºC and a molecular weight of 279.9.

Structurally it is composed of a phenyl group, a piperidine
group, and a cyclohexyl ring. Structure activity relationship
data indicate that the electron-dense region in the area of the
aromatic ring and the cyclohexyl moiety are required for producing behavioral effects. Binding to receptors by PCP and its
derivatives probably occurs in the thermodynamically most
stable conformation with an axial phenyl group. The phenyl
equatorial group has found to produce low binding capability.

The second most commonly abused member of the dissociative group and the only legal member is ketamine hydrochloride which is manufactured under the trade name Ketalar by
Parke Davis Laboratories as an anesthetic agent (Figure 33-1).
It has a 2-O-chlorophenyl-1-2-methylaminecyclohexanone configuration. The third most commonly used member of this group
and the second most commonly abused drug is phenylcyclohexylpyrrolidine (PHP). It is popular to use because in addition to
having all the side effects and effects of PCP, it is also difficult
to detect in routine urinalysis. Its structure is 1-(1-phenylcy-
clohexyl)-pyrrolidine. Other commonly abused analogs are cy-
clo hexamine (PCE), N-ethyl-1-phenylcyclohexylamine: TCP,
1-(1-2-thienylcyclohexyl)piperidine and PCC, 1-piperidinocy-
clohexancarbonitrile. Replacement of the phenyl group with
thienyl enhances central activity (Figure 33-2). Aliphatic analogs have lesser central potency. Compounds with a three-
carbon chain are the most active. The presence of an unsaturated bond has been shown to also further enhance central activity.

METABOLISM AND EXCRETION

Effects of PCP are perceived instantaneously when injected,
within 30-60 sec after inhalation, 1-5 min after smoking or
snorting, and approximately 20 min after ingestion. The half-
life of PCP has a range of between 11 and 89 hr, but effects
have been reported to last for as long as 5 days. Phencyclidine
is a weak base with a dissociation constant of 8.5-9.5 with high
lipid solubility, and is rapidly absorbed from the gastrointestinal tract. It is ionized at a pH of 6.5. Since the ionic form of
PCP does not readily pass lipophyllic tissue, it accumulates in
the stomach and the urine. It is, however, readily absorbed

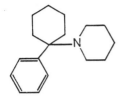

Phencyclidine (PCP)
1-(phenylcyclohexyl)
piperidine

Ketamine
2-(o-chlorophenyl)-2-methyl-
amine cyclohexanone

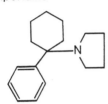

PHP
1-(1-phenylcyclohexyl)
pyrrolidine

TCP
1-(1-2-thienylcyclohexyl)
piperidine

PCC
1-piperidinocyclohexane-
carbonitrile

Cyclohexamine (PCE)
N-ethyl-1-phenylcyclohexylamine

Figure 33-1   The Dissociatives.

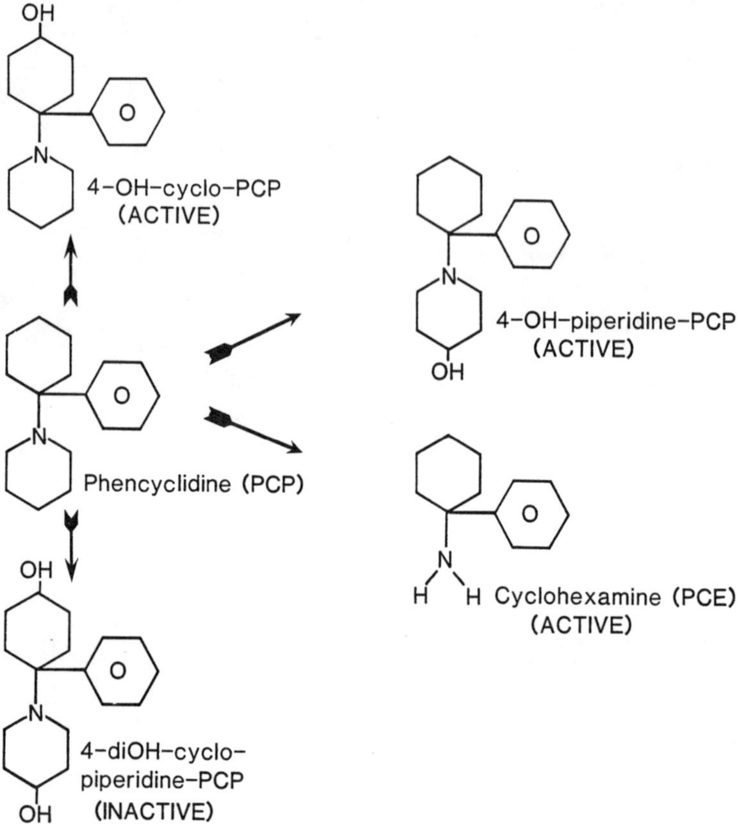

Figure 33-2   Metabolites of phencyclidine.

from the intestines into the systemic and enterohepatic circulation. The presence of enterohepatic circulation gives the appearance of frequent remissions and exacerbations.

After administration of PCP, most urinary and fecal excretion is complete within 72 hr. Less than 5% of phencyclidine is found in the feces, implying a relatively minor role for biliary excretion. About 50% of urinary compounds can be identified as either PCP or enzymatically hydrolyzable conjugates of hydroxymetabolites. Total clearance of PCP averages 0.38 liters/min while nonrenal clearance averages about 3.5 liter/min. Phencyclidine is metabolized principally by the liver into glucornide and hydroxylated forms. Phencyclidine has also been found in the perspiration with concentration here being seven times that of plasma.

Phencyclidine pyrolysis produces 1-phenylcyclohexene. Both phenylcyclohexene and PCP have been found in the smoke of marijuana and parsley cigarettes containing PCP. About 40% of all PCP smoke is absorbed. It is trapped within the membranes of the mouth or lung or bronchial tissues. Once trapped here, due to its basicity it can be released to the systemic circulation. Metabolic disposition of smoked PCP is the same as by other routes.

Approximately 35% of PCP is free in the plasma and capable therefore of crossing the blood-brain barrier. It binds strongly to alpha-1-glycoprotein and less strongly to albumin. High-density lipoproteins have not been shown to play an important role in PCP binding.

RECEPTORS

Phencyclidine produces a wide variety of effects which have been shown to be due to their action at numerous types of neuro-receptor sites. These sites have included mascarinic and nicotinic receptors as well as gamma-aminobutyric acid (GABA)-nergic, dopaminergic, serotonergic, and putative PCP-specific receptor sites. The more significant receptor sites will be discussed below.

ACETYLCHOLINE

Phencyclidine has the typical structure of most atropinic agents. It has a cationic head, a phenyl group, and a large hydroxy group. It has been shown to be a powerful noncompetitive inhibitor of nicotinic receptor sites in the sympathetic nervous system. It also acts peripherally at the skeletal muscle to block potassium channels and the linkage between the potassium channel and the cholinergic receptor site. This blockade of the potassium channel also reduces acetylcholine-induced secretion of catecholamines in the adrenal glands. Calcium-induced configurational changes can decrease PCP affinity to nicotinic receptors. Physostigmine can also reverse PCP-induced inhibition of skeletal muscle or adrenal potassium channels.

Centrally PCP is competitive with acetylcholine at muscarinic sites. The interference with the receptor site and its potassium ionophor seen in the nicotinic receptor has not been reported to occur in the muscarinic receptors of the central nervous system. At lower dose levels of PCP, that is about 5-10 mg, atropinic effects appear to predominate. These include a free-floating dissociative reaction with mild elevations of blood pressure. Pupils generally are constricted with the pathognomonic horizontal/vertical nystagmus. Deep tendon reflexes are hyperactive in both upper and lower extremities with mild rigidity or ataxia. The patient usually is flushed with warm dry skin. Treatment for this state usually involves observation of vital signs. If the patient's dissociation becomes clinically significant, the intoxication can be treated as an atropinic toxicity. Physostigmine salicylate 2 mg intramuscularly attenuates behavioral effects and will decrease the frequency of a resting tremor or vertical nystagmus. It will also treat any anxiety, tension, conceptual disorganization, and excitement that may be present. Phencyclidine use, of course, is not without risk. It can cause a number of cholinergic side effects such as bradycardia, bronchial secretions, and convulsions.

DOPAMINE

The association of PCP ingested in quantities of 10-20 mg or more with florid psychoses has indicated an involvement of the dopamine (DA) neurotransmitter system. This hypothesis has been strengthened by the fact that PCP suppresses serum prolactin levels and enhances amphetamine-induced stereotype. Phencyclidine inhibits dopamine (DA) accumulation by uptake in vesicles and synaptosomes in a manner similar to amphetamine. It also interacts with presynaptic potassium channels to increase the release of DA. Predominant sites of action seem to be located at the DA-2 presynaptic receptor sites in the corticostriatal neurons. Phencyclidine acts as an amphetaminelike sympathomimetic causing increased release of stored DA.

Because of the major role DA plays in generating PCP psychosis the treatment is similar to that in a schizophrenic psychosis. Neuroleptic agents having strong DA-2 receptor

specificity are indicated. These include all members of the butyrophenone group. Clinical literature has reported efficacious
treatment with haloperidol 5 mg intramuscularly q 20 min for
psychosis. Haloperidol has predominant DA-2 receptor-specif-
ic actions and produces more complete reversal of the psychosis than the phenothiazines, molindones, or loxapenes.

OPIOIDS

The dissociatives, especially PCP and ketamine, were thought
to produce opiate actions due to their anesthetic effects. In
squirrel monkeys, ketamine produces similar responses to
shock-maintained behavior as does morphine. Methadone has
been reported to suppress PCP-induced behavior in rats. In
addition, PCP-induced cross-tolerance to morphine occurs in
humans and over 10 different types of other mammals. In early
clinical trials of PCP, psychotic reactions were controlled with
either meperidine or morphine. Controlled clinical trials have
also shown meperidine to be superior to numerous antidotal
agents in the treatment of phencyclidine psychosis.

Behaviorally, PCP has been shown to affect both m - and
sigma-opioid receptors. SKF 10,047, the putative sigma-agon-
ist developed by Smith, Kline and French Laboratories, mini-
mized the effect of PCP on dogs with lesioned spinal cords.
The mu-agonist, morphine, increased metenkephlin-induced
PCP ataxia while naloxone blocked it. In receptor studies, PCP
blocked binding of naloxone, a relative mu-antagonist, and also
blocked binding of morphine, a relative mu-agonist. SKF 10,047
also has been shown to selectively displace PCP binding in the
brain. Acute PCP intoxication is associated with decreased
metenkephlin in the striate bodies, medulla oblongata, pons,
and midbrain in the human subject. Chronic use of PCP has also been shown to increase striatal metenkephalin.

Recent controlled clinical trials have shown meperidine, a
synthetic opiate, to be superior to all commonly used PCP antidotal agents. Injections of meperidine have been shown to be
superior in antipsychotic efficacy to hydroxyzine, diazepam,
physostigmine, and chlorpromazine. It was also found to be
equal to haloperidol in terms of therapeutic efficacy. The action
of meperidine is a delayed one. Chlorpromazine and haloperidol
usually produced greater initial symptom relief especially within the first half-hour. By the end of 1-2 hr of treatment, meperidine has been shown to be equal or superior to all agents thus
reported. In clinical situations PCP psychosis can be treated
with meperidine 50 mg intramuscularly q 20 min to a total dose
of 200 mg. This delayed but greater efficacy has led some

authors to hypothesize that dopaminergic activity, at least in PCP psychosis, could possibly be modulated by an upstream opioid mechanism.

THE PUTATIVE PHENCYCLIDINE RECEPTOR

It had been postulated that a specific PCP receptor exists within the rat brain. Its binding is saturable and reversible. When PCP binds to muscarinic and opioid receptors, both muscarinic and opiate agonists and antagonists have been ineffective in displacing PCP bound to the putative PCP receptor. Phencyclidine binds to its own receptor with an affinity that is two orders of magnitude greater than the affinity for either muscarinic or opiate receptors. When PCP was given experimentally to rats, 0.15% was bound to the opiate receptors and 0.22% to muscarinic receptors, while 99.63% was bound to the PCP receptor. Replacing the phenyl ring of PCP by a 2-thienyl ring produces a compound with increased affinity for the PCP-receptor as well as increased central potency. Phencyclidine also displaces SKF 10,047 binding to the sigma opioid receptors suggesting that both PCP and sigma-opiates interact at the same receptor sites. Phencyclidine receptors have been found to be primarily distributed in the cortex and hippocampus.

SYMPTOMATIC TREATMENT

When an unconscious PCP-intoxicated patient presents to the emergency room, the treatment is the same as that of any comatose patient: maintain the airway with proper ventilation, monitor cardiac status, protect the patient from harm, and remove the intoxicating agent. In addition, cardiac monitoring should be done due to the possibility of atropinic arrhythmias that can occur with PCP. If the intoxicated patient is conscious, decrease the external stimuli and protect the patient from harm to himself or others. If he is extremely agitated, avoid physical restraints which when coupled with PCP skeletal muscle exertion and PCP-induced anesthesia, can lead to skeletal muscle damage, rhabdomyolysis, and resulting renal damage. If the patient is seen within 6 hr after oral ingestion, gastric lavage is indicated. Gastric excretion should be removed by continuous drainage via nasogastric tube. A charcoal slurry may help decrease reabsorption from the small intestine. The dosage of activated charcoal is usually 10-20 times the amount that it is expected to absorb. To remove PCP from the alimentary tract, sodium sulfate, 0.3 g/kg via the tube helps promote fecal excretion in ionized form.

In all cases of PCP intoxication, acidification and elimination are key procedures. Urinary acidification should be avoided only when a urine toxicology screen shows the presence of barbiturates or salicylates. Acidification in mild cases of intoxication is produced by oral ingestion of ascorbic acid 1000-2000 mg every 6 hr accompanied by ingestion of cranberry juice, a source of hippuric acid. In moderate to severe intoxication, ammonium chloride 2.75 mEq/kg in 60 ml 0.9% saline can be given through a nasogastric tube or intravenously 1-2% in 0.9% saline solution. Once a urinary pH of 5.5 or lower is achieved, furosemide 40 mg intramuscularly in an adult and 1.0 mg/kg in a child should be given for quick diuresis. Maintain hydration and electrolyte balance to insure a urine flow of 1-2 ml/kg/hr.

BIBLIOGRAPHY

Albuquerque, E. X., Aguayo, L. G., Warnick, J. E., et al.: Interactions of phencyclidine with ion channels of nerve and muscle behavioral implications. Fed Proc 42:2854-2859, 1983.

Castellani, S., Giannini, A. J., and Adams, P. M.: Effects of naloxone, metenkephlin and morphine on phencyclidine-induced behavior in the rat. Psychopharmacology 78:76-80, 1982.

Castellani, S., Giannini, A. J., and Adams, P. M.: Physostigmine and haloperidol treatment of acute phencyclidine intoxication. Am J Psychiatry 131:5080510, 1982.

Castellani, S., Giannini, A. J., Boeringa, J. A., and Adams, P. M.: Phencyclidine intoxication: assessment of possible antidotes. Clin Toxicol 19:313-319, 1982.

Giannini, A. J., and Castellani, S.: A case of phenylcyclohexylpyrrolidine (PHP) intoxication treatment with physostigmine. Clin Toxicol 19:505-508, 1982.

Giannini, A. J., and Price, W. A.: Antidotal strategies in phencyclidine intoxication. Int J Psychiatr Med 14:315, 1984.

Giannini, A. J., and Price, W. A.: The dissociatives. Med Psychiatry (in press).

Giannini, A. J., and Price, W. A.: Management of phencyclidine intoxication. Res Staff (in press).

Giannini, A. J., Eighan, M. S., Loiselle, R. H., Giannini, M. C.: Comparison of haloperidol and chlorpromazine in the treatment of phencyclidine psychosis. J Clin Pharmacol 24:118, 1984.

Giannini, A. J., Price, W. A., Loiselle, R. H., and Giannini, M. C.: Comparison of chlorpromazine and meperidine in the treatment of phencyclidine psychosis: role of the opiate receptor. J Clin Psychiatry 24:202-204, 1984.

Giannini, A. J., Kalavsky, S., Loiselle, R. H., Giannini, M. C., and Price, W. A.: Possible role of the DA-2 receptor in phencyclidine psychosis. Neurosci Abstr 9:33, 1983.

Giannini, A. J., Nageolte, C., Loiselle, R. H., Price, W. A., and Malone, D. A.: Modulation of dopamine-induced PCP psychosis by pimozide and haloperidol. Clin Pharmacol (in press).

Giannini, A. J., Price, W. A., Giannini, M. L., Loiselle, R. N., Malone, D. A.: Treatment of phenylhexlpyrrolidine (PHP) with haloperidol. Clin Toxicol (in press).

Giles, H. G., Corrigall, W. A., Khouw, V., and Tillman, T. F.: Plasma protein binding of phencyclidine. Clin Pharmacol Ther 31:77-82, 1982.

Greifenstein, F. E., and DeVault, M.: A study of cyclohexyla-mine for anesthesia. Anesth Analg 37:283-294, 1958.

Kalii, A.: Structure-activity relationship of phencyclidine derivatives. Psychopharmacol Bull 16:54-57, 1980.

Kamenka, J. M., and Geneste, P.: Confirmation behavior of phencyclidine and biological activity. Psychopharmacol Bull 16:77-79, 1980.

Peterson, R. C., and Stillman, R. C.: Phencyclidine an overview. Natl Inst Drug Abuse Res Monogr Ser 21:1-17, 1978.

Snyder, S. H.: Phencyclidine. Nature 285:355-356, 1980.

Verebey, K., Kogan, M. J., and Mule, S. J.: Phencyclidine induced stereotypy in rats: effects of methadone. apomorphine and naloxone. Psychopharmacol 75:44-47, 1981.

RECOMMENDED READINGS
AND INDEX

RECOMMENDED READINGS

Barchas, J.D., Berger, P.A., and Ciaranello, R.D.: Psychopharmacology from Theory to Practice. Oxford University
Press, New York, 1977.

Barr, M.L.: The Human Nervous System: an Anatomical
Viewpoint. Harper & Row, Hagerstown, MD, 1976.

Cooper, J.R., Bloom, E.E., and Roth, R.H.: The Biochemical
Basis of Neuropharmacology, 3rd ed. Oxford University Press,
New York, 1982.

Fields, W (Editor): Neurotransmitter Function. Stratton-
Intercontinental, New York, 1977.

Giannini, A.J., and Black, H.R.: Psychiatric, Psychogenic,
and Somatopsychic Disorders Handbook. Medical Examination
Publishing, Garden City, 1978.

Giannini, A.J., and Gilliland, R.H.: Neurologic, Neurogenic,
and Neuropsychiatric Disorders. Medical Examination Publishing
Garden City, 1978.

Giannini, A.J., Slaby, A.E., and Giannini, A.J.: Overdose and
Detoxification Emergencies. Medical Examination Publishing,
Garden City, NY, 1982.

Goldberg, R.C.: Anxiety. Medical Examination Publishing
Company, Garden City, NY, 1982.

Lipton, M.A., DiMascio, A., and Killman, K.A. (Editors):
Psychopharmacology: a Generation of Progress, Raven Press,
New York, 1978.

Merikangas, J.R. (Editor): Brain-Behavior Relationships. D.C.
Health, Lexington, MA, 1981.

Petersen, R.C. (Editor): The International Challenge of Drug
Abuse, NIDA Research Monograph. National Institute of Drug
Abuse, Rockville, MD, 1978.

Post, R.M., and Ballenger, J.C. (Editors): The Neurobiology of Manic-Depressive Illness. Williams & Wilkins, Baltimore, (in press).

Schoolar, J.C., and Claghorn, J.L.: The Kinetics of Psychoactive Drugs, Brunner-Mazel, New York, 1978.

Usdin, E., and Hanin, I. (Editors): Biological Markers in Psychiatry and Neurology. Pergamon Press, Oxford, 1982.

Usdin, E., Kopin, I.J., and Barchas, J. (Editors): Catecholamines: Basic and Clinical Frontiers. Pergamon Press, Oxford, 1979.

Wells, C.E., (Editor): Dementia, 3rd ed. F. A. Davis, Philadelphia, 1982.

INDEX